Contemporary Leadership Behavior

C0-ARE-266

Phyllis Fischer

Contemporary Leadership Behavior

SELECTED READINGS

EDITED BY

Eleanor C. Hein, *R.N., Ed.D.*

PROFESSOR,
UNIVERSITY OF SAN FRANCISCO SCHOOL OF NURSING,
SAN FRANCISCO

M. Jean Nicholson, *R.N., M.S.N.E.*

ASSISTANT PROFESSOR,
UNIVERSITY OF SAN FRANCISCO SCHOOL OF NURSING,
SAN FRANCISCO

Little, Brown and Company
Boston

Copyright © 1982 by Eleanor C. Hein and M. Jean Nicholson

First Edition

All rights reserved. No part of this book may be reproduced in any
form or by any electronic or mechanical means, including
information storage and retrieval systems, without permission in
writing from the publisher, except by a reviewer who may quote
brief passages in a review.

Library of Congress Catalog Card No. 82-82682

ISBN 0-316-35447-3

Printed in the United States of America

DON

Contents

Contributing Authors

Jo Ann Ashley, R.N., Ed.D.
Formerly Professor, Wright State University School of Nursing, Dayton, Ohio

Marilyn Bagwell, R.N., B.S.N., M.A.
Assistant Professor, Arizona State University College of Nursing, Tempe

Elaine E. Beletz, R.N., Ed.D., F.A.A.N.
Assistant Director of Nursing, Brooklyn Hospital, New York

Bonnie Graczyk Castrey, R.N., B.S.N.
Commissioner, Federal Mediation and Conciliation Service Agency, Santa Ana, Calif.

Robert T. Castrey
Management/Labor Arbitrator (Private Practice), Huntington Beach; formerly Commissioner, Federal Mediation and Conciliation Service, Santa Ana, Calif.

Margaret Colangelo, R.N., M.S.
Professor Emeritus of Nursing, Riverside City College, Riverside, Calif.

Dorothy F. Corona, R.N., M.S.N.
Associate Professor, College of Nursing and Allied Health, University of Texas, El Paso

Nancy A. Couillard, R.N., C.C.R.N.
Clinical Nurse, Johns Hopkins Hospital, Baltimore

Leah L. Curtin, R.N., M.S., M.A.
Editor, *Nursing Management,* Cincinnati; formerly Director, National Center for Nursing Ethics, Cincinnati

Christy Z. Dachelet, M.S.
Coordinator of Corporate Planning, Methodist Hospital, St. Louis Park, Minn.; formerly Health Projects Coordinator, University of Rochester School of Nursing, Rochester, N.Y.

Nancy P. Greenleaf, R.N., D.N.Sc.
Assistant Professor, University of South Maine School of Nursing, Portland

Margaret Smith Hamilton, R.N., M.S.
Formerly Clinical Instructor, Boston College School of Nursing, Boston

Eleanor C. Hein, R.N., Ed.D.
Professor, University of San Francisco School of Nursing, San Francisco

Ada Sue Hinshaw, R.N., Ph.D., F.A.A.N.
Professor and Director of Research, University of Arizona College of Nursing; Associate Director of Nursing for Research, University Hospital, Arizona Health Sciences Center, Tucson

Linda Hughes, R.N., M.S., C.C.R.N.
Assistant Professor of Nursing, Oklahoma Baptist University, Shawnee; Staff Nurse, Coronary Care Unit, Baptist Medical Center, Oklahoma City

Ada Jacox, R.N., Ph.D.
Professor of Nursing, University of Maryland, Baltimore

Beatrice J. Kalisch, R.N., Ed.D., F.A.A.N.
Titus Distinguished Professor of Nursing and Chairperson, Parent-Child Nursing, The University of Michigan School of Nursing, Ann Arbor

Philip A. Kalisch, Ph.D.
Professor of History, Economics and Politics of Nursing, The University of Michigan School of Nursing, Ann Arbor

Mary F. Kohnke, R.N., Ed.D., F.A.A.N.
Program Director, Delivery of Nursing Service, Division of Nursing, New York University, New York

Phyllis Beck Kritek, R.N., Ph.D.
Associate Professor and Director, Center for Nursing Research and Evaluation, University of Wisconsin School of Nursing, Milwaukee

Margaret Levi, Ph.D.
Associate Professor of Political Science and Public Affairs, University of Washington, Seattle

Claire Manfredi, R.N., Ed.D.
Assistant Professor, University of Rhode Island College of Nursing, Kingston

Ann Marriner, R.N., Ph.D.
Professor and Associate Dean, Indiana University School of Nursing, Indianapolis

Geoffry McEnany, R.N., B.S.N.
Clinical Nurse III, Adult Inpatient and Research Service, Langley Porter Psychiatric Institute, University of California, San Francisco

Dalton E. McFarland, Ph.D.
University Professor and Professor of Business Administration, University of Alabama, Birmingham

Jeanne Margaret McNally, R.N., Ph.D.
General Administrator, Sisters of Mercy, Belmont, N.C.

Mary T. Meng, R.N., M.S.
Vice President—Administration/Director of Nursing, Rochester General Hospital, Rochester, N.Y.

J. Randolph New, D.B.A.
Assistant Professor of Management, University of Baltimore, Baltimore

M. Jean Nicholson, R.N., M.S.N.E.
Assistant Professor, University of San Francisco School of Nursing, San Francisco

Dorothy Ozimek, R.N., Ed.D., D.Sci.
Chairperson, Department of Nursing, Fairleigh Dickinson University, Rutherford, N.J.

Stephanie Farley Pardue, R.N., Ed.D.
Associate Professor, University of Texas School of Nursing; Clinical Associate, Nursing Service, University of Texas Medical Branch, Galveston

Patricia Chehy Pilette, R.N., M.S.
Co-Director, Humanistic Nursing Consultant Services, Boston; Associate, Comprehensive Counseling Associates, Westboro, Mass.

Winifred J. Pinch, R.N., B.S.N.Ed., M.Ed.
Assistant Professor, St. Anselm College, Manchester, N.H.

Marilyn M. Rawnsley, R.N., D.N.Sc.
Associate Professor of Nursing, University of Massachusetts, Amherst

Nancy D. Sanford, R.N., M.S.
Independent Practitioner in Nursing Education; Board Member, Santa Clara County Health Systems Agency, Santa Clara, Calif.

Dorothy L. Sexton, R.N., Ed.D.
Associate Professor and Chairperson, Medical-Surgical Nursing Program, Yale University School of Nursing, New Haven, Conn.

Nola Shiflett, R.N., M.S.N.
Instructor, Department of Nursing, Gadsden State Junior College, Gadsden, Ala.

Roxane Spitzer, R.N., M.A., F.A.A.N.
Assistant Administrator for Nursing, University of Illinois Medical Center, Chicago

Gertrud B. Ujhely, R.N., Ph.D.
New York State Certified Clinical Nurse Specialist in Psychiatric and Mental Health Nursing, Jungian Analyst (Private Practice); formerly Professor and Director of Graduate Program in Psychiatric Nursing, Adelphi University, Garden City, N.Y.

Connie N. Vance, R.N., Ed.D.
Assistant Professor, Division of Nursing, New York University, New York

Mary B. Walsh, R.N., M.S.N.
Associate Professor, The Catholic University of America School of Nursing, Washington, D.C.

Lynne Brodie Welch, R.N., Ed.D.
Associate Professor of Nursing, Lienhard School of Nursing, Pace University, Pleasantville, N.Y.

Helen Yura, R.N., Ph.D., F.A.A.N.
Professor and Graduate Program Director, Department of Nursing, Old Dominion University, Norfolk, Va.

Preface

Books on leadership in nursing share one common message: the skills of leadership are essential to professional nursing and must be acquired and used effectively if nursing is to be acknowledged as an autonomous profession. This book is no exception to that theme.

This book grew out of an unsuccessful search for one volume that included the concepts we believe are vital to the practice of leadership. We use the phrase "the practice of leadership" purposely, for we believe that every professional nurse's nursing practice *is* the practice of leadership. The intent of this book, therefore, is functional—to help professional nurses enhance the practice of leadership by drawing to their attention the contemporary leadership behaviors that must be incorporated into their nursing practice if that practice is to be effective.

The readings in Part I, The Culture of Nursing, were selected to remind the reader how long and how extensively we have been conditioned *not* to think and *not* to act both socially and professionally. Whether shaped by that elusive and powerful force known as public opinion or carefully taught by generations of parents, we have become trapped inside fortresses of security that others have built and in which (at times all too willingly) we reside, captives of past experiences and past behaviors. The readings selected for Part I point out that each time we do nothing to learn how to breach these fortresses, we continue to exhibit the self-limiting behavior that keeps nurses from realizing greater professional status.

The theories of leadership in Part II have been chosen to help nurses become familiar with some of the theories that can serve as a basis of their practice. The underlying premise of nursing leadership in this book is that it is an interactional process between a nurse and a patient, directed toward the achievement of health care goals. Followership, self-esteem, and values are three leadership attributes selected for inclusion in Part II: followership, because it acts as an interdependent, legitimizing agent of leadership; self-esteem, because it acts as our power base as we consciously give ourselves appreciative self-definition instead of accepting others' stereotypic definitions; and values, because they are the means by which we explore what we believe about leadership and why. These attributes are pivotal to all subsequent leadership behaviors.

Contemporary leadership behaviors highlight Part III. The leadership behaviors selected for Part III—assertiveness, advocacy, mentoring, power, politics, collective action, change, and conflict resolution—are ideas that have existed in all human endeavors throughout history. They become contemporary when they converge at a particular time in response to fast-moving and far-reaching events. The present rapid changes within the health care delivery system mark such a time. The impact of these changes upon our profession will have far-reaching consequences for all of us if we continue to sit back safely cocooned in the notion that exercising leadership is someone else's responsibility. The readings selected for Part III stress, in one way or another, that leadership is an activity, either individual or collective, directed toward excellence in practice and the advancement of nursing as an autonomous profession.

Finally, the readings selected for Part IV serve as an introduction to the assessment and understanding of basic organizational structure. They will be particularly relevant for nurses who have not had courses in organizational behavior or managerial psychology. With or without such background, however, nurses must know the components of organizational structure if they are to use their leadership behavior effectively within the system. These two elements, leadership behavior and knowledge of organizational structure, are the focus of the final chapter in Part IV, which recounts one nursing student's attempt to effect a change within a health care facility.

Although the parts in this book are arranged in a certain sequence, they can be read in any order. Within each part, readings dealing with theoretical material generally precede those of a practical nature. Wherever possible, readings that illustrate or demonstrate various aspects of leadership were placed at the end of a particular section or part. Each part concludes with a series of discussion questions designed to stimulate thought and the exchange of ideas.

Several criteria guided the selection of readings for this book. First, we wanted the readings to be drawn exclusively from the nursing literature and written by nurses. With one or two exceptions, we were able to meet this criterion. Second, we wanted readings that were written with practicing professional nurses in mind, not those who function primarily in administrative roles. Although books for nurses holding administrative positions are proliferating, and they make a significant contribution to nursing literature, few books, if any, address themselves to nurses who need to learn to develop leadership behavior in the immediacy of their nursing practice. We discovered that this goal was not completely possible as we had hoped; several readings do assume an audience in administrative positions. We included them, nevertheless, because we felt that the points made were applicable to the practice area. This discovery did, however, illustrate the need for a book such as this. Third, we wanted readings that struck a balance between the theoretical and the practical. For the most part this balance has been achieved, although it has become apparent that writings of a more practical nature are needed on the various topics in this book. Finally, we attempted to include readings that were published recently. There were exceptions, however. The few readings with a pre-1979 publication date have a primarily theoretical focus. Because the content has not changed appreciably since their publication, we felt they continued to be relevant and timely. We appreciate the cooperation of the various journals and authors in granting us permission to use their material.

Contemporary Leadership Behavior is intended for all professional nurses committed to improving the practice of their leadership behaviors. This goal is as applicable to nursing students approaching graduation, who use this book as a text, as it is to professional nurses in practice for several years, who use it as a resource for their continuing education. The purpose of this book is not to divide or limit its readers by their educational background but to bring together *all* nurses who have as their aim excellence in the practice of leadership.

E. C. H.
M. J. N.

I The Culture of Nursing

This is a bewildering time for nurses. We are asked to prepare a foundation for the future of our profession, but we have no plan to guide us. We are asked to build its structure, but we have no mortar for the bricks. We are asked to furnish its interior but we do not know how to begin. There is no design to follow, no clear picture of what could be—only an elusive image waiting to be defined, acknowledged, and accepted.

Professional nursing has a fleeting image of the future awaiting definition, acknowledgment, and acceptance. Culture has shaped nursing in the same way it shapes every facet of human endeavor. Every idea we have, every value we hold, and every belief we cling to is determined to some extent by our cultural heritage. Through its pervasive influence, we are provided with a pattern for living to which all of us are unconsciously and inexorably bound. The culture of nursing has an equally pervasive influence on our professional behavior, behavior we have unquestioningly acted out as significant members of the largest group of health care givers in our society. What definition the image of nursing has, has been shaped by past myths that have been idealized and distorted by another powerful source of influence—public opinion.

Public opinion evolves from information that is distilled and disseminated through the mass communication media whose role is to preserve our cultural heritage by controlling and thus limiting the ways to carry out its norms and expectations. What we must be and how we must act are reflections from the various forms of media images to which we are all exposed. What we really are and could be as individual human beings are not viable images for the mirrors of our culture. We are locked in a mirror reflecting one picture, condemned to mold ourselves to a vision that is not of our making. What more complete images of ourselves we try to see must be seen through cracks in the mirror and are all too fragmented. The effect of this form of social control has taken its toll on our personal and professional role behavior. Without a true picture of ourselves, we cannot go forward to plan our own future; without understanding what behaviors we have unquestioningly adopted and, in contrast, those we need to acquire, we cannot build a lasting structure of professionalism; without understanding that we have been carefully taught not to help each other, and what we must now do to help each other, we cannot begin to impress on public opinion the uniqueness and value of our professional practice.

The readings in Part I provide us with a vantage point from which to look back at our cultural heritage. From this unique position, we are reminded of those fixed images that have stamped our personal and professional conduct and can look ahead to those that are yet to be realized. What is worth salvaging is a decision each of us must make. Molding a new image is the challenge before us. The task involves risk, but without risk our foundation for the future will continue to be unplanned, unstructured, and unfurnished.

1 The Public Image of the Nurse

Linda Hughes

THE SCOPE and function of nursing practice have expanded over the past century, yet nurses continue to be bound by myths, traditions, and archaic ideas about their role in health care delivery. Although many nurses are now assuming independent and innovative roles in health care, the public continues to view the physician as the sole authority and as the primary provider of health care. Nursing potential has not been fully recognized or utilized by the public, and this has led to wasted nursing talent and inadequate care for society.

A historical study was recently conducted to determine the public opinion of the nurse and the nursing profession during the period 1896 to 1976 [1]. Data from popular magazines, novels and newspapers were obtained to formulate generalizations and identify themes that emerged during that period. The mass media have not only reflected but have also directed public opinion about the nurse and the nursing profession. From a historical perspective, the image of the nurse that has been projected through the mass media has been a distortion of reality, grounded in mythical beliefs and traditional ideas that for too long have gone unchallenged and unquestioned by the general public and by many nurses. The public image of the nurse may account, at least partially, for the failure of the public to fully utilize the services of the nurse in health care delivery.

HISTORICAL STUDY OF PUBLIC OPINION

Social and cultural changes evolve slowly and the effects of these changes are felt over a long period of time. Examination of historical records can give the researcher the advantage of discovering significant truths about human nature and social action. "The historian's advantage is that he is apt to see the whole Gestalt of circumstances which serves as a matrix for the ensuing behavior" [2, pp. 34–35]. For this reason, the historical study of public opinion is valid. Indeed, the concept of public opinion was identified by a historian over 2,000 years ago: "Thucydides, in his *History of the Peloponnesian War* organized his book around three closely related but different themes, the distribution of public opinion, the processes of opinion formation, and the impact of opinion upon government decisions" [3, pp. 117–118].

In his essay on the study of public opinion, Benson defined the historical approach to be "the use of procedures to secure data from documents that the researcher locates and selects but does not create, directly or indirectly. By selecting documents and . . . interrogating their author, historical researchers generate data designed to answer questions about past public opinion" [3, p. 109].

Reprinted from *Advances in Nursing Science*, by Linda Hughes, by permission of Aspen Systems Corporation, © April 1980.

Garraghan also discussed the value of documents in generating ideas about public opinion: The historian, he wrote, is able to "construct clear and distinct ideas or images of persons, events, institutions, and other things about which the document informs us" [4, p. 330].

SOURCES

Standard sources utilized by historians often do not reflect the opinion and popular ideas held by the mass population. Opinions expressed in newspaper and magazine editorials cannot always be assumed to reflect the opinion of the general public. The historian is well advised to look for data about public opinion in other sources such as school books, pulp fiction, comic books, fan magazines, novels, and popular magazines [5].

Vincent characterized the concept of public opinion as elusive and one that requires the researcher to utilize many and varied sources in order to make accurate and valid generalizations. He also pointed to the difficulty of determining exactly what public opinion was at a given time. He cautioned that "a large portion of the mass accepts its opinions from others"—and that those "others" may be a small but vociferous minority [6, pp. 281–282].

The ability of the historian to know and understand the men and women of the past is dependent upon the traces left behind. The historian must utilize every possible method of historical inquiry to come to the highest attainable degree of truth about the past. The following statement, by a historian, points out the importance of making inferences and generalizations in the study of public opinion.

[T]he men and women who have left records were not the common people; they were the literate, the people in positions of power and influence of one kind or another. They were, in brief, not representative of the entire population, though certainly they may have been representative of their own class or group. The problem of knowing the ordinary man . . . is compounded by the scant records in which those people set forth their feelings and concerns. The historian is often left to infer from the records of literate people what the ordinary man thought about himself and about those who directed the course of his actions by domestic and diplomatic decisions [5, p. 58].

NURSING "POORLY UNDERSTOOD"

Nurses have recognized the necessity of public understanding and cooperation in elevating the status of the nursing profession and initiating changes within the health care system. In 1928 the *American Journal of Nursing* requested its readers to define the major professional aim for the coming year. Public cooperation and understanding of the nursing profession was identified by many of the respondents as the major aim toward which the nursing profession should address itself. As one nurse commented, "the task of obtaining community understanding and, through it, community cooperation is indeed a challenge for, as nurses and as a profession, we are still poorly understood. For the most part, the community does not consider nursing an essential service for which it has a responsibility" [7, p. 52].

Despite an additional 52 years of evolution, the nursing profession is still poorly understood. Kinlein, describing the inception of her independent nursing practice, observed in 1977: "In the minds of the public, nursing was an adjunct to medicine, and any time they approached a nurse for care, or a nurse approached them to give care, the need had flowed from the medical condition of the person . . ." [8, p. 43]. Kinlein's observation about the publicly perceived close tie between nursing practice and medical practice bears a remarkable similarity to a comment made 100 years ago. The leaders of *Nineteenth Century* were told in 1880 that "Nursing is doctoring. . . . Any one who will set himself to define the function of the nurse as distinct from that of the doctor will very soon find himself involved in absurdity" [9, p. 1092].

Public opinion, though elusive, is a powerful factor influencing the consumer's utilization of nursing care. In light of the current public dissatisfaction with the health care system, nursing has the opportunity to assume a more beneficial role in health care delivery. To ensure more efficient and effective utilization of nursing care, the public must be cognizant of and receptive to the actual and potential role of the nurse in health care. Historical study can provide insight into factors that have influenced past public opinion toward the nursing profession. This knowledge can facilitate the nursing profession's development in the future.

DEFINITION OF TERMS

The following terms were defined for the purpose of studying public opinion regarding the nurse and the nursing profession.

Historical development—the chronological series of events, nursing and nonnursing, that have had a direct bearing upon the nursing profession.

Historical method—the effective gathering of source materials about past ideas of groups, appraising them critically, and presenting an interpretation of the results obtained.

Public opinion—a persistent, general orientation of society toward some individuals, groups or institutions which may or may not be based upon legitimate, correct or informed knowledge.

Nurse—one who provides preventive, curative or rehabilitative care to an individual or a group of individuals for the purpose of obtaining economic, educational or emotional remuneration. (This definition is based on the public's perception of the nurse and is not necessarily consistent with the nursing profession's definition.)

METHODOLOGY

The author used the historical method of research to analyze the problem. The collection of data was limited to literature obtainable in libraries of the southwestern United States. *Readers' Guide to Periodical Literature*, 1896 through 1976, was used to obtain data from secular magazines pertaining to the nurse and the nursing profession. The *New York Times*, 1895 through 1976, was sytematically examined to obtain data about the nursing profession. The author also examined selected lay novels pertaining to the nurse and the nursing profession. These data were analyzed to provide an understanding of the public view of the nurse and her role. The author then drew inferences, generalizations and conclusions regarding public opinion of the nurse and the nursing profession.

To determine a relationship between nursing practice and the public opinion of the nurse, the author examined the professional organ of the American Nurses' Association, the *American Journal of Nursing*, 1900 through 1976, as well as the professional organ of the National League of Nursing, *Nursing Outlook*, 1953 through 1976. Major trends within nursing practice were identified along with specific major social, legislative and economic factors that have influenced nursing practice. On the basis of these findings, the author determined the effect of nursing practice upon the public opinion of the nurse.

OVERVIEW OF FINDINGS
WOMAN'S WORK

The public consistently identified nursing as "work peculiarly suited to the dainty, delicate-minded woman" [10, p. 974]. Indeed, the nursing role and the mothering role were seen as historically interrelated. Innate maternalism and womanly qualities were publicly viewed as essential characteristics of the ideal nurse. Since women were mothers, it naturally followed that women were better suited for the nursing role than men both psychologically and emotionally. The public assumed that all women had a natural affinity for nursing work and that providing care for the sick came as second nature to any woman. As one nurse observed in 1883, the public "consider[s] hardly any training at all necessary for our nurses . . . the generality of people think that any woman can nurse" [11, p. 310].

VICTORIAN ROOTS

Training schools for nurses were established and a professional association for nurses in the United States was developed during the closing years of the Victorian Era. Victorian ideology "defined women's proper social roles in narrow and restricted ways. . . . women's actions had to be consistent with moral sensibility, purity, and maternal affection, and no other code of behavior was acceptable" [12, p. 14]. Victorian ideology dictated that women exhibit specific womanly qualities and subordinate all personal interests and activities to the maintenance of the home and the family [12, 13]. Educational and career opportunities for women were restricted because endeavors in these areas were believed to detract the woman from the execution of her responsibilities as a wife and mother. Women were expected to be passive, conservative, submissive and obedient to masculine authority. Society viewed competitiveness, aggressiveness, independence and initiative as masculine attributes. Such attributes were considered unattractive when exhibited in a woman. Women hesitated to engage in activities that could make them appear "unladylike" and thereby detract from their womanliness. Social respectability was stressed in Victorian ideology, and the vast majority of women made every effort to earn and maintain respectability by their actions and their manner.

Nineteenth-century women were not always the passive, submissive and pure creatures of popular idealizations, but neither were they ever completely free from this stereotype. Its most pervasive and effective form of control was through the social and individual demand for respectability. . . . [13, p. xix].

VIRTUE PERSONIFIED

As a predominantly woman's profession, nursing was deeply influenced by Victorian ideas about women and their proper place in society. The public image of the ideal nurse mirrored the public image of the virtuous woman [12, 13, 15]. Nurses were depicted in the secular literature as the epitome of true womanhood and the embodiment of all good womanly qualities. As the readers of *Good Housekeeping* were told in 1915, nursing is "that very high development of the qualities known as 'womanly' . . . [the nurse] seems to be a sort of embodied womanhood raised to the nth power [16, p. 736].

In light of the restrictions historically placed upon women in terms of their roles outside the home, equating nurses with true womanhood in the public literature served to tell women, in effect, that nursing was one occupation in which they could utilize their potential without compromising their social respectability. In fact, many articles written about nursing in the popular literature encouraged women to enter the nursing profession precisely because it *was* a woman's profession and nursing was one field in which women could rise to top positions and be well compensated for their achievements. Outlining the advantages of nursing as a suitable occupation for women, one nurse commented in 1904 that nursing "is also unique to being perhaps the only profession unreservedly assigned to women . . . in which they occupy all the higher positions. In every other line of life women either struggle in ineffectual competition with men or occupy the subordinate and less well-paid posts" [17, p. 310].

In 1915 a lay writer informed the public that a nursing career was available to women simply because men allowed it. This writer again commented on the absence of competition from men: "it is still a tussle to get a footing at all [in other leading professions] because of 'Keep Off the Ladder' signs posted in masculine handwriting. But here is a profession to which nobody nowadays denies women full access" [16, p. 729].

Thirty years later this theme was repeated in an effort to recruit women for nursing during World War II. Women were told: "The opportunity . . . to advance to posts of responsibility in nursing is relatively great because of the size of the field and lack of competition from men" [18, p. 18].

These statements in relation to a predominantly woman's profession cast insight into the secondary role which women historically were forced to assume. They reveal that competition with men was seen as useless and hardly worth the woman's efforts. Competitiveness was not a womanly quality and nursing was obviously seen as an avenue for women to realize their potential without appearing unwomanly.

UNWHOLESOME REPUTATION

Advertising nursing as a virtuous and womanly occupation had a beneficial effect, at least initially, upon the nursing profession. Before the establishment of training schools for nurses in this country, nurses had a particularly unwholesome reputation. Criminals, prostitutes, and intemperate and immoral women were commonplace among the ranks of those calling themselves nurses. By the very nature of the work, nursing was seen as menial labor barely befitting consideration by domestic servants. Women who were forced to earn a living and who were unable to secure any other form of work engaged in nursing.

In *Martin Chuzzlewit*, published in 1844, Dickens provided a representative example of the "professional nurse" of the time in the fictitious character of Sairey Gamp: "it was difficult to enjoy her society without becoming conscious of a smell of spirits . . . she took to [her profession] very kindly; insomuch, that setting aside her natural predilections as a woman, she went to a lying-in or a laying-out with equal zest and relish" [19, p. 302].

The sick who fell subject to the administrations of these "Sairey Gamps" were victims more often than they were recipients of nursing care. Dominated by women of such questionable reputation, nursing did not attract any respectable or well-qualified women. An English nurse provided the following summation of pre-Nightingale nursing:

. . . nursing . . . was at a low ebb; arduous and ill-paid, neither religious nor professional, it only attracted people who were quite unfit for any other occupation, often drunken and brutal, almost invariably inefficient. Particularly feeble paupers were . . . made night nurses,

because the pittance so earned would enable them to buy better food than the ordinary workhouse fare [20, pp. 587–588].

Nurses in the United States were of no higher caliber than those of England. Prior to 1873 the trained nurse did not exist in this country. Any woman who desired to nurse the sick could do so; indeed, many women were coerced into nursing work. One physician wrote that, prior to the trained nurse, "some of the nursing in Bellevue Hospital . . . was done by drunken prostitutes who in the Police Court were given the option of going to prison or to hospital service. No wonder they were often found in drunken sleep under the beds of their dead patients whose liquor they had stolen" [21, p. 71].

Nursing work was not only confined to women of questionable reputation, but convalescent patients also provided much of the nursing care in the early hospitals. One New York physician reminisced: "when I was an interne in a large hospital in 1875 . . . nurses were far inferior to the average domestic servant. Not a few of them had been patients who when convalescent had been elevated to the position of nurses. Some of them were faithful souls and did their best, but most of them had a fondness for Sairey Gamp's teapot and smelt of Sairey Gamp's tea" [22, pp. 164–165].

CHANGING THE PUBLIC IMAGE

With the establishment of training schools in the United States, the public image of the nurse underwent a slow process of change. Early nursing educators were intent upon upgrading the social status and the public image of the nurse. These early nurses attempted to keep the temperamentally unfit out of the profession by carefully screening applicants to training schools and rigidly enforcing a standard of exemplary behavior in pupil nurses. As one hospital manager reported in 1908, "no matron would choose her probationers from applicants with marked physical blemishes . . . she would wisely give preference to those who were personally pleasing" [23, p. 824].

The power of the public press also served to facilitate the improvement in the image of the nurse by publicly placing the nurse on a compatible social level with the good Victorian woman. Elevating the social status of the nurse enhanced the ability of the nursing profession to attract women of a higher quality for nursing work. Had nursing not come to be positively viewed by the public as a womanly occupation, many respectable and intelligent women never could have been induced to enter the nursing profession.

Thus defining the ideal nurse as an example of true womanhood in the public literature did exert a positive influence upon the nursing profession. However, the close public correlation between the ideal nurse and the true woman had some damaging effects upon the profession as well. Longstanding social beliefs about women and their role in society became the foundation for several mythical beliefs that were associated with the nursing profession. The confining image of the nurse which developed on the basis of social beliefs about women hampered the growth of nursing as a profession and promoted restrictions in the scope of nursing practice [24, 25].

THE IDEAL NURSE

The mass media created a mythical image of the ideal nurse, and the public historically expected all practicing nurses to adhere to that image. Many popular magazines depicted the nurse as little more than a "starched white figure moving romantically in hospital wards and operating rooms" [26, p. 74]. The ideal nurse was portrayed in lay publications as pretty, preferably young, cool and calmly efficient, clean and crisp in her uniform, and possessing a pleasing personality.

EMPHASIS ON PERSONALITY

The personality of the nurse was given a great deal of emphasis in the public literature. The personality characteristics of the ideal nurse paralleled the personality characteristics of the good Victorian woman. Womanly qualities were stressed as essential to the successful performance of the nursing role. In 1942, for example, *Occupations* ran an article, directed to high school students, which summarized the qualities of the ideal nurse as "neatness, tact, reliability, good judgment, poise, accuracy, dependability, honesty, common sense, and emotional stability. A nurse should also be loyal, conscientious, and cooperative. She should have initiative, dignity, imagination, and a timely sense of humor. She should be alert . . . [and] interested in her patients . . ." [27, p. 280].

While these qualities provided an excellent description of a fictitious nurse like Cherry Ames, they neither accurately nor realistically described actual nurses engaged in day-to-day nursing practice. Given the best of circumstances, it would be difficult for any person to display all of these qualities consistently, since situations and interactions are never static.

Much of the popular literature implied that if the nurse had a pleasing personality, then her mental capabilities were of secondary importance. As the public was told in 1941, "the personality and appearance of the nurse reacts subtly but genuinely upon the sick person" [28, p. 9]. While that is true, the intellectual and technical abilities of the nurse react subtly with the sick person as well. However, the public literature tended to stress the nurse's personality almost to the point of negating the intellectual and educational requirements of nursing practice.

In light of the importance placed upon the personality of the nurse, the implication was often made that education could not compensate for the absence of pleasing personality characteristics in the nurse. The public was told that "No amount of training will make a coarse-minded woman a dainty nurse" [10, p. 974]. Arguing that state registration of the nurse would not improve the quality of the practicing nurse, a hospital administrator made the following assertion in 1902: "far more attention is paid to and value put upon the character of the nurses than on their success in the technical part of their training" [29, pp. 772–773]. In 1956 *Reader's Digest* repeated that statement when it reported that "The responsiveness of a nurse comes more from her personality than from her formal education . . ." though the nurse was required to "perform delicate tasks and exercise the kind of judgment that until recent years were the exclusive prerogatives of doctors" [30, p. 82].

While a pleasing personality is essential for any professional person seeking to serve the public, this qualification alone could hardly be considered adequate to aid the nurse in exercising judgment, day in and day out, upon which the patient's life could depend. The inconsistency of statements such as these was not, however, seriously questioned by the public, primarily because the public had a limited understanding of the role of the nurse in patient care.

OVERLOOKING ABILITIES AND KNOWLEDGE

Nurses have had their role defined to the public in terms of the performance of rote and repetitive tasks. In 1955 *Look* defined the functions of the nurse as "giving injections, back rubs and bed baths, [and] making a neat hospital bed" [31, p. 62]. As recently as 1971 *Life* reported that, as a student nurse, one "learns the right way to take a blood pressure, read thermometers—and even empty a bedpan" [32, p. 47]. Given this limited view of the role of the nurse in health care, it is little wonder that the public failed to recognize intellectual abilities and a sound knowledge base as necessary requirements for excellence in nursing practice.

Intellectual abilities again assumed a secondary place in light of the qualification of physical fitness for nursing work. Besides being dainty, delicate minded, and womanly, the nurse was expected to be a hard worker. Physical strength and stamina were consistently seen as basic requirements for the ideal nurse. Women were told in 1915 that to be considered eligible for nurses' training they must be "guaranteed sound of body by a physician, sound of morals by a clergyman, and sound of teeth by a dentist" [16, p. 732]. In 1943 potential applicants for nursing schools were told that they would have to "pass a rigid physical test, probably intelligence and aptitude tests" [33, p. 67].

A BEDSIDE VOICE

Even the timbre of the nurse's voice was given consideration by the public. In a letter to the *American Journal of Nursing* in 1906 a former patient encouraged nurses to cultivate a soft speaking voice because "a well-modulated voice is a blessing" in the sick room [34, p. 104]. In 1917 *Literary Digest* quoted a physician as saying that upon the nurse's voice depended much of her usefulness, and that "if she has not a good 'bedside' voice by inheritance and home-training, she should proceed to acquire it at all costs" [35, p. 27].

UNREALISTIC EXPECTATIONS

The image of the ideal nurse projected through the mass media was a figment of public imagination. This image created an unrealistic expectation of the practicing nurse. The nursing profession historically faced public criticism because actual nurses often failed to measure up to the idealistic standard that was projected through the mass media. In addition, the public image of the ideal nurse did not advance the ability of the profession to gain public support for needed improvements in legislation and education for the practicing nurse.

NURSING AS A CALLING

For centuries the responsibility for providing nursing care to the sick poor was assumed by religious orders. The early association between nursing and religion resulted in the public identification of nursing as a charitable and merciful gesture to humankind. This belief about nursing continued after it became a secular occupation for women. Many nurses and the general public alike historically equated nursing with a religious calling that required its followers to display the qualities of devotion, dedication, obedience to authority, willing self-sacrifice, and self-effacement. Ethel Fenwick, first president of the International Council of Nurses, elaborated upon the woman's motivation in choosing the nursing profession as a career: "I believe that a large proportion [of nurses] adopt this calling from the highest motives and the heart-felt desire to fulfil the Divine command to tend the sick" [36, p. 326].

Nonnursing groups often expressed the opinion that, in the absence of the religious motivations Fenwick described, no nurses could hope to attain any measure of success in their work. As one hospital manager concluded in 1902, "it will never be possible to have perfect nursing without willing self-sacrifice" [29, p. 772].

In working for reforms to elevate the economic and professional status of the profession, nurses were often judged as being selfish, self-centered, and failing to live up to the religious instincts that were felt to be natural to their calling. Nurses were often viewed as subject to "small feminine vanities," believed to be "strangely out of place when allied with a calling concerned with issues so grave" [23, p. 824]. Typifying the attitude of many of his colleagues, one hospital administrator blatantly declared that nurses must subordinate themselves to the duties of their calling. In his words,

. . . nursing is a calling demanding of its followers, if they are to excel, a measure of self-obliteration which to minds dominated by ideas of personal advantage and advancement may appear foolishness, but is essential to the true nurse. This does not mean that the woman who takes up nursing must be necessarily indifferent to matters affecting her own health and well-being. . . . But she must be capable of giving them their rightful, which is a secondary, place [23, p. 825].

The natural and inevitable result of viewing nursing as a calling led to the belief that, for their labors, nurses received heavenly rather than earthly rewards. Isabel Stewart, a prominent nursing educator, concluded in 1927 that nurses had been persuaded to believe that the "only satisfactions . . . ever expect[ed] in nursing are the satisfactions that come through self-sacrifice" [37, p. 538]. An article run in *Good Housekeeping* in 1961 summarized this belief in this way: "despite long hours, low pay, and more grind than glamour, the moments when [the nurse's] compassion and skill help relieve a patient's suffering more than compensate for the drawbacks of her profession" [38, p. 35].

The correlation between nursing and a religious calling and the resultant belief that willing self-sacrifice was essential to nursing practice provided the justification needed to support the low pay and long hours of labor that historically characterized the nurse's employment. Of greater importance, this belief was supported by male-dominated groups within the health care system, groups that exerted external control over the practice and the education of the nurse. By advocating this belief, these groups attempted to provide legitimate rationalization for the exploitation of women's labors in the health care system.

MYTHICAL THEMES ASSOCIATED WITH THE NURSING PROFESSION

The public image of the nurse has been intricately related to several mythical beliefs that have been projected to the public as repeated themes throughout the history of the nursing profession. Mythical beliefs have a powerful influence on society in part because of their adherence to cultural beliefs and also because they are generalized to an entire society or group within society. Despite the connotation of the term falsity, myths exist because the majority of society believe in their authenticity and validity. By responding to consciously and unconsciously held beliefs and values, myths transmit their validity and justify their existence and their perpetuation.

THE BORN NURSE

The public has historically viewed nursing work as a special area in which women could excel because of their innate "womanliness." As a result of this belief, the need to educate women for nursing work was publicly minimized. Maternal instincts and womanly qualities were God-given, and a woman was born with them or without them. Even after training schools were established in this country, the belief existed that the nurse was born, not made; thus leading to the assumption that no amount or kind of training could instill in a woman the essential qualities of the ideal nurse. As a hospital manager asserted in 1902, "No training, whether the hours be long or short, will endow a young woman with gifts which Nature has failed to bestow upon her. . . . Maternal instincts and nursing instincts are much the same, and women are born with them or without them" [29, pp. 771–772].

The argument that the nurse was born and not made was used throughout nursing's history as justification for limiting the educational preparation of student nurses. Nursing education in the United States developed as a manifestation of apprenticeship training. Training schools for nurses were affiliated with a specific hospital. Student nurses functioned as the nursing service department of the hospital. Following a specified time of service, the student nurse received a diploma from the training school and was discharged from the hospital as a graduate trained nurse. Student nurses, in effect, traded their labor on the hospital wards for their training as a nurse.

Hospital administrators were quick to recognize the economic value of the hospital-based training school for nurses. Staffing the hospital wards with student nurses provided a plentiful and inexpensive source of labor. Moreover, admitting women to the training school every six months or every year provided the hospital with a fresh group of workers to staff the hospital wards. In fact, in many training schools, student admission occurred year-round depending on the labor needs of the hospital. If one student nurse dropped out, another was readily admitted.

Functioning as the nursing service department of the hospital, the vast majority of student nurses did not receive the educational opportunities needed to adequately prepare them for nursing work. The educational needs of the student nurse assumed a secondary place in light of the nursing service needs of the hospital. Many training schools for nurses offered no semblance of an education for their students. Student nurses worked as many as 105 hours a week; lectures, of which there were few, were offered in the evening after a full day of work; classroom and laboratory facilities were virtually nonexistent; and few schools provided even one paid instructor [25].

Nonnursing groups, especially hospital administrators, who had an economic investment in the type and amount of training student nurses received, were the primary advocates of the born-nurse myth. Defending the limited educational preparation of the student nurse, one hospital authority stated in 1908 that "no amount of training will transform a probationer wanting in personal suitability into a good nurse. . . . Inefficiency in a nurse is much more often due to want of character than to a lack of intelligence or a capacity to learn the mere technicalities of her art . . ." [23, p. 830].

The born-nurse myth appeared in the popular literature in relation to the educational preparation of the nurse as recently as 1968. *Look*, reporting on an apparent nursing shortage, reported that the "aggravating factor" was the recommendation made in 1965 by the American Nurses' Association that the baccalaureate degree should be the basic requirement for beginning entry into professional nursing practice. "Your ability to like people depends on your basic personality," opined an anonymous hospital authority. "Love and concern are God-given; they're not handed out with a college degree" [39, p. 29].

The born-nurse myth contributed to the difficulties faced by the nursing profession as attempts were made to improve the educational opportunities available to prepare women for nursing work. Although nursing educators repeatedly argued that nurses were only as good as their education, they had little impact upon a belief that had been ingrained in the minds of the public for the better part of the century. The propagation of the born-nurse myth has been a persuasive argument used to thwart the attempts of the profession to elevate nurses' educational and professional standards. Following a study of medical education in 1910, standards for medical education were developed and medical schools were quickly established in the university setting. As a general rule, however, collegiate affiliations for nursing education were not established until some 40 years later.

THE NEW ROAD TO MARRIAGE

Marriage and motherhood have been the traditional societal expectation of women. Since nursing has traditionally been predominantly a woman's profession, it was inevitable that the marriageability of nurses would receive the attention of the public, especially young women seeking to enter the profession. The promise of marriage as an attractive fringe benefit of nursing work pervaded popular literature. Articles published about nursing, geared to the young woman, often implied that becoming a nurse would improve one's chances for marriage, especially marriage to physicians. Nursing was defined as the "new road to matrimony" in 1897 [40, p. 31], and 70 years later, *Mademoiselle* advised young women "in search of a physician-husband" that they "would do well to conduct the search in hospital corridors, for a homely nurse is more likely to marry a young physician or medical student than is a homely secretary or teacher" [41, p. 134].

While an attractive salary, fringe benefits, and opportunities for career advancement have been the usual selling features for most vocations, marriage was the primary selling feature for the nursing profession in the popular literature. Particularly during the war years when the need for nurses was especially great, advertising the improved marriageability of nurses went into high gear. Recruitment campaigns conducted especially during World War II promised women that if they became nurses and volunteered for overseas duty they could expect romantic encounters that could well culminate in marriage. Based on an interview with a nurse recruiter during World War II, the *New York Times* informed women that on overseas military bases marriages were occurring at the rate of four per day [42]. Women were told that "nurses were never inclined to be old maids very much. Why, most nurses can hardly avoid marrying doctors . . ." [43, p. 4].

Many women, having been conditioned to view nursing work as a temporary and, at best, stopgap occupation, entered nursing with little desire to maintain a long-term commitment to the profession. Nursing schools historically trained thousands of women, many of whom remained in nursing work for only a short period of time. Moreover, many nurses were satisfied to tolerate the low pay and poor working conditions that throughout history have plagued the working nurse because they viewed their employment as temporary and anticipated eventual withdrawal from nursing practice.

NURSE AS PHYSICIAN'S HELPMATE

The public has viewed nurses as being wedded to physicians. Nursing practice, in the minds of the public, has been and continues to be subordinately linked to medical practice. The public has for many years watched nurses faithfully carry out physicians' orders, respond to physicians' demands and idiosyncrasies, prepare patients and the sickroom for physicians' visits, and clean up after physicians following their departure from the sickroom. As a result, the public has believed that the physician is the "master and controller of both nurse and patient" [44, p. 1105]. In a more recent era, *Today's Health* reported on flight nurses in Vietnam with the observation that "romance is flourishing. . . . To date, five nurses have married men they met at war, and almost all others are being energetically courted" [45, p. 60].

Women were also told that undergoing nurse's training would be excellent preparation for marriage and motherhood. Women had nothing to lose by completing nurses' training because, whether they chose to practice as nurses or not, they could use the knowledge gained to aid them in their role as wives and mothers. For a nominal tuition and "three years of interesting work, [the woman] could buy herself . . . perfect preparation for marriage and motherhood" [46, p. 116].

As mentioned before, Victorian ideology dictated that women not assume careers that could interfere with the execution of their responsibilities as wives and mothers. Consistent with this ideology, the subtle implication was made throughout the popular media that, after marriage, women were no longer expected to remain in active nursing practice. Marriage provided a legitimate exit from the profession. Several "true" stories about nurses were published in the popular literature which depicted the ideal nurse who, though deeply gratified by her service to humanity, planned to marry and retire from the profession [47, 48]. As recently as 1960 *Today's Health* reported that "if later [nurses] should trade their caps for a wedding ring, what better preparation would there be for marriage and motherhood?" [49, p. 66].

This image of the nurse led to the assumption that nurses functioned only under physician supervision. The public has viewed nurses as being totally dependent upon physicians to guide everyday nursing practice. Indeed, the public has been led to believe that any action by a nurse that had not been approved by a physician could result in harm to the patient. The public was told that "A fundamental principle of the nurse's existence is that she gives nursing care only under the direction of a licensed physician. . . . Infringement, with the best intentions in the world, may lead to misunderstanding, harm, even danger to the patient . . ." [50, p. 206].

To the detriment of the public and the nursing profession alike, the public has never identified nursing care as separate and distinct from physician care. In fact, the public has historically assumed that the major role of the nurse is to aid physicians in their efforts to provide medical services. The public has never equated nursing care with health care, rather it has viewed nursing care as a watered-down version of physician care. The nurse has been seen as an extension of the physician, performing simple medical procedures in the sickroom. As an editorial in the *New York Times* stated in 1921, the nurse "is trained to exercise judgment and assume responsibility in many minor matters, and so enables her chief to devote himself more fully to the major functions of his profession" [51, p. 14]. This notion was repeated 55 years later when nurse practitioners were defined as "trained assistants and [physician] surrogates" whose function was to "free the highly trained modern physician from . . . routine and often repetitive tasks" [52, p. 532].

The mythical belief in the nurse's subordination to the physician, projected through the popular media, has led to public depreciation of the role of the nurse in health care. Nursing care has always existed with or without physician supervision. The failure of the public to recognize this has had a damaging effect upon the growth of nurses as professional practitioners and upon the utilization of nurses to their fullest potential in health care.

EDUCATING THE PUBLIC

The need for public education has been dramatically demonstrated by the media's interpretation of the recent expansion of many nurses into more independent and health-oriented roles. For example, in the words of two popular magazines, nurses in expanded roles are performing "routine tasks that we've come to associate with physicians" [53, p. 21], tasks that "bore more M.D.'s, yet take up so much of their expensive time" [54, p. 35]. The public continues to view the nurse as dependent upon physician supervision and unable to function without medical direction. As recently as 1975 *McCalls* reported that independent nurse practitioners "generally have to be associated with doctors in some way since, despite their independence, they are really an extension of good medical service" [54, p. 35].

Nursing care continues to be equated with the performance of tasks and, for the most part, is not associated with the use of decision-making skills and independent thinking. Reporting on the development of an independent nurse practitioner program in 1966 *Time* quoted a physician to say that the nurse "doesn't have to know the specific difficulty . . . she simply has to know enough to say to herself . . . This one is for the doctor" [55, p. 71].

Any profession that seeks to serve the public must concern itself with public opinion. Public opinion has been and continues to be a powerful tool to promote change in society. The nursing profession has been aware of the need to maintain a well-educated and informed public. The American Nurses' Association, for example, declared 1978 as the Year of the Nurse and conducted a nationwide campaign to educate the public to the role of the nurse in health care.

To be beneficial, however, public education must be a constant process that gives the public consistent and repetitive exposure to the nursing profession. Although some nurses have utilized the public press, they have been well in the minority. Lack of journalistic knowledge and insecurity in their literary ability have kept many nurses from attempting to communicate with the public through the press. As a result, nursing's efforts to educate the public have proved to be haphazard, thus ineffectual.

The importance of establishing a positive public image is especially great at this time in history. Debates about the crisis in health care are common and many of the inadequacies of the present health care system are being publicly exposed. As consumers of health care, the public is expressing dissatisfaction with the high cost and the poor quality of services available to them. This social climate will inevitably lead to changes in the health care delivery system.

Because of the nursing profession's intimate association with the existing health care system, changes in this system will have a direct bearing on nursing practice. Public opinion of the nurse has had and will continue to have an effect on the ability of the nursing profession to provide a unique and beneficial service to the public. The general public is the consumer of health care, and its demand for and utilization of nursing services will determine the extent to which nurses will function in nontraditional roles in the future. For example, the ability to function as professional practitioners mandates that third party payment and direct reimbursement for nursing services be established. This form of reimbursement must compensate nurses for more than just the performance of tasks and the execution of the physician's orders.

If the nursing profession believes that it has a valuable service to offer in the area of health care, this must be communicated to the public through the mass media. There is no one more capable or better qualified to inform the public of contributions the nursing profession can make in the area of health care than nurses themselves. By openly communicating with the public, nurses can dispel the myths that have long surrounded the nursing profession and begin to project an image that accurately and positively reflects what nursing is. As one nurse commented half a century ago, "we have unequalled opportunities for service and instruction. . . . Whether we justify our existence, whether we convince the public that we are really essential, rests with us" [56, p. 819].

REFERENCES

1. Hughes, L. "Nursing and the Public: Images and Opinions of the Profession 1896–1976." Master's thesis, Texas Woman's University 1978.
2. Ware, C. *The Cultural Approach to History* (New York: Columbia University Press 1940).
3. Benson, L. *Toward the Scientific Study of History* (Philadelphia: J. B. Lippincott Co. 1972).
4. Garraghan, G. *A Guide to Historical Method* (Westport, Conn.: Greenwood Press 1940).
5. Stephens, L. *Probing the Past* (Boston: Allyn and Bacon 1974).
6. Vincent, J. *Historical Research* (New York: Franklin Reprints 1974).
7. Roberts, A. "Aims for 1928." *Am J Nurs* 28:1 (January 1928) p. 52.
8. Kinlein, M. L. *Independent Nursing Practice with Clients* (Philadelphia: J. B. Lippincott Co. 1977).
9. Sturges, O. "Doctors and Nurses." *Nineteenth Century* 7:40 (June 1880) pp. 1089–1096.
10. Rae, L. "The Question of the Modern Trained Nurse." *Nineteenth Century* 51:304 (June 1902) pp. 972-974.
11. Craven, F. "Servants of the Sick Poor." *Nineteenth Century* 13:74 (April 1883) pp. 667, 668.
12. Rothman, S. *Woman's Proper Place* (New York: Basic Books 1978).
13. Hymowitz, C. and Weissman, M. *A History of Women in America* (New York: Bantam Books 1978).
14. Vicinus, M. *A Widening Sphere* (Bloomington, Ind.: University Press 1977).
15. Kalisch, P. and Kalisch, B. *The Advance of American Nursing* (Boston: Little, Brown and Co. 1978).
16. Comstock, S. "Your Daughter's Career: If She Wants to Be a Nurse," *Good Housekeeping* 61:6 (December 1915) pp. 728–736.
17. Ferguson, H. "State Registration of Nurses." *Nineteenth Century* 55:324 (February 1904) pp. 310–317.
18. "Says U.S. Will Have 48,000 Nurses in '48 with Post-War Jobs for All." *New York Times* (June 11, 1945) p. 18.
19. Dickens, C. *Martin Chuzzlewit* (New York: Dutton Press 1968).
20. Moss, M. "The Evolution of the Trained Nurse." *Atlantic Monthly* 91:1047 (May 1903) pp. 587–599.
21. Worchester, A. *Nurses and Nursing* (Cambridge: Harvard University Press 1927).
22. Bristow, A. T. "What Registration Has Done for the Medical Profession." *Am J Nurs* 3:3 (December 1903) pp. 161–167.
23. Rawlings, B. "Nurses in Hospitals." *Nineteenth Century* 64:381 (November 1908) pp. 824–836.
24. Bullough, B. "Barriers to the Nurse Practitioner Movement: Problems of Women in a Woman's Field" in Bullough, B. and Bullough, V., eds. *Expanding Horizons for Nurses* (New York: Springer Publishing Co. 1977) pp. 307–318.
25. Ashley, J. *Hospitals, Paternalism, and the Role of the Nurse* (New York: Teachers College Press 1976).
26. Stafford, J. "Operation Nurse." *Science Newsletter* 51:5 (February 1, 1947) pp. 74–75.
27. Madison, L. "What I Want to Be." *Occupations* 30:4 (January 1952) pp. 280–281.
28. McLaughlin, K. "Needed: More Nurses." *New York Times Magazine* (March 9, 1941) p. 9+.

29. Holland, S. "The Case for Hospital Nurses." *Nineteenth Century* 51:303 (May 1902) pp. 770–779.
30. Reynolds, Q. "Young Women in White." *Reader's Digest* 69:415 (November 1956) pp. 79–83.
31. "Twin Nurses." *Look* 19:9 (May 3, 1955) p. 62.
32. "A Man in Blue Dons Nurse's White." *Life* 70:18 (May 14, 1971) pp. 47, 48.
33. Hawes, E. "There's a Career in Nursing." *Woman's Home Companion* 70:1 (January 1943) pp. 66, 67.
34. "The Nurse from a Patient's Point of View." *Am J Nurs* 7:2 (November 1906) p. 104.
35. "The Nurse's Voice." *Literary Digest* 55:19 (November 10, 1917) p. 27.
36. Fenwick, E. "Nurses a la Mode." *Nineteenth Century* 41:240 (February 1897) pp. 325–332.
37. Stewart, I. "Educating Nurses." *Survey* 58:10–12 (August 15–September 15, 1927) pp. 537, 538.
38. Markel, H. "Student Nurse." *Good Housekeeping* 153:1 (July 1961) p. 32 +.
39. Berg, R. "Where Did All the Nurses Go?" *Look* 32:2 (January 23, 1968) p. 26 +.
40. Priestley, E. "Nurses a la Mode." *Nineteenth Century* 41:239 (January 1897) pp. 28–37.
41. Hoffman, R. "The Angel of Mercy Is Dead." *Mademoiselle* 66:2 (December 1976) p. 134 +.
42. "Col. Clement Hails Army Nurses in Pacific: Homemaking Skills in Jungle Is Stressed." *New York Times* (May 17, 1944) p. 22.
43. "Higher Learning Urged for Nurses." *New York Times* (December 8, 1940) sec. 2, p. 4.
44. Lonsdale, M. "Doctors and Nurses." *Nineteenth Century* 7:40 (June 1880) pp. 1105–1108.
45. Martin, L. "Angels of Vietnam." *Today's Health* 45:8 (August 1967) p. 16 +.
46. Mayor, M. "How to Get Nurses Galore." *Reader's Digest* 56:334 (February 1950) pp. 116–118.
47. Acuille, J. "I Had to Grow Up—in a Hurry." *Woman's Home Companion* 82:10 (October 1955) pp. 36–38.
48. Villet, B. "More than Compassion." *Life* 72:14 (April 1972) p. 68.
49. Conley, V. "R.N.—Those Magic Initials." *Today's Health* 38:12 (December 1960) p. 38 +.
50. Deming, D. "Nursing by Leg Power." *Survey* 63:4 (November 15, 1929) pp. 205, 206.
51. Editorial Comment. "Nursing as a Profession." *New York Times* (May 19, 1921) p. 14.
52. Birenbaum, A. "New Health Practitioner in Primary Care." *Intellect* 105:2374 (April 1976) pp. 532-534.
53. Safran, C. "Their Patients Call Them Supernurses." *Today's Health* 53:7 (July–August 1975) p. 20 +.
54. "The New Family Doctor Is a Nurse." *McCalls* 103:1 (October 1975) p. 35.
55. "Where Doctors Don't Reach." *Time* 88:4 (July 22, 1966) p. 71.
56. "Minutes of the Proceedings of the Thirteenth Annual Convention of the Nurses' Associated Alumnae of the United States." *Am. J Nurs* 19:10 (July 1910) pp. 817–819.

2 Feminine Attributes in a Masculine World

Winifred J. Pinch

AS A GROUP nurses often lack power and prestige, and therefore, the rights and responsibilities to carry out their professional role. Power groups, such as hospital administrators and physicians, have in the past had a larger degree of control over the practice of the profession of nursing than nurses themselves. The profession today is in part a product of that history, and in order to change, an understanding of this perspective is necessary.

The prototype for professional nursing evolved from the mother's role in the family and the mother's duties in situations of illness, injury, and death. The work of deaconesses and religious orders that promoted loving care, charity, devotion, and similar virtues also exerted a formative influence. (While there is nothing inherently wrong with such behaviors, in our society they are not usually rewarded economically or politically. Autonomy, competition, and aggression are. They lead to power and the ability to create and promote significant changes in society.)

Much later, Nightingale's nonsectarian reform movement gave nursing the potential for autonomy. Training schools were established, a suitable occupation was developed, and efficient nursing service was provided outside the financial control of established institutions such as hospitals and religious groups. Nightingale did not view nursing as subservient to the medical profession but instead as a useful, desirable occupation for women beyond marriage and managing a home.

By contrast, training schools for nurses in the United States were founded by hospital administrators as the least expensive means of providing nursing care [1]. Not only did the role of nursing evolve from the mother's role in the family, but the family itself served as a model for care in the hospital. Nurses, who were women, were to provide efficient, economical care to patients, be loyal to the institution, and function in the role of the mother, attending to the household chores and meeting the needs of the physician.

The majority of hospital staff members prior to 1950 consisted of student nurses [2]. Graduate nurses were employed for supervisory or administrative positions. The larger sphere of employment for graduate nurses was outside the hospital, in community health nursing. Even those positions were competitive with students, who were also available at cheaper rates for private home care. Thus, abundance and competition characterized the scene and provided the foundation for a division between education and practice.

Apprenticeship education became firmly established. Criticism of the role of the nurse or the hospital system could now appear to be analogous to an attack on the family—a blow to

Copyright © 1981, American Journal of Nursing Company. Reproduced, with permission, from *Nursing Outlook*, October, Volume 29, Number 10.

the very heart of the American social system. Some individuals with accurate, perceptive visions of the future anticipated the stranglehold that an apprenticeship system would produce on nursing. Leaders in the early 1900s recognized the system as supporting persistent conditions of extreme exploitation [3]. Education, however, was controlled by the commercial interests of hospitals, and the commercial basis of delivering health care was in turn a major impediment to the realization of improved patient care under control of the professional nurse [4].

Identification of two major tasks by nursing leaders in the early 1900s led to the creation of two major nursing organizations. The hospital-based task of improving the education and the working conditions of students led to the formation of the American Society of Superintendents of Training Schools for Nurses of the United States and Canada (later the National League for Nursing). The community-based task of protecting graduates in their work setting, attaining legal status, and arresting competition from partially trained individuals became a primary duty of the Nurses Associated Alumnae of the United States and Canada (later the American Nurses' Association) [5]. The conflicts and misunderstandings created by this division haunt nursing to this day as educators and practitioners wrestle with their differences instead of recognizing the strength in what is common to each.

BIASED PREMISES

But a more far-reaching effect results from the socialization and educational processes to which nurses, 98 percent of whom are female, are exposed. In the educational process, which in part is an attempt to explain our development, roles, and functions in society, there is a strong bias that favors the male. Theories of developmental psychology, including moral development, for example, take the male as their model of the mature adult and fail to legitimize women's experiences.

The bias that pervades these theories promotes a concern for autonomy and achievement. Autonomy in our society is closely related to power, which can be seen as a prerequisite to rights. If moral developmental theories are used to evaluate individual growth and to provide guidelines for educational method and content, we must be aware of their premises. Gilligan identifies Freud, Piaget, Erikson, and Kohlberg as appropriate starting points to begin to recognize how we have been perceiving the world through the eyes of men [6]. There is a common theme in these developmental theories: the confirmation and promotion of emotional dependency and responsibility for people in women. At the same time, individuality, autonomy, and natural rights are promoted in men [7].

Erikson's eight-stage theory has been widely integrated into nursing content. Gilligan examines his account of human development and states that the crucial stage to investigate is the fifth: the adolescent identity crisis [8]. During this stage a coherent sense of self must be formed to span puberty and adulthood in order to have the capacity to work. But, Gilligan asks, does this description apply equally to boys and girls? In evaluating Erikson's work, Gilligan says no, the sequence for women is different:

> . . . *the girl holds herself in abeyance as she prepares to attract the man by whose name she will be known, by whose station she will be defined . . . for men, identity precedes intimacy and generativity in the optimal cycle of human separation and attachment. For women these tasks seem to be fused instead. Intimacy precedes, or rather goes along with, identity as the female comes to know herself as she is known, through her relationships with others [9].*

Erikson may have observed differences in the development of women, but these differences go unrecognized as the norm proposed in his history. Optimal development is identified with separation and individuation.

Attachments or the lack of autonomy are viewed as developmental impediments and are traits that are usually seen as characterologic deficiencies in women [10].

The theories of all of these men are related since the later theorists built upon the work of their predecessors. Erikson frequently refers to the work of Freud and Piaget, quotes from Freud abound in Piaget, and Kohlberg credits Piaget as exerting considerable influence upon his own thinking and actual development of his theory. Therefore, it is relevant to examine the earlier theorists' views of women and to look at current research as well.

Piaget in his *Moral Judgment of the Child* mentions girls only as an aside and makes one remark in the contents and three brief entries in the index. Boys receive no specific mention because "the child" is assumed to be male [11]. Piaget conducted a naturalistic study of the rules of games. Girls accepted rules if they were repaid in the process of playing the game. They were more tolerant, made more exceptions, and were reconciled to innovations, although Piaget defined this as being more pragmatic. Boys become increasingly fascinated with a legal elaboration of rules and became involved in the rules as much as the game. Rules were drawn up to resolve conflict and devised so that a fair process of playing the game developed as well. Piaget considered rule development essential for moral development and found these abilities more apparent in boys [12].

Freud, too, can be seen as projecting a masculine image. His theory of psychosexual development was built around the experiences of the male child that culminated in the Oedipal complex and its resolution. He struggled to resolve the contradictions posed for his theory by the female's differing configurations of sexuality and differing dynamics of early family relationships. He finally concluded, however, that the differences were responsible for what he considered woman's developmental failure. Freud attempted at one point to say that women envied something that they did not have (penis envy), but he had difficulty explaining the strength and persistence of the female pre-Oedipal attachments to the mother. Oedipal resolution did not occur in females as it did in males, and therefore, he concluded, women did not develop a superego as did men. This, Freud said, created a difference in the level of ethically normal action: in the realm of ethical thinking, women are more influenced by feelings of affection and hostility than are men [13].

Kohlberg's theory of moral development has been gaining more and more prestige. Previously he was given no more mention than an endnote in some psychology books. Now whole chapters and books on moral development, psychology, and educational psychology are built around his work. Women were completely absent from his original research sample. Yet he developed and proposed a universal theory of moral development from his data. Criticism can also be aimed at his selection of the characteristics of justice, equality, and rights—the old rationalist, enlightenment values—as the epitome of moral development. If the emphasis was instead on responsibility and obligation, the definition of moral stages and the scores of some, notably women, might be modified. Kohlberg identifies a strong interpersonal bias in the moral judgments of women, which leads them to be considered as typically at the third stage of his six-stage developmental sequence [14]. Obviously, this places women lower by three stages than the optimal stages of moral reasoning.

HOW TO KILL A MOCKINGBIRD

It is interesting to note the large number of nurses who are using Kohlberg's theory in research at the doctoral level, accepting his premises and conclusions, and implementing changes in the educational processes of nurses based on that research. Are we accumulating evidence and supporting hypotheses that serve only to undermine or negate our position in society as a whole and our profession in particular?

Considerable psychological data have been accumulated to support the proposal that morality is viewed differently by women than by men. The destructive aspect of this alleged difference is that the male perspective is considered to be superior, better, or preferred.

In fairy tales, myths, legends, and literature, as well as in psychology, man's context is the world, woman's, the relationship to people. We have been bombarded with these models from infancy. The princess is frequently put into a deep sleep or imprisoned at the onset of puberty and confined to this state until Prince Charming comes along to rescue her. This implies a moratorium on development of the female in every sphere, until she has a partner for life and can be fulfilled through her association and identification with a male. In addition women have been viewed as the root of evil in myths and legends, most notably, Pandora and Eve.

CITIZENS WITHOUT RIGHTS

Frequently, women are not considered as individuals within common political and legal parameters. Though officially they are citizens in almost every country of the Western world, real economic and social equality are denied them. Modern arguments, strikingly parallel to thoughts spanning centuries of Western political history, continue to justify unequal treatment of women—the denial of rights that are taken for granted by men.

The use of generic terms "man," "mankind," and "he" by philosophers does *not,* in fact, always refer to the human race as a whole. "Human nature" as described by Aristotle, Aquinas, Locke, and Rousseau was meant as *male* human nature only. Such philosophers who have "regarded the family as a natural and necessary institution," defined women by their sexual, procreative, and child-rearing functions within it. This has led to differences in the code of morality and definitions of rights between men and women [15].

Still very much in evidence today is woman as wife and mother within the family. In Western philosophical thought, it has been historically asked "What are men like?" "What are women for?" [16]. Elaborate theories have been developed in which "men were seen as mature and complete individuals and women were seen as inseparable from sexual and family roles—mothers, housekeepers, and caregivers, *naturally* subject to men [17].

If philosophy is a search for truth, and these views represent the truth as major philosophers have seen it, major political, economic, and educational ramifications follow. Women become victims of such thinking in every aspect of their lives, including the professional one.

CONFLICTING ATTRIBUTES

So basic are these assumptions in the socialization of women to the female role, that it becomes very difficult to separate the traditional female role from the role of nurse. Women are typically seen as being responsible for the caring functions of humankind, expected to alleviate trouble and discomfort [18]. Tact, gentleness, awareness of the feelings of others, and the expression of tender feelings are the "goodness" of women [19]. These same attributes also contribute positively to the care of patients. It is the kind of care that patients want and need and that nurses want to be able to give. Perhaps it is also hindering the widespread acceptance of nursing as a profession.

How can one professionalize the nurturing role of mother or caregiver? These functions are not easily amenable to rigorous scientific definition and description. Incongruence develops as nurses foster the development of these traits in relationships with patients while struggling for identification and enhancement of characteristics needed to be effective in relationships with administrators and government. This is the sort of double-bind that engenders schizophrenia.

Thus, history and socialization combine to produce situations that result in moral dilemmas for the nurse and a conflict of rights. The conflict, however, is a conflict of power related to professional roles and territoriality.

Solutions to the problem demand changes of basic societal assumptions. As has been noted, "an expanded conception of adulthood that would result from the integration of the 'feminine voice' in developmental theories" and "a more balanced conception of human development" are in order [20, 21]. Envision the "different" attributes and characteristics of women valued as much as those that have been traditionally identified with men.

Such an integration and recognition, however, will not just happen by itself, and it will take more than the efforts of a few scholars giving recognition to the importance of the distinguishing characteristics of half the population. Leaders are needed with power, prestige, and autonomy to promote and emphasize the value of these characteristics. The need for power and prestige is fundamental. Presently, assertiveness, even aggression, autonomy, and independence are characteristics that are rewarded with the power to make changes. These attributes must be cultivated and implemented to promote the values of caring, gentleness, and responsibility more fully. In the end, hopefully, a balance of both sets of attributes will become the norm of healthy adulthood for men and women.

As nurses responsible for the practice of the profession and for the education of future practitioners, we must be alert to the influence of our own history and our personal socialization upon the issues of rights and power.

A large proportion of professional nurses are uncommitted, uninterested, and divided in relation to their profession; many are confused and frustrated in their professional role. We have little understanding of the significance of such a position for personal growth and in turn the growth of the profession. We have the potential for creating a dynamic influence on our government and society if we first understand and remedy our own social position. When we comprehend the ambiguity of the rights issue and grasp the full implications of the issues of power and prestige, we will be able to vitalize our efforts in every direction.

There are several great barriers to transcend. However, the task is not impossible. If we begin with education and reeducation of our members, continue with renewed and vigorous support for our organization, then we can move out to work for public recognition for our profession. At that point, we will be well on our way to becoming a more powerful and influential force in society today.

REFERENCES

1. Ashley, J. A. *Hospitals, Paternalism and the Role of the Nurse.* New York, Teachers College Press, Teachers College, Columbia University, 1976, p. 9.
2. Ibid., p. 55.
3. Ibid., pp. 48–49.
4. Ibid., p. 72.
5. Ibid., pp. 95–96.
6. Gilligan, C. Woman's place in man's life cycle. *Harvard Educ. Rev.* 49:432, Nov. 1979.

7. Ibid., p. 445.
8. Ibid., pp. 436–437.
9. Ibid., p. 437.
10. Gilligan, *op. cit.*, p. 437.
11. Piaget, J. *The Moral Judgment of the Child.* New York, The Free Press, 1933, p. 408.
12. Ibid., pp. 77, 82.
13. Gilligan, *op. cit.,* p. 433.
14. Gilligan, C. In a different voice: women's conceptions of self and morality. *Harvard Educ. Rev.* 47:484, Nov. 1977.
15. Okin, S. M. *Women in Western Political Thought.* Princeton, N.J., Princeton University Press, 1979, p. 9.
16. Ibid., p. 10.
17. Robb, C. Vive la difference. *Boston Globe Mag.* Oct. 5, 1980, pp. 11, 76.
18. Piaget, *op. cit.*, p. 72.
19. Gilligan, C. In a different voice: women's conceptions of self and morality. *Harvard Educ. Rev.* 47:484, Nov. 1977.
20. Ibid., p. 481.
21. Gilligan, C. Woman's place in man's life cycle. *Harvard Educ. Rev.* 49:431, Nov. 1979

3 Socialization and Resocialization of Nurses for Professional Nursing Practice

Ada Sue Hinshaw

THE DELIVERY of health care to clients involves a number of professions and paraprofessions in complex, interactive, collaborative relationships. Each of the professions has delineated roles and defined standards for how individuals in a particular role should act or behave. However, due to changes in health care delivery systems, technology, and shifting manpower distributions, these interactive professionals work in roles that have fluid boundaries and are consistently changing. For example, the need for increased manpower to deliver primary health care and provide basic health assessment has led to the development of the expanded role concept in nursing and numerous programs to educate persons for these positions. The continuing knowledge and technology explosion has stimulated, at the basic level, curriculums based on general principles, concepts, and theories which have wide applicability in practice. At the graduate level, the expansion of knowledge has led to the development of clinical specialist programs in various fields. Registered nurses who have completed their basic educational programs are confronted with a constant need to engage in continuing education. Nurses who are returning to professional practice after an inactive period are appalled by the immense changes that have occurred, not only in terms of the knowledge and skills that are presently required but also the differences in role expectations and standards.

From the perspective of the profession, the fact that there are constantly evolving and changing nursing practitioner roles requires that there be continual redefinition of standards and sets of value and behavior expectations as a mechanism for assuring the quality of care that will be delivered. Such continual redefinition of role standards includes mechanisms for reviewing and monitoring the standards and the educational programs which prepare the practitioners; it stimulates the need for various types of credentialing programs.

From the perspective of nursing professionals, the practitioners' continually changing roles confront them with a career pattern of socialization and resocialization. According to Ritzer [1972], the constant change accompanying resocialization for career roles is closely associated with the generation of conflict. Thus, professional nurses who are experiencing continual change in their roles can expect to confront conflict as a natural and predictable phenomenon.

The purpose of this paper is to examine the socialization and resocialization processes which professional nurses experience and to discuss several major factors that influence the processes and their product—the professional nurse.

Reprinted with permission from *Socialization and Resocialization of Nurses for Professional Nursing Practice*, National League for Nursing Booklet Number 15-1659, 1977.

PROCESS OF SOCIALIZATION/RESOCIALIZATION

Adult socialization is a process through which individuals prepare for the life roles that they will enact in their society. It is useful to define socialization as the process of learning new roles and the adaptation to them, and as such, continual processes by which individuals become members of a social group. As Kramer [1974] notes, operationally, the concept of socialization refers to a period of time individuals spend learning the necessary knowledge and skills and undergoing the self-identity and internalization process to prepare themselves for a specific role. Kramer also states that acquiring the necessary knowledge and skills for occupational roles is among the most important socialization/resocialization process adults experience.

According to Rosow [1965], standards for the socialization process are drawn from the norms of a given target system and a specific role and set of values in that system. The objectives of socialization are twofold: to inculcate the novice or person being socialized with both a basic set of role values and consequent behaviors. Thus the socialized individual is expected to internalize certain accepted beliefs and also display defined appropriate behaviors [Rosow, 1965].

From the perspective of professional nursing, the adult socialization/resocialization processes focus on providing the values and behaviors basic to the delivery of quality client care. Standards for the socialization/resocialization processes are drawn from the norms of service professions and guide the specific role of professional nurses. The processes ultimately provide both the values and behaviors required for nursing practice.

Several characteristics of adult socialization need to be noted. They are recurring, consist of sequential interactive stages and assume that individuals undergoing socialization will adopt an active role. Since resocialization is a process in which new roles or sets of expectations are learned, it occurs with entry into each new position or assignment in a social system, such as in a service profession. Schien's [1971] model for the structure of a career suggests that one enters a career pattern with the intent of changing roles or assignments several times and functioning in several positions. There is generally an initial formal socialization into the basic role set one has chosen but as a career advances, each change in role position requires a degree of resocialization.

This paper will first examine a general model of socialization and then consider several models descriptive of the initial nursing socialization and resocialization experiences.

A GENERAL MODEL OF SOCIALIZATION

Several authors suggest that the course of socialization is a complex, multiform chain of events which ideally expose novices to those experiences that will prepare them for particular types of social participation. For analytical purposes, socialization can be viewed as a sequential set of phases or "chain of events." A general model (Fig. 3-1) has been adapted from Simpson [1967] which consists of three phases:

  I. Transition from anticipatory expectations of role to specific expectations of role as defined by societal group
 II. Attachment to significant others in the social system milieu/labeling incongruencies in role expectations
III. Internalization, adaptation, or integration of role values and standards

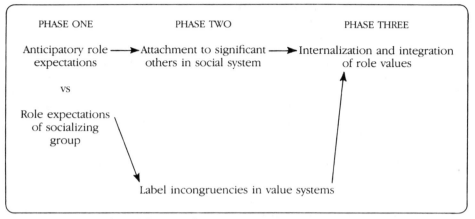

PHASE ONE   PHASE TWO   PHASE THREE

Anticipatory role ⟶ Attachment to significant ⟶ Internalization and integration
expectations   others in social system   of role values

vs

Role expectations
of socializing
group

Label incongruencies in value systems

Figure 3-1. A general model of socialization. (Adapted from Simpson, 1967.)

A word of caution: a staged socialization model deliberately glosses over the details of processes which are tied to specific sets of socializing conditions. The model is presented as a way of gaining a frame of reference from which to consider several empirical processes of socialization and resocialization.

PHASE I: TRANSITION OF ANTICIPATORY ROLE EXPECTATIONS TO ROLE EXPECTATIONS OF SOCIETAL GROUP

During the first stage individuals shift their imagery of the role from the anticipated conception to the expectations defined by incumbents who are setting the standards for them [Rosow, 1965]. With the process of adult socialization, it must be assumed that the individuals entering the social system or the profession have already learned a number of roles and values which give them a perspective for evaluating new roles. Furthermore, the individuals are assumed to have an active part in being socialized into a new role which in this stage means they have chosen to learn the new role expectations and thus have deliberately chosen to enter into the socialization or resocialization process.

PHASE II: ATTACHMENT TO SIGNIFICANT OTHERS/LABEL INCONGRUENCIES

Phase II has two components: individuals will attach themselves to significant others in the social system and simultaneously will label encounters with incongruencies between what they anticipated their new role would be and what it is as presented by the significant others. The significant others generally evolve from the social system in which the individuals are currently accountable. For example, in the initial professional socialization experience this tends to be a group of faculty who are seen as role models for the values and behaviors of the new role. In a work setting, significant others refer to specific colleagues or immediate supervisors who are selected as role models. In both cases, the individuals chosen are ones who are influential in the role setting of the new individual. This is a crucial point since if successful outcomes for this stage of socialization/resocialization depend on the existence of appropriate role models, then both educational programs and work settings are confronted with the problem of how to identify and provide such models.

As new individuals learn the expectations set by the social group or profession and form relationships with role models who personify the values and behaviors, a point is reached in socialization where people are able to label or articulate that these role expectations are not what they had anticipated. This stage is often accompanied by strong emotional reactions to the conflict generated as individuals are confronted with two or several sets of expectations which may or may not be congruent and must decide how to resolve the situation. The ability to successfully resolve the conflict is related to the existence of role models in the setting who exhibit appropriate behaviors that illustrate how to integrate conflicting systems of standards and values. Thus the two aspects of this phase, identification with significant others and use of role models to resolve conflict, are strongly interactive.

PHASE III: INTERNALIZATION OF ROLE VALUES/BEHAVIORS

The third phase in the socialization/resocialization process involves an individual's internalization of the values and standards of the new role. Several major aspects of this phase must be considered: (1) to what degree are values and standards internalized and (2) by what processes did he or she in socialization resolve the incongruencies in role expectations.

Kelman [1961] has defined three levels of opinion change. Individuals, in the process of forming new opinions or values, may be identified as illustrating one or a blend of these levels. One level of value orientation is that of *compliance*. At this point, the individual has not accepted the set of values or expectations as his or her own but enacts the expected behavior in order to get positive responses from others around him. The second level of opinion or value change is that of *identification*. In socialization, one selectively adopts certain role behaviors that are acceptable to him and are a part of how he or she would like to be perceived. This does not necessarily include an acceptance of the values, only the behaviors. The third level of opinion/value change is labeled *internalization*. At this point the individual accepts the norms and standards of the new role because he or she believes in them and they have become a part of their own value system.

TO SUMMARIZE

The socialization process will have brought the new individual to one of these points of opinion and value change. How individuals at each point of compliance, identification, and internalization will react in later resocialization experiences is a question for discussion. As Kramer [1974] notes, compliance behavior can be expected "to be abandoned" when it no longer generates positive responses and identification behavior will change as identified role models or influential people change. Does this mean that any socializer not reaching maximum socialization or internalization can be expected to readily capitulate these professional values and behaviors in another setting? If so, how can such capitulation be countered?

The second aspect of this last phase concerns how individuals handle incongruencies in role expectations. Moving from the second phase where labeling or deliberate acknowledgment of incongruencies occur, do the individuals merge or integrate two sets of role expectations, which would suggest both sets of expectations are maintained and used at appropriate times, or is the conflict in the incongruency so great that the individual chooses to opt out in some manner. How incongruencies are handled either by the individual or the socializing system they are involved with is crucial to one's ability to achieve a high level of socialization or internalization of values.

This section of the paper has presented a general model of socialization/resocialization in order to provide a common frame of reference for the following discussion. In nursing, two major socialization/resocialization processes have been described by researchers: (1) the initial adult socialization era in which lay people are socialized into our profession through a formal education process and (2) the resocialization process that occurs as graduates leave their formal educational programs and enter work settings for the first time. What occurs during these two socialization/resocialization processes is crucial to the development and maintenance of professional values in nursing practice.

INITIAL PROFESSIONALIZATION EXPERIENCE

In the initial professionalization experience, individuals learn both the cultural content of a new role, i.e., its skills, required knowledge, values and behavioral modes, *and* they acquire a degree of identification with the role [Simpson, 1967]. A number of papers and investigations have described this process. For the purpose of this discussion, Davis's [1966] classical description of the doctrinal conversation process among nursing students will be utilized. This process focuses on the transition of changing values and imagery of a role from that of a lay person to that of a professional nurse, which according to Hughes [1958] is the most crucial and problematic aspect of becoming a professional. There are six stages in Davis's doctrinal conversion model (Fig. 3-2).

STAGE ONE: INITIAL INNOCENCE

Individuals enter a professional program with an image of what they expect to become and of how they "should" act or behave. Davis [1966, p. 239] suggests that individuals enter nursing with a service orientation of "actively doing in relationship to a worthy purpose." This image of active service includes a "means-end manipulation of tools and procedures in order to insure successful outcomes" for sick people. In contrast, the professional educational imagery of the nurse is generally of one who (1) defines clients in terms of health and maintaining health, (2) views the relationship between the nurse and clients therapeutically and analytically, (3) approaches technical mastery of tools and procedures from the viewpoint of knowledge principles that guide their use, (4) uses critical inquiry processes to creatively manipulate knowledge in relation to clients' concerns and (5) accepts responsibility/accountability for patient-care decisions. These are major values stressed by professional nursing.

Behavior which is based on the lay imagery of someone who is being socialized is not positively reinforced, and pressures are present for that person to behave in ways that he or she does not yet comprehend, e.g., instead of being praised for bed bath technique he is asked to analyze the interaction with the patient to whom the bath was given. This confrontation of different expectations results in disappointment and frustration for the socializing individuals. These negative feelings seem to be denied through the immediate "honeymoon" period with the educational programs but begin to be expressed soon after the first faculty-student evaluation conferences occur.

GENERAL MODEL	DAVIS'S MODEL OF DOCTRINAL CONVERSION
PHASE ONE Anticipatory role expectations vs Role expectations of socializing group	STAGE ONE Initial innocence STAGE TWO Incongruencies labeled
PHASE TWO Label incongruencies in value system Attachment to significant others	STAGE THREE "Psyching out" STAGE FOUR Role simulation
PHASE THREE Internalization and integration of values and expectations	STAGE FIVE Provisional internalization STAGE SIX Stable internalization

Figure 3-2. Empirical model: Socialization into a professional role.

STAGE TWO: LABELED RECOGNITION OF INCONGRUITY

The formal evaluation process seems to provide the framework for allowing students to verbally articulate their concerns. In that process it becomes evident to them that they are not alone but share a basic set of value incongruencies with their peers. The process of verbally sharing concerns leads to collectively labeling what the incongruencies are. As Davis notes, this is a problematic stage because those being socialized have only a vague insight into the ideological rationale of the professional/educational value system but are being pressured to produce behavior based on that system. Will they? Can they? Do they want to?

STAGES THREE AND FOUR: "PSYCHING OUT" AND ROLE SIMULATION

For individuals who want to continue with nursing their next steps must be to begin to identify what behaviors they are expected to exhibit and to role model such behaviors. In Davis's terms this becomes a matter of "psyching out" the faculty. It is at this point that the rudimentary cognitive framework for the internalization of professional nursing values and standards begins to take shape. He suggests that the more the role simulation is done successfully the more the individual believes the behavior to be authentic and part of him. Thus, the behaviors become part of the individual's own repertoire for how to act. One problem in this stage is important to note, a feeling of moral discomfort occurs, of not being "true to oneself" and "playing a game," which results in individual guilt and ego alienation. How will this influence later ability to adhere to professional values under different conditions?

STAGES FIVE AND SIX: PROVISIONAL AND STABLE INTERNALIZATION

In stage five the persons being socialized vacillate between commitment and performance of new behaviors attached to the professional imagery and behaviors reflecting their lay imagery. Two factors reinforce their use of the new imagery model: (1) an increasing ability to comfortably use the language of the profession and (2) an increasing identification with positive professional role models, in this case, faculty.

In stage six, the imagery and behavior of the individual reflect the professionally/educationally approved model. It is important to emphasize that socialization is not completed with this stage but is only relative or specific to the educational institution through which the individual has progressed.

In essence, professional socialization has only begun with the initial process. The questions to consider now are: What happens once the new graduate leaves the formal educational system and enters the work setting? In what ways are the values and behaviors acquired applicable, influenced, changed, or integrated? Which values and behaviors are operational? What new values and behaviors must be acquired?

RESOCIALIZATION INTO A WORK SETTING

The resocialization process that has received extensive discussion occurs as new professionals leave their initial formal educational programs and enter various work settings. Since nurses traditionally enact their professional roles as employees in organized work settings, such as hospitals, community health agencies, neighborhood health centers, etc., they are faced with how to operationalize professional values in these settings and how to integrate into their behavior and values certain role expectations of the agencies. This issue has been labeled "the professional-bureaucratic conflict." The label acknowledges the existence of two dominant value systems, which may require the nurse to have two sets of behaviors.

The professional work system focuses on the entirety of a service activity which is based on a systematic body of knowledge acquired through extensive study. The initiation, evaluation, and control of such activities are accounted for through self-responsibility and peer review. In essence, the judgments and actions of professionals are guided by the rules and standards of their parent profession and ultimate accountability and loyalty are to that formal colleague group. In contrast, the bureaucratic work system consists of an extensive division of labor around sets of task activities that can be handled by standardized rules and regulations and on-the-job technical training. The control and evaluation of the employees' actions generally reside with the higher levels of administrative hierarchy. Scott summarizes the areas of normative conflict that can be generated when professionals function in organizations: resistance to bureaucratic rules, standards and supervision; and inability to give the organization primary loyalty.

With both the initial socialization process and the process of resocialization into a work setting, the generation of conflict is an expected phenomenon. With professionals' initial socialization process, conflict occurs due to differences between the lay and professional/educational images; however, the clear expectation for conflict resolution is for value transition to occur with the professional image becoming dominant. In the case of the resocialization of the new professional into an organized work setting, the conflict is again anticipated; however, expectations for its resolution are different. It is not the expectation or desire of either the profession or the work setting that professional values be changed to work-bureaucratic values. The organization employed the new graduate in order to utilize his or her recently acquired professional behaviors and standards. Concurrently, the profession requires that graduates have a commitment to the delivery of client care based on its values and standards in order to assure quality. Thus, transition to one set of values is not a desired or expected goal in the resocialization process. Resolution of value and role conflict must

PHASE ONE
    Anticipatory role expectations
                vs
    Role expectations of socializing group
PHASE TWO
    Attachment to significant others
    Label incongruencies in value system
PHASE THREE
    Internalization and integration
    of role values and expectations

STAGE ONE
    General principles to specific skills
STAGE TWO
    Social integration
STAGE THREE
    Moral outrage
STAGE FOUR
    Conflict resolution

Figure 3-3. Empirical model: Socialization of professional into an organizational role.

encompass instead an integration or adaptation of the two value systems, professional and bureaucratic.

Based on her research, Kramer [1974] describes a postgraduate resocialization model (Fig. 3-3). In essence this socialization process focuses on operationalizing or integrating the "shoulds" and general knowledge and skills acquired in educational programs with the performance of behaviors specific in the work setting. There are four stages in the grounded model generated from her data.

STAGE ONE: SKILL AND ROUTINE MASTERY

New graduates bring to the work setting universal principles for how to function and how to behave and are confronted with the demands of the work setting to function in a specific manner with their knowledge and skill. Initially the graduates feel incompetent and frustrated, which generates the immediate solution of "throwing" themselves into mastery of specific skills and techniques. Note: competent, efficient delivery of procedures and techniques to clients is a value basic to both the professional and bureaucratic systems. It is not an area likely to generate conflict. The successful application of general knowledge principles to specific procedures and skills is congruent with both systems and will elicit positive feedback from both. The problem is, What is occurring with other values? How does a focus on specific skill mastery affect the new graduate's priority-setting with patient care criteria not involving skills, or how does such a focus affect the graduate's attention to patient interaction and a patient's response to the skill? As the graduates recognize the number of skills to be mastered will they fixate at this stage and thus be unable to refocus their attention on other aspects of care?

STAGE TWO: SOCIAL INTEGRATION

The major concern with this stage is "getting along with co-workers and becoming one of the group." This probably requires having mastered the skills and being perceived as "a competent and efficient nurse." This step involves not only forming interpersonal relationships but also gaining entrance to the "backstage" reality of the work setting. This entails being "let in on" how to act and behave as the others do, e.g., how to react to a client's family, how to talk to new interns, how to treat or respond to unusual client requests. This stage brings new graduates to the point of choosing to enact backstage behaviors, remaining with skill mastery or starting to apply more of the knowledge and orientation that was gained in the initial socialization process. To choose the latter may alienate the colleague group in which social integration has been achieved.

STAGE THREE: MORAL OUTRAGE

In this stage the incongruencies between the professional/educational imagery of how nurses "ought to" behave and the manner in which behavior does occur in the work setting becomes labeled and acknowledged. The new graduates feel frustrated, angry, and betrayed by both their professional education and new work positions; their perception is that they were not prepared adequately (they were not really told how "it would be") and now people won't let them use their preparation. It is a crucial point with the conflict phenomenon because the graduates are not perceiving rationally, they are using a great deal of emotional energy and in general are experiencing both a developmental and situational crisis in the socialization/resocialization process. Questions that must be asked are: How could the graduates have been prepared for this point? How could they have been given the opportunity to discuss possible alternatives for how to cope with the situation? Who in the work setting is available to intervene during this crisis? Otherwise as Kramer and Baker [1971] note in their article "The Exodus: Can We Prevent It?" professional nursing pays a high price for unsuccessful resolution of this crisis from the perspective of both educational and work-setting programs.

STAGE FOUR: CONFLICT RESOLUTION

In this stage, Kramer suggests a typology for how graduates evaluate and resolve the conflict between value systems. Individuals will either capitulate their behaviors or their values or integrate the two dominant work systems, professional and bureaucratic. Those who choose behavioral capitulation, change their behavior but keep their values. Operationally, these graduates are those who leave the organized service setting and either return to educational settings or leave nursing altogether. A second type of conflict resolution is value capitulation in which the values of the bureaucratic system are accepted and the professional/educational values are capitulated. This is labeled "going native." A third type of resolution is to capitulate both values and behaviors and simply conform enough to maintain a working position. A fourth type of resolution Kramer labels biculturalism [1974, p. 162], which is suggested to be the healthiest and most successful resolution of conflict:

In this approach the nurses have learned that they possess a value orientation that is perhaps different from the dominant one in the work organization, but that they have the responsibility to listen to and seek out the ideas of others as resource material in effecting viable integration of both value systems. They have learned that they are not just a target of influence and pressure from others, but that they are in a reciprocal relationship with others and have the right and responsibility to attempt to influence them and to direct their influence attempts.

In essence, these new graduates are able to identify and utilize the values and behaviors of both the professional and bureaucratic work systems in a politically astute manner.

RECURRING NATURE OF SOCIALIZATION/RESOCIALIZATION PROCESS

The initial socialization into the profession through formal educational programs and the immediate resocialization process as graduates enter work settings are the two major aspects of socialization that have been discussed and investigated in nursing. Yet, as Schien [1971] notes, socialization/resocialization is a process strand that occurs and recurs through an entire career. At any point that individuals change their career goals, or change career status or move the work setting in which they are functioning, role expectations will also change. Educational institutions witness the resocialization process when RNs with diplomas return to acquire degrees, when inactive nurses return for refresher courses and when nurses with baccalaureate degrees return to obtain clinical specialist degrees, or administrative or teaching knowledge and skills [Brophy, 1974]. Service organizations see the resocialization process occurring when nurses change positions within the work setting and each time nurses move from educational systems with new skills and knowledge to operationalize in the organized work system [Woodrow and Bell, 1971; Johnson, 1971].

Questions that must be considered are: What are the general factors that influence the trajectory of the socialization/resocialization process? How can the influence of these factors be predicted?

FACTORS THAT INFLUENCE THE SOCIALIZATION/RESOCIALIZATION PROCESSES

There are several major factors that influence the trajectory of the socialization/resocialization processes. The seven areas that this paper will present are:

The formality of the initial socialization setting
The professional orientation of the work setting
The diversity of role expectations confronting individuals in work settings
The legitimation of the parent profession
Existence of role models
The dominant sex makeup of the profession
Ethnicity of the person being socialized.

Several questions may be raised in terms of how each of these seven areas influence the socialization/resocialization issues. An interesting, creative approach for stimulating questions is the application of a matrix technique in studying the influence of certain contextual factors on a process (Fig. 3-4). This technique has the advantage of illustrating all logical intersections between the factors and the process of socialization/resocialization. However, it has the disadvantage of any two-dimensional space technique in that it does not allow for enough complexity. The technique is illustrated here because it may be valuable in helping to see the many points at which the factors and processes interrelate.

FORMALITY OF INITIAL SOCIALIZATION SETTING

The first factor, formality of the initial socialization setting, is defined as the degree to which the educational setting is segregated from the "on-going" work context [Van Naanen, 1975]. Van Naanen suggests that formal settings concentrate more on universal attitudes than on specific acts and thus the greater the separation of the initial educational program from the organization "work-a-day" reality, the less the ability of new graduates to carry over or

Phases of Processes	Formality of Initial Socialization Setting	Professional Orientation of Work Setting	Role Diversity	Legitimation of Profession	Existence of Role Models	Dominant Sex Makeup	Ethnicity of Person Being Socialized
I. Anticipatory role expectations vs role expectations of socializing group							
II. Attachment to significant others							
III. Label incongruencies in value system							
IV. Internalization and integration of values and expectations							

Figure 3-4. Matrix technique: Intersection of factors with phases of socialization/resocialization processes.

generalize the knowledge and skills learned in the socialization setting. This is one factor that underlies the phenomenon of the professional-bureaucratic conflict. In the formal socialization process, nurses are educated in systems of higher education. While they are exposed to experience in the organized work setting, it is as students accountable to faculty. Thus their role expectations, consequent reward systems, and their role models are derived primarily from that educational system.

The role and positional expectations of the organized work system will vary from those learned in the educational setting and conflict is a predictable consequence when the two systems merge. Where in the initial educational experience could students be helped to anticipate (as Kramer suggests): (1) the difference in values, (2) alternatives for how to cope with such differences and (3) alternatives for how to cope with the conflict generated. How in nursing departments can role models be provided that show behaviors that illustrate integration between the two value systems? Can colleague groups of new and integrated role model employees be utilized to discuss conflict in values and ways to resolve it?

PROFESSIONAL ORIENTATION OF THE WORK SETTING

A second factor, the professional orientation of the work setting, influences how nursing is practiced. Service organizations, such as health care agencies, in general differ from bureaucratic organizations. By definition such organizations facilitate the provision of services to clientele. The nature of tasks is different; the activities tend to be more nonroutine, unpredictable and exceptional. Such tasks require the employment of professionals who possess the knowledge and expertise from their educational background to handle them [Georgopoulos and Mann, 1972]. The tasks do not as readily allow for standardization or for division of labor. The inability to standardize the organization's tasks and the need to utilize professionals have consequences for the decision structure of organizations, generally resulting in decentralization of authority.

The professional bureaucratic orientation will vary in work settings where nurses function. If work settings have a strong professional orientation, what is the influence on a new graduate's ability to operationalize professional nursing values and behaviors, in contrast to a strong bureaucratic orientation? If a work setting has a strong professional orientation, will there be an increased number of integrative role models available to nursing students and new graduates? In an organized work setting with a strong professional orientation is there a stronger colleague support group for operationalizing professional values and behaviors in response to nonroutine, unusual client activities? Furthermore, if nurses wish to increase the professionalization of their work settings, what mechanisms can be used? Does the primary care organization of nursing practice, the employment of an all RN staff, the employment of only RNs with baccalaureate degrees, or the instigation of quality assurance and peer review programs increase the professionalism of a work setting? What is the influence of any of these mechanisms on an individual practitioner's ability to operationalize values and behaviors in the work setting?

ROLE SET DIVERSIFICATION

A third factor, diversity of role expectations, influences socialization and resocialization. Role set designates the total complement of relationships in which a person becomes involved by virtue of occupying a particular social position. A role set is considered more or less diversified to the extent that it involves the maintenance of a variety of role relationships [Snoek, 1966]. Role senders are persons in complement roles who communicate and both hold and enforce certain relevant role expectations. Professional nurses are involved in a complex system of communication and role complements, i.e., the client, physicians, peers, nursing administrators, allied health workers, representatives of other services in the organized work setting, etc. These people complement the role of professional nurses and have certain expectations of them. Snoek's research suggests "the greater the diversification of a role set, the greater the possibility of intrarole conflicts, because each class of role senders is apt to develop expectations that are more attuned to its own organizational goals, norms, values than to the requirements of the position holder's role" [Snoek, 1966, p. 364]. Nursing has recognized this source of conflict for many years; from a theoretical perspective the care-cure-coordinate classification system was one attempt to organize several major sets of role expectations for analytical purposes. Empirically, the result of Oakes and Hinshaw [1976] testing three theoretical models predicting patient, MD and nurse expectations of quality nursing care, indicated that the sets of expectations differ markedly. This multiple set of role expectations is another logical point for the generation of conflict. How does this diverse set of expectations influence the orientation of a professional socializing to the work setting? The role senders have varying levels of status in the setting. How does this influence the operationalization of professional nursing values? Is there an opportunity either in educational programs or work settings to confront the tension generated by such diversity and discuss alternatives for its resolution?

LEGITIMATION OF PARENT PROFESSION

A fourth factor is the degree of legitimation of the parent profession. One of the stages a profession experiences as it matures is public legitimation of its right to use its knowledge base and skills autonomously [Caplow, 1966]. Nurses recognize that certain aspects of their role in an organized work setting are more legitimated than others. The instrumental or skill mastery aspects are well accepted by a number of role senders—clients, nursing colleagues, MDs, etc. Other aspects of the nursing role as defined by the profession may not be as well legitimated in the work setting, e.g., independent decision making, counseling of clients' families, etc. The greater the degree of nonlegitimation by major role senders toward certain role functions, the greater the resistance to enacting those functions. If this hypothesis holds, then what is the influence of nonlegitimation on certain values and standards of new professionals when they attempt to implement them in the work setting?

EXISTENCE OF ROLE MODELS

A fifth factor that both Davis [1966] and Kramer [1974] discussed as influencing socialization/resocialization concerned the existence of role models in the socializing system. Recall that Kelman's [1961] taxonomy for stages of internalization of new opinions/values suggested the presence of role models as crucial to the identification stage. Davis's work substantiates that point. He states that students in their initial socialization process require behavioral role models in order to learn the desired professional behaviors. Once the behaviors become part of them then they are better able to internalize the values/standards. Faculty were able to serve as role models for the professional imagery behaviors. Kramer's description of the postgraduate theory of resocialization also substantiates the need for role models. Since

Kramer is concerned with the new graduate, she suggests that the role models must not only hold high professional standards but also be able to operationalize those standards in the work setting. Successful operationalization is strongly influenced by the existence of bicultural role models. Thus, the data from both researchers indicate role models are needed in forming new values and opinions, the identification phase. Can such role models be provided for individuals involved in the socialization/resocialization processes? How can integrative role models be identified in both educational and work settings? Kramer's 1974 study suggests that there is not a high proportion of such role models so how can they be utilized most effectively? In schools, as anticipatory models? In work settings, as work-a-day reality models?

Dominant Sex Makeup of Profession

The fact that nursing is primarily a profession of females influences the socialization/resocialization process in several ways: (1) the way in which the professional role is defined and enacted, (2) the degree of career commitment given to the professional role and (3) the manner in which major role senders interact with nurses. Davis and Oeleson [1966] contend that the socialization process is considerably influenced when the characteristics of the person being socialized vary from the traditional profile of being male, Anglo, and middle class. For example, from their study of female nursing students, it was evident that socialization occurred differently because their identity with the role required an integration of professional role values and expectations with the emerging values and behaviors of becoming an adult female. Thus the professional role as ultimately enacted was and is a merger or integration of the adult female and professional nursing roles. Obviously, as role senders react to the female professional nurse they are responding to both aspects of the role. Questions to consider are: Are female professional nurses deliberately aware of how the two roles interact? Are they able to analyze the behaviors that flow from each role set? Are they able to deliberately identify problems in role interaction that flow from being female and then are they able to change those behaviors for constructive purposes?

A major issue is career commitment and retaining professionals on active status. Cleland [1976] notes that a vast number of women are socialized into nursing but remain in practice only a short time. This is an expensive drain on both educational and working resources. How might individuals with long-term career commitments be identified? Wouldn't it be less expensive to educate selectively? As researcher Douglas T. Hall notes, women in society who choose to follow careers that are separate from their home and family defined roles are confronted with interrole conflict. How does this source of tension influence an individual's level of commitment to a career? How would it influence one's ability to internalize professional values and standards? Would such interrole conflict drain energy so that only compliance or identification with professional roles could be achieved? Cleland [1976] suggests that anticipatory guidance during the initial socialization program is required to assist new professionals to understand that they are entering a dual career life-style. How can these two careers, professional and personal, be integrated? How can a support system be generated to allow both to flourish? How can a basic orientation be conveyed during the socialization/resocialization processes that a professional career commitment is expected of females just as it is of males?

ETHNICITY OF PERSON BEING SOCIALIZED

A seventh factor influencing socialization/resocialization that remains relatively unmentioned in nursing research literature is the ethnicity of individuals being socialized. As noted earlier, whenever one of the major characteristics of the traditional profile changes, i.e., male, Anglo, middle class, it can be predicted that the socialization process will differ. Obviously, different cultural value systems will integrate with professional value systems in unique ways. What integrated sets of values will emerge as different cultural values combine with professional nursing values? What behavior patterns will be evident with different value integrations? How will specific socializing/resocializing techniques need to change to maximize socialization and its relevancy under varying cultural systems?

INFLUENCING FACTORS IN TOTAL

The above section of the paper spoke to the influence of several major factors on the socialization/resocialization process. Many questions were posed. The several areas initiated for discussion require refinement and elaboration. It is important to note the interactive quality of the factors influencing the socialization/resocialization processes. Other factors also need consideration; one that comes to mind is, How does the level of opinion change (compliance, identification, or internalization) in a person being socialized influence later progression through additional resocialization experiences?

The basic theme that is evident from the examination of the seven factors is the degree of tension or conflict that seems to be a natural and predictable consequence at several points in the socialization/resocialization processes. Nurses are consistently confronted with conflict between their professional values and the bureaucratic values of employing organizations, the diverse set of expectations of those working with them in complement roles, and the life roles external to their professional careers. Discussion needs to be directed to the identification and development of models and strategies for coping with and resolving conflict. Kramer [1974] has spearheaded this work with her research on anticipatory guidance and immunization against value and behavioral capitulation in work settings. But many questions still require investigation. What aspects of anticipated conflict can be predicted? Can support systems be established in the initial educational programs and in the work settings for discussing and reinforcing the use of strategies and models for coping with conflict? New professionals need to be confronted early and consistently with not only the identification and existence of conflict but also with situations in which they must develop strategies for coping with conflict.

IN SUMMARY

A general model of socialization and resocialization of nurses for professional nursing practice has been presented, including discussion of the phases of these processes and empirical examples that outline the initial socialization of the professional and the resocialization that occurs with passage from formal education programs to the work setting. While the importance of these two points in a professional nurse's career were not denied, this paper has also emphasized the continual recurring nature of the socialization/resocialization processes. Several major factors that influence the trajectory of the processes or the effectiveness of their products, professional nurses, were considered: the formality of the initial socialization setting; professional orientation to the work setting; role diversification; existence of role models; legitimation of the parent profession; dominant sex makeup of the profession; and the ethnicity of the person being socialized.

Many questions have been posed in this paper. It was intentional. A great deal of writing is evident on specific aspects in the socialization/resocialization issues. I have attempted here to encompass those aspects and ask questions that will stimulate further thought. The continued professionalization of nursing care delivered to clients depends on nursing's ability to successfully address the issues and questions related to the socialization/resocialization processes.

REFERENCES

Caplow, Theodore. "The Concept of Professionalization," H. M. Vollmer and D. L. Mills (Eds) *Professionalization.* Englewood Cliffs, N.J.: Prentice-Hall, Inc., 1966, p. 19.

Cleland, Virginia, Alan R. Bass, Norma McHugh, and Jocelyn Montano. "Social and Psychologic Influences on Employment of Married Nurses," *Nursing Research,* 25:2, March-April 1976, p. 90.

Davis, Fred. "Professional Socialization as Subjective Experience: The Process of Doctrinal Conversion among Student Nurses," Sixth World Congress of Sociology Paper, Evian, France, September 1966.

Davis, Fred, and Virginia Oeleson. "Status Differences and Professionalization," H. M. Vollmer and Mills (Eds) *Professionalization.* Englewood Cliffs, N.J.: Prentice-Hall, Inc., 1966, p. 34.

Hughes, Everett C. *Men and Their Work.* Glencoe, Ill.: The Free Press, 1958, p. 119.

Johnson, Nancy D. "The Professional-Bureaucratic Conflict," *Journal of Nursing Administration,* May–June 1971, p. 31.

Kelman, H. "Processes of Opinion Changes," *Public Opinion Quarterly* 25:1, 1961, p. 57.

Kramer, Marlene. *Reality Shock: Why Nurses Leave Nursing.* St. Louis: C. V. Mosby Co., 1974.

Kramer, Marlene, and Constance Baker. "The Exodus: Can We Prevent It?" *Journal of Nursing Administration,* May–June 1971, p. 15.

Oakes, Deborah, and Ada Sue Hinshaw. "Patients', Nurses' and Physicians' Perceptions of Quality Nursing Care," Paper in Progress, University of Arizona, 1976.

Rosow, Irving. "Forms and Functions of Adult Socialization," *Social Forces,* 44, 1965, p. 35.

Schien, Edgar. "The Individual, the Organization, and the Career: A Conceptual Scheme," *The Journal of Applied Behavioral Science,* 7:4, 1971, p. 401.

Simpson, Ida Harper. "Patterns of Socialization into Professions: The Case of Student Nurses," *Sociological Inquiry,* 37, Winter 1967, p. 47.

Snoek, J. Diedrick. "Role Strain in Diversified Role Sets," *American Journal of Sociology,* 71:4, January 1966, p. 363.

Van Naanen, John. "Police Socialization: A Longitudinal Examination of Job Attitudes in an Urban Police Department," *Administrative Science Quarterly,* 20, June 1975, p. 207.

Woodrow, Mary, and Judith A. Bell. "Clinical Specialization: Conflict Between Reality and Theory," *Journal of Nursing Administration,* November-December 1971, p. 23.

4 Nursing's Bid for Increased Status

Christy Z. Dachelet

SOCIOLOGISTS can document the hierarchical status system in the medical establishment and the public can discern it, but it is the health care team members who must deal with it and its implications, daily.

Perhaps most acutely aware of the status hierarchy is the health practitioner working closest with the physician—the nurse. The general status disparity and concomitant income differential between the two has not gone unnoticed by the nursing profession. It has been cited as a social factor causing "structured-in conflict" between nurses and physicians [Peeples and Francis, 1968].

Today the nursing profession is challenging for a higher rung in the status hierarchy. It is making a bid for increased professional status and for the accompanying material, personal, and professional awards, increased prestige and status command. The purpose of this article, therefore, is to examine selected characteristics of the nursing profession that either impede or support its progress toward realization of its goal.

The activities of nurses individually, and of the nursing profession collectively, toward this end are not occurring in a vacuum. On the contrary, the activity is occurring in the ordered hierarchical bureaucracy of the health care organization; a bureaucracy in which the physician and medical profession have laid firm claim to the position at the top of the pyramid. Consequently, it is appropriate to direct attention later in this article to the response of physicians and the medical profession to nursing's challenge to the status quo.

An argument might well be made that the quality of patient care rendered is the important issue and that, in fact, a hierarchical status system is dysfunctional to that end. Be that as it may, the intent of this writer is not to arrive at a value judgment as to the appropriateness of a hierarchical status system. The reality is that such a system exists, and it is nursing's challenge within that system that is being examined.

EMERGENCE OF NURSING'S CLAIM TO INCREASED PROFESSIONAL STATUS

Nursing's bid for a "higher rung on the ladder" is a timely topic for consideration. This is a period of heightened, change-oriented activity within the greater health care system. New organizational structures for delivering health services are being developed and implemented, more equitable financing mechanisms debated, and a new genre of health manpower emerging. Numerically, nursing represents the single largest group of health professionals providing patient care [NCSNNE, 1970], and "nursing power as a productive force"

From *Nursing Forum*, Volume 17, Number 1, 1978. Pp. 19–43. Reprinted with permission from Nursing Publications, Inc., 194-B Kinderkamack Road, Park Ridge, New Jersey 07656.

has been cited as "the single most important factor maintaining our health care systems today" [Ashley, 1973]. It would clearly be folly for planners, administrators, physicians, or government to proceed to restructure elements of the health care system without regard for the internal changes in nursing. Of course, nursing, as it realigns its position, must be mindful of the changes occurring within the greater health care system. But, if for no other reason than sheer numerical strength, the system will be required to make some accommodations to nursing.

A second factor that gives this topic import is the relevance of the nurse-physician relationship to patient care. As pointed out, nursing's bid will have consequence for this relationship. Duff and Hollingshead [1968, p. 37] examined the interrelationship between patient care and the elements of the social environment in which that care is provided. They cited the nurse-physician relationship as, "an integral part of the patient care process." Pellegrino [1964, p. 12] referred to the "delicate" nurse-physician relationship. Granting that the interrelationship of the two is an influential factor in the therapeutic function of the hospital, he advised that, "each profession should seek resolution of jurisdictional or status problems which adversely affect the care which patients receive and their responses to illness."

Finally, the topic of nursing's bid for increased status and its rewards is particularly timely for this neo-feminist period. Many authors have recognized the parallel and non-coincidental relationship between the women's movement and nursing's present activity [Roberts and Group, 1973; Cleland, 1971; NCSNNE, 1973; Lamb, 1973]. It is Lamb's [1973, p. 328] thesis that the Women's Rights Movement and nursing are "inextricably bound together." Cleland [1971, p. 1542] articulated the relationship between the status of women and the status of nurses. She stated, "our most fundamental problem is that we are members of a woman's profession in a male dominated culture." This premise will be cited later as one of the factors having implications for nursing's bid.

A REVIEW OF THE LITERATURE

A review of literature points up the variety of words being suggested to define the emergent position of the nurse. It is not significant that this position is being described in relation to the practitioner as the top of the hierarchy. Bates [1972] spoke of a "collegial" relationship; Cohen [1973] spoke of "collaborative co-professionals"; Lysaught [NCSNNE, 1973] referred to "congruent roles," and Aradine and Pridham [1973] spoke of "interdependent" practitioners.

Shirley Smoyak [1974], an articulate spokesperson for the nursing profession, called for nurse-physician "equality in such dimensions as status, power, prestige and access to information. . . ." Her remarks appeared in the official newspaper of the American Medical Association, and not without the expected rebuttals [American Medical News, 1974].

Schlotfeldt [1974], another nursing leader, writing on the professional status of nursing stated:

. . . The time is long overdue for nurses to assert their professional prerogatives and with confidence communicate and demonstrate the nature and value of their contribution . . . the time is long overdue for nurses, without embarrassment, to declare the scope of their responsibilities, demonstrate their competencies and expect appropriate rewards—not only those that are intrinsic to their work, but also those that include recognition and compensation commensurate with their contribution to the health care system.

As one would expect, it is nursing's academic leadership that is in the fore calling for increased status for the practitioners. It is important to consider though whether the rank and file nurse is in agreement with the goals of the leadership. This is especially significant in nursing, a profession in which the 3 percent of the practitioners who hold masters or doctoral degrees tend to be spokespersons for over 600,000 staff nurses [Sadler, Sadler et al., 1972].

What becomes obvious in interviews with staff nurses is that these nurses see themselves caught in the middle. On the one hand, nursing leadership is telling them to become involved in health teaching, nursing assessment, and other psychosocial oriented activities; this being the nursing practice that nursing leadership sees as the role of the "professional" nurse and the role which will lead to increased status for the profession. However, many staff nurses, particularly the diploma program graduates, do not feel confident in this role, and are not even convinced of its importance. On the other hand, paraprofessionals are being hired to do the technical tasks which staff nurses do feel are important and in which they feel themselves proficient. One staff nurse said in a personal interview that the profession's leadership is "telling us not to do things that are below our status, but to me those are the things nurses do." The schism between professional and technical nursing is one of the factors impeding nursing's bid for increased status that will be considered further.

Nursing is basing its claim for increased status on the premise that medicine and nursing are two separate, distinct, professions each with an equally valuable skill to offer and each sharing a common goal. Nursing is emphasizing its expertise in "caring, comforting, counseling, and helping patients and families to cope with their health care problems" [Smoyak, 1974]. Physician's expertise is acknowledged in diagnosing illness and curing disease.

This is a subtle distinction, a distinction between health care and medical care which must be understood and accepted as legitimate by the public and physicians if nurses are to succeed in their bid for increased status. The public and physicians must be convinced that nursing skills are not merely easier medical skills; that health care and medical care are not interchangeable terms. Thus, a significant part of nursing's organized effort to increase its status is based on defining its unique role, describing and demarcating that area of expertise, skill, and knowledge over which it would be acknowledged as the authority and, perhaps, most critically, establishing the legitimacy of that role in the eyes of the public and physicians.

FACTORS HAMPERING NURSING'S BID FOR INCREASED STATUS

In this and the following section, a survey of the factors influencing nursing's bid for increased status will be presented. These factors were identified through a review of the literature and through personal interviews. Although, as presented here, the factors tend to be described as if independent elements, in reality they are closely interrelated, and tend to reinforce one another.

THE SOCIALIZATION PROCESS OF NURSES

The socialization process, which begins very early in nursing students' educational experience, has served to stifle the initiative, creativity, and academic potential of the human resources of the profession. Compare these descriptions of the products of medical education and nursing education. John H. Knowles, M.D. [1969], now President of the Rockefeller Foundation, described a medical graduate:

At the end of four years, he is a highly individualistic person, cloaked with the charismatic robes of the profession, trained to take immediate action with the individual patient and to expect immediate rewards, with his knowledge firmly grounded in science.

Rita de Torneyay [1971] described the nursing education process:

We have socialized nursing students to the submissive role. We have helped students to be tactful and diplomatic to the point of obscuring their collaborative role. We have so filled nursing students with the fear of making a mistake that they are low risk takers. Along with fostering this fear of making mistakes, we socialize our students to depend on physicians and to be reluctant to accept responsibility and accountability for their own actions.

Further, consider this recollection of Marsha R. Murphy [1973], a nurse with doctoral preparation:

I remember the first time I saw the cheerful binding on our medical surgical text. My first thought was that it was abducted from a sixth-grade social studies classroom. I glanced at the medical text which lay near it—dignified and scholarly. It had no cover illustrations of smiling interns and calm chiefs-of-staff poised mannequin-like against the background scenes of medical-surgical experience. I was already beginning to feel quite inferior to persons who read those regal medical books. It was impossible to believe I would ever be their colleague.

Many authors have recognized [cf. Kushner, 1973; Wilson, 1971] the implications of this socialization process on the nurse. The nurse trained little more than a decade ago lives not only with a sense of dependence and subservience to the physician, but also with a marked sense of intellectual nonworth. She was taught the art of communicating recommendations to the physician in such a way as to disguise the fact that she was actually contributing something intelligent to the management of patient care. Indeed, she was a participant in the too familiar doctor-nurse game described by Stein [1967].

If the profession is to realize increased status, its practitioners must overcome the influences of this socialization process—indeed the process must be substantially modified.

THE FORMAL EDUCATION PROCESS OF NURSES

The formal education process that has been traditional to nursing since Florence Nightingale has disserved the profession. Again, one can draw a comparison between medical education and nursing education. The academic rigors, demanding scholarship, and scientific inquiry that have typified post-Flexner medical education were absent from nursing education too long. Schlotfeldt [1965, p. 103] points out the detriment to nursing of an educational process that focuses on "learning how to do rather than learning how to know." To the extent that the nursing education process is technique oriented, hospital-based, and of relatively short duration, the profession will be hampered in its bid for increased recognition.

THE SCHISM BETWEEN "TECHNICAL" AND "PROFESSIONAL" NURSING

The schism between "technical" and "professional" nursing was alluded to earlier as an internally divisive element in the nursing profession. The wide range in educational background, occupational commitment, and skill level represented among the approximately 1.5 million "nurses" is largely responsible for the lack of consensus on goals within nursing. Graduates of masters, baccalaureate, and associate degree programs, diploma programs, L.P.N. programs, and nurse aide programs are all indiscriminately referred to as "nurses."

In an attempt to distinguish levels of nursing practice, the American Nurses Association [ANA, 1965] issued a position paper which set forth a distinction between professional and technical nursing—a distinction based on educational preparation. Minimum preparation for the professional nurse was set at the baccalaureate level; minimum preparation for the technical nurse was set at the associate degree level.

It is questionable how successful nursing leadership will be in its efforts to implement this distinction. The unfortunate fact is that in our society the very words "professional" and "technical" connote a status level and relative worth of a contribution. Associate nursing degree programs are growing markedly faster than baccalaureate programs [ANA, 1976], and these graduates generally see themselves as "professional" nurses. Researchers [Alluto, Hrebriniak, et al., 1971] who have studied the differential socialization of nurses in the three educational pathways to the R.N. (i.e., diploma, associate, and baccalaureate programs) found the graduates exhibited similar degrees of commitment to the profession, to their employing organization, and to their clinical specialty. These researchers concluded,

It would be difficult to justify such a distinction [i.e., the distinction proposed by the ANA between a professional and technical nurse] on the basis of existing levels of commitment to nursing among students, and [the] findings suggest the associate degree and diploma graduates will strongly resist any attempts to professionally differentiate between them and baccalaureate graduates.

The unresolved internal conflict between technical and professional nursing does not bode well for any unified effort to raise the status of the occupation group. But perhaps of even greater detriment to the effort is nursing leaderships' inability to rally rank and file nurses to the "cause." Economist Eli Ginzberg [1974] remarked, "nursing leadership has never been able to pull their troops with them." Friedson [1973, p. 21] succinctly pointed out the difficulties facing nursing leadership, which is dedicated to professionalization, as it strives to "mobilize a heterogeneous and shifting corps of often casual and transient skilled workers." Nursing leadership is not unaware of where its battles must be fought. Schlotfeldt [1965] said, "The struggle to wrest nursing from the clutches of those who would keep it a field of servitude, rather than a field of professional service, must first be won within the ranks of nursing itself."

THE PUBLIC IMAGE OF NURSING—THE LACK OF PERCEPTION OF THE SKILL LEVEL OF NURSES

It is somewhat of a paradox that at the same time nursing is making a bid for increased recognition, the occupation is in a professional identity struggle. It is no surprise then that the profession has not been able to project a consistent image to the public or to other health care providers. "The public's view of nursing is somewhat vague and largely undifferentiated . . ." [NCSNNE, 1970, p. 58]. The public's perception seems generally to be that anyone, or at least any female, can provide basic nursing service.

It was noted above that nursing must establish the legitimacy of its role if it hopes to realize increased recognition. Nursing is emphasizing the psychosocial components of its role. Caring, comforting, counseling are the profession's bywords. But, will the public and physicians accept that as legitimate, marketable service? Friedson [1973, p. 11–12] pointed out that for a consulting, personal service occupation to succeed, the public must believe in the competence of the practitioners and must believe they have a skill and knowledge that can be effectively applied to practical problems. To the extent that the public does not have this awareness of nursing's service or confidence in nursing or does not see a "rational and pragmatic material advantage" the public will not consult the nurse. One physician interviewed responded with her view on the public acceptance of the role nursing is carving out for itself. She stated, "Nurses are economically naive. The public just won't buy that kind of nursing care. The public isn't interested in all that psychosocial stuff."

The findings of a study reported by Shortell [1974] have implications for nursing. He examined occupational prestige differences within the medical profession to determine possible explanations for the existence of prestige differences among medical specialties. He found the highest prestige was accorded medical specialties in which the physician "actually does something to the patient and the patient is a 'passive recipient' of the action." Lesser prestige went to specialists who "tell the patient what to do and the patient acts as a 'cooperator.'" Least prestige was accorded specialties characterized by "mutual cooperation" or "partnership" relationship between physician and patient.

Shortell's findings suggested that the degree of control the physician had over the patient's outcome was closely related to the specialties' prestige ranking. Over 50 percent of the respondents indicated they based their rating of occupational prestige on the "degree of skill" possessed by the physician.

To the extent that nursing emphasizes a caring, comforting, facilitating role it tends toward the mutual cooperation, partnership nurse-patient relationship. If the findings of Shortell's study are applicable to nursing, it is likely that patients will not accord nurses the same degree of prestige they accord practitioners who "actively do something to" them.

This does not mean that the psychosocial role of the nurse is not a legitimate or valuable part of patient care. However, what will determine the nurse's prestige is how her role is perceived by her patients and coworkers. Psychosocial care is elusive; there is no instrument to adequately measure it. The sophisticated skills required for the performance of this aspect of nursing care will be less obvious to the patient and may be perceived to be of relatively little significance to the clinically oriented physician.

Indeed, part of the skill in providing this sophisticated nursing care is that the care and facilitating are provided unobtrusively. It is ironic but quite possible that to the extent the nurse is effective as a nurse the profession will be accorded less prestige.

THE CONSEQUENCE OF A PREDOMINANTLY FEMALE PROFESSION

Many authors have cited [cf. Lamb, 1973; Heide, 1973; Babich, 1968; Shetland, 1971; Cleland, 1971] the direct relationship between the status of the nursing profession and the female image of the profession. The status of nursing is inextricably bound to the status of women. It will not be possible for the profession to realize first class status while society accords second class status to the majority of its practitioners. One feminist author stated,

Our oppression as women health workers today is inextricably bound to our oppression as women. Nursing, our predominant role in the health system, is simply a workplace extension of our roles as wife and mother. . . . Doctors are the bosses in an industry where the workers are predominantly women. Take away sexism and you take away one of the mainstays of the health hierarchy.

An important consequence of nursing's predominantly female image is that the profession is excluded from policy and decision-making roles—roles society reserves for males. This consequence is critical to a profession whose goal is to increase its status. There is a direct, self-evident relationship between status and power. And, the attainment of power is a direct result of skillful maneuvering at policy-making levels.

Group and Roberts [1974] portrayed university nursing faculty as powerless pawns of a male-dominated authoritarian structure. The informal communication networks that lead to power positions and the techniques of maneuvering for power are too frequently not understood by nursing's leadership. If nursing is to increase its status, it must not only understand the intricacies of power, but it must aggressively exercise that power to its advantage in a system which equates power with prestige.

FACTORS ENHANCING NURSING'S BID FOR INCREASED STATUS

Contraposed to the above are several factors that will enhance nursing's bid for increased prestige. Again, although isolated as distinct elements, they are interrelated.

CHANGES OCCURRING IN THE EDUCATIONAL PROCESS

Friedson [1973, p. 55] pointed out the positive correlation between increased length of training, increased formality of training, the proximity of that training to the university, to position in the labor hierarchy. Nursing educators have recognized this and are moving on all three fronts.

The minimum educational level for a professional nurse has been set at the baccalaureate degree by the American Nurses' Association definition. The report of the National Commission for the Study of Nursing and Nursing Education [1970] concurred with the position taken by the ANA in 1965, that nursing education should occur in institutions of higher education. In this past decade the number of hospital-based diploma schools of nursing has decreased markedly, from 727 in 1968 to 494 in 1973. During this same period the number of associate degree programs increased from 340 to 574, and the number of baccalaureate programs increased from 235 to 305. The percent of the total number of nursing students admitted to diploma programs decreased from 72.0 percent in 1964 to 29.6 percent in 1973. During the same decade the percent of students admitted to baccalaureate programs increased from 21.4 percent in 1964 to 36.6 percent in 1973 [ANA, 1976, pp. 79–81].

The enrollment trend in masters and doctoral programs in nursing has been upward over the past decade. There was a 17 percent enrollment increase between the 1971–1972 academic year and the 1972–1973 academic year at the masters level. The number of students completing doctoral nursing programs, while small, doubled from 27 to 49. This is obviously a healthy indication for a profession anxious to increase its status. An equally healthy sign for the profession is that most of the graduate students are preparing for advanced clinical practice (over 57 percent) or teaching (27 percent). Only about 7 percent are preparing for supervision or administration. Information on the functional purpose of 9 percent was unspecified [ANA, 1976, pp. 81–85]. This reverses an earlier trend that had nurses with advanced credentials leaving direct patient care for administration or supervisor positions.

The quality of the education the nurse is receiving is also increasing. Scholarship, decision-making, and scientific inquiry are no longer unpopular. In an interview, a prominent nurse educator at the University of Rochester School of Nursing described the curriculum revisions which are occurring within the university-based schools of nursing. As described, such curriculums promise to offer programs that teach more than how to do. They emphasize learning how to find out.

THE TREND TOWARD RESEARCH IN NURSING PRACTICE

Closely related to the emphasis on higher quality educational programs for nurses is the trend toward research in the profession. This is particularly in evidence as nursing preparation moves into the university community. Emphasis on research is a well recognized step taken by professions as they move for a higher station in the hierarchy. It is part of the legitimizing process—part of gaining acceptance in academe.

Nursing is stressing the need for research into the science of the practice of nursing. That is, the need to test theories fundamental to that practice. Presenting observations on the professional status of nursing, Schlotfeldt [1974] focused on the role of nursing research and posited that nursing research has come of age. She said,

No longer do nurse investigators and theorists self-consciously speak of their commitment to science; they now with self-confidence and pride proclaim their obligation to advance, verify and continuously restructure the expanding body of knowledge known as nursing science.

INCREASED APPRECIATION OF NURSING SKILLS

A rather bleak picture was painted in a previous section of the public image of nursing and the lack of recognition of the nurses' skills. There is reason to believe, however, that changes are occurring which will have positive implications for the profession's image.

The site for providing primary and secondary health care is moving away from the hospital. Increasingly the hospital is being seen as the site for tertiary, acute care. Medical practitioners will undoubtedly continue to dominate in this setting. However, the new health care delivery facilities that are developing are affording nurses the opportunity to demonstrate their skills. Community health centers, health maintenance organizations, family planning clinics, and community mental health centers are found to be focusing on preventive care, health education, health counseling, well baby care, supportive care . . . that is, nursing care.

Increasingly, patients will be seen by nurses who will be "doing something to them." On some visits the patients may see only the nurse. The public perception of what a nurse does will become clearer as she is seen in action—as she is seen making decisions, writing orders, assessing health status, and managing patient care. The public will see her in a collegial relationship with the physician. The blurred image of the nurse will come into focus, and with the clearer view of the nursing role will come increased appreciation of her contribution to health care.

A small number of nurses have gone a step farther and have established independent fee-for-service nursing practices [Murray, 1972; Rafferty and Carner, 1973; Greenidge, Zimmen, et al., 1973]. These nurses saw the hospital bureaucracy as preventing their realization of a sense of professional autonomy. In choosing independent practice, these independent practitioners accepted full responsibility for the quality of the nursing care provided and for the consequences of their actions. Whether or not independent nursing practice spreads is not the significant issue; what is more important to note is the new mood found among nursing professionals.

REVISION OF NURSE PRACTICE ACTS

The need for defining nursing (health) care as distinct from physician (medical) care was described above. Until nursing can carve out and control a fairly discrete area of work and can practice without dependency on physicians, an increase in the status of the profession is doubtful. Recognizing this, state nurses' associations have taken action to legitimize the changing role of the nurse via licensure statutes.

During the past few years in over thirty states nurse practice acts have been introduced for revision or amendment to bring the legal definition of practice in line with the emergent role of the nurse. The New York State Nurse Practice Act of 1972 made a substantive change in the definition of nursing practice and has been cited as a model [Kelly, 1974]. The act included the phraseology:

. . . [professional nursing practice] is defined as diagnosing and treating human responses to actual and potential health problems through such services as case finding, health teaching, health counseling and provision of care supportive to or restorative of life and well being. . . .

Nursing faced strong opposition to the passage of this bill from physicians opposed to the use of the words "diagnosis" and "treatment."

Nursing leadership clearly recognized the importance of the Act to the profession. A president of the New York State Nurses' Association [Peck, quoted in Sadler, Sadler, et al., 1972] said, "Enactment of this definition is a landmark achievement; nursing's unique and historic function has finally been acknowledged and legitimized. . . ." *The NYSNA Legislative Bulletin* [1971, p. 1] said, "The intent of the bill is to clearly delineate the elements of nursing practice and to specify the independence of the *nursing* function. . . ." Clearly, practice acts, although not a total answer, are an important part of the armamentarium of a profesion moving to raise its status.

CHANGING THE FEMALE IMAGE OF NURSING

Recognizing the relationship between the status of females and the status of a female occupation, several writers have recommended that males be encouraged to enter the nursing profession [Cleland, 1971; Silver and McAtee, 1972; Duff and Hollingshead, 1968, pp. 384–385]. Admission figures show that the number of males in nursing programs has increased from 3.5 percent in 1969 to 6.1 percent in 1972 [ANA, 1974, pp. 70–73].

It has been posed that males, career oriented and not culturally assigned to the child-raising role, will change the transient worker image of the occupation. Silver and McAtee [1972] are of the opinion that males would effect an improvement in the occupation (which they advocate not calling "nursing") by their insistence on higher salaries, increased professional recognition, better working conditions, better utilization of their skills, acceptance of the professional aspects of nursing, and more reciprocal relationships with physicians.

As pointed out previously, if nursing is to realize increased professional status it must legitimize its role as a vital part of the health care system. When males and females are attracted to the profession it is a positive sign that the legitimacy and importance of the role is recognized.

THE FEMINIST MOVEMENT

Of the predominantly female occupations, perhaps none stands to gain more from the feminist movement than nursing. The feminist movement offered nurses another view of themselves and their role. Nurses became aware that they could be independent and decisive, that they could exercise judgment, apply their knowledge, and become involved in policy and decision making. The impact of the feminist movement was recognized by several nurses interviewed. One said,

I grew up in the '50s and '60s—an oppressive, stifling time for females. I am only now beginning to believe in myself as a person and as a competent nurse with something to offer to the management of patient care. I don't think this generation of nursing students will have to cross that hurdle.

Another nurse said,

I think nursing knew it wanted to go somewhere as a profession. We [nurses] had the concepts just waiting to be developed. The feminist movement gave us something to cling to, something to rally around.

A study of 120 medical nurse-practitioner students and 31 physicians at the University of Rochester also lends support to the assertion that in this neo-feminist period nurses are overcoming ingrained psychological barriers [Sullivan, 1978]. When tested, using the Edwards Personal Preference Schedule, these nurses showed a noteworthy shift in identified needs. Whereas nurses had traditionally scored high on "order," "deference," and "endurance," they scored highest in the needs of "heterosexuality," "dominance," "intraception," "change," and "achievement." These findings of the shift in needs of nurses and the high degree of similarity between the needs of nurses and physicians suggest an emerging assertiveness on the part of nurses and a trend toward similarity of need patterns with primary care physicians.

There is no question but that this period of neo-feminism affords nursing the opportune environment in which to realize a bid for increased status as a practice profession.

THE RESPONSE OF THE MEDICAL PROFESSION TO NURSING'S CHALLENGE TO THE STATUS QUO

This article has examined the nursing profession at a time when it is challenging for a higher rung on the status hierarchy. In the opening remarks, the physician-dominated hierarchical system in which nursing is making its bid for increased status was described. To come full circle these concluding remarks contain some observations on the responses of physicians to nursing's challenge. The evidence to be presented is admittedly piecemeal and is intended only to suggest some factors that will play a role in shaping physicians' attitudes.

One might consider first the description often applied to physicians—omnipotent, authoritarian, directive, individualistic, decisive, and dominant. It is readily apparent that these adjectives do not suggest a tolerance for the collegial, partnership, and co-equal relationships nurses are promoting.

Just as nurses are products of their educational and socialization process, so are physicians. For physicians the process is one of producing a self-perception of omniscience and omnipotence [Kane and Kane, 1969]. The physician completes a long rigorous, educational sequence. It is unlikely he will look favorably on less rigorously prepared practitioners challenging his authority, decisions, or status.

There is evidence that physicians do not understand or appreciate the significance of nursing care. Kane and Kane [1969] reported on a study which was designed in part to assess the physician's perception of the need for other skills in addition to his own in caring for a patient population in eastern Kentucky. The results showed 82 percent of the respondents disclaiming need for assistance from other health professionals. Bates [1970] provided evidence that support a position that physicians give little recognition to the contribution of other health care team members. Furthermore, even if the physician recognizes the nursing function, he may not regard it as significant as his. One physician [*American Medical News,* 1974, p. 6] stated, "The level of knowledge and ability involved in diagnosing and curing patients is qualitatively higher than 'caring, comforting, and counseling' (all of which physicians do, as a matter of course)."

Another factor that will play a role in shaping physicians' attitudes is the physician's sense of responsibility for the patient's care. The physician faces a dilemma when confronted by the nursing profession seeking independence and autonomy. The physician is imbued with a sense of ultimate moral-legal responsibility for the patient. To handle this responsibility he seeks total control over all matters that affect the patient's safety. It is not likely he will relinquish control until this responsibility is shared legally.

Economic self-interest also will affect physician attitudes. Bates [1972] acknowledged that competition for the health-care dollar will play a role in shaping nurse-physician relationships. Two nurses opening independent practice [Rafferty and Carner, 1973] spoke of their services being offered in "the competitive market place." Levy [1966] pointed out that as one of the last remaining private entrepreneurs "the issue of who performs what health services must carry very real economic implications" for the physician.

It is interesting to consider "evidence" that might predict the response and the attitude of those in the medical profession toward nursing's challenge to the status quo, nursing's bid for co-equal status. There are positive and negative signs. One physician, although not sympathetic to the move, stated he understood nursing's intent. He stated [*American Medical News,* 1974, p. 6]:

We seem to live in an age where everybody is obsessed with power, especially those who think they don't have enough of it. The reasonable sounding arguments used by [nurses] can't obscure the fact that, in the final analysis, they are making a power play.

A clue that organized medicine is not inclined to encourage talk of nurse-physician collegueship was a remark made during an interview by a physician who has been actively involved in efforts to foster collegial nurse-physician relationships. He explained that he found papers on nurse-physician relationship welcomed by editors of the nursing literature, but found editors of medical journals generally unreceptive to papers on this subject.

On the positive side is the functioning of a National Joint Practice Committee established in 1972 and co-sponsored by the American Nurses Association and the American Medical Association. The committee of 16, eight nurses and eight physicians, was established "to discuss and make recommendations concerning the congruent roles of the physician and nurse . . ." [NCSNNE, 1970, p. 89]. One of the objectives of the NJPC is:

to address the traditional problems which affect nurse-physician relationships . . . to . . . examine the issues that affect collaborative nurse-physician relationships, such as sex, social class and professional status. . . ." [NCSNNE, 1973, p. 100]

In 1973 this group undertook to accumulate information on the joint practice of nurses and physicians in primary care. In 1977, the Commission [NJPC, 1977] presented its findings from twenty-four selected case studies. The selected examples demonstrated instances where relationships of mutual respect and trust have been established and where relationships of collaborative, collegial practice were realized.

CONCLUSION

The nursing profession continues its bid for a position of increased status, prestige, recognition, and power in the health system hierarchy. It is doing so with increasing self-confidence, determination, and openness. It is too early to predict success or failure. The health care system as a whole is in a period of transition. Changes are occurring not only in interprofessional relationships but also in modes of delivering services and in the attitudes of consumers. It is left for the observer of perhaps twenty years hence to reflect upon the events of this decade and assess the impact and effect of nursing's bid for increased professional status.

REFERENCES

Alluto, Joseph A., Laurence G. Hrebriniak, and Ramon Alonso, "A Study of Differential Socialization for Members of One Professional Occupation," *Journal of Health and Social Behavior*, 12:140–147, 1971.

American Medical News, Letters to the editor, March 4, 1974, Chicago: American Medical Association.

American Nurses' Association, *Educational Preparation for Nurse Practitioners and Assistants to Nurses*, Kansas City: The Association, 1965.

American Nurses' Association, *Facts About Nursing*, 1972–1973 edition, Kansas City: The Association, 1974.

American Nurses' Association, *Facts About Nursing*, 1974–1975 edition, Kansas City: The Association, 1976.

Aradine, Carolyn R., and Karen F. Pridham, "Model for Collaboration," *Nursing Outlook*. 21:655–657, 1973.

Ashley, JoAnn, "This I Believe: About Power in Nursing," *Nursing Outlook*, 21:637–641, 1973.

Babich, Karen Sue, "The Perception of Professionalism: Equality," *Nursing Forum*, 7:14–20, 1968.

Bates, Barbara, "Doctors and Nurses: Changing Roles and Relations," *New England Journal of Medicine,* 288:129–134, 1970.

Bates, Barbara, "Nurse-Physician Dyad: Collegial or Competitive," in *Three Challenges to the Nursing Profession*, selected papers from the 1972 ANA convention, 5–11, 1972.

Cleland, Virginia, "Sex Discrimination: Nursing's Most Pervasive Problem," *American Journal of Nursing*, 71:1542–1547, 1971.

Cohen, Raquel E., "The Collaborative Co-professional: Developing a New Mental Health Role," *Hospital and Community Psychiatry*, 24:242–244, 1973.

Coser, Rose Laub, *Life in the Ward*, East Lansing: Michigan University Press, 1962.

de Torneyay, Rita, "Two Views on the Latest Health Manpower Issue: Expanding the Nurse's Role Does Not Make Her a Physician's Assistant," 71:974–977, 1971.

Duff, Raymond S. and August B. Hollingshead, *Sickness and Society*, New York: Harper and Row, 1968.

Ehrenreich, Barbara, and Deirdre English, *Witches, Midwives and Nurses: A History of Women Healers*, Oyster Bay, New York: Glass Mountain Pamphlets (undated).

Friedson, Eliot, *The Profession of Medicine*, New York: Dodd, Mead, and Co., 1973.

Ginsberg, Eli, Informal remarks at the Joseph C. Wilson Day, University of Rochester, Rochester, New York, October 30, 1974.

Greenidge, Joselyn, Ann Zimmen, and Mary Kohnke, "Community Nurse Practitioners—A Partnership," *Nursing Outlook*, 21:228–231, 1973.

Group, Thetis M., and Joan I. Roberts, "Exorcising the Ghosts of the Crimea," *Nursing Outlook*, 22:368–372, 1974.

Heide, Wilma Scott, "Nursing and Women's Liberation: A Parallel," *American Journal of Nursing*, 73:824–827, 1973.

Kane, Robert L., and Rosalie A. Kane, "Physicians' Attitudes of Omnipotence in a University Hospital," *Journal of Medical Education*, 44:684–690, 1969.

Kelly, Lucie Young, "Nursing Practice Acts," *American Journal of Nursing*, 74:1310–1319, 1974.

Knowles, John H., "The Rationalization of Health Services," in *Views of Education and Medical Care*, Knowles, J. H. (Ed.), Cambridge, Mass.: Harvard University Press, 1968. Quoted in Kane, R. L. and R. A. Kane, 1969.

Kushner, Trucia D., "The Nursing Profession: In Critical Condition." *Ms* 11:72 + , 1973.

Lamb, Karen Thompson, "Freedom for Our Sisters, Freedom for Ourselves: Nursing Confronts Social Change," *Nursing Forum*, 12:328–352, 1973.

Levy, Leo, "Factors which Facilitate or Impede Transfer of Medical Functions from Physicians to Paramedical Personnel," *Journal of Health and Human Behavior*, 7:50–54, 1966.

Murphy, Marsha R., Quoted in Kushner, T.D., 1973.

Murray, Louise, "A Case for Independent Group Nursing Practice," *Nursing Outlook*, 20:60–64, 1972.

National Commission for the Study of Nursing and Nursing Education (Jerome P. Lysaught, Director), *An Abstract for Action*, New York: McGraw-Hill, 1970.

National Commission for the Study of Nursing and Nursing Education (Jerome P. Lysaught, Director), *From Abstract Into Action*, New York: McGraw-Hill, 1973.

National Joint Practice Commission, *Together: A Casebook of Joint Practices in Primary Care*, Berton Roueché (Ed.), Chicago: Educational Publications and Innovative Communications, 1977.

New York Legislative Bulletin, 4: February 16, 1971.

Peeples, Edward H., and Gloria M. Francis, "Social Psychological Obstacles to Effective Health Team Practice," *Nursing Forum*, 7:28–37, 1968.

Pellegrino, Edmund D., "Ethical Implications in Changing Practice," *American Journal of Nursing*, 66:110–112, 1964.

Rafferty, Rita, and Jean Carner, "Nursing Consultants, Inc.—A Corporation," *Nursing Outlook*, 12:232–235, 1973.

Roberts, Joan T., and Thetis M. Group, "The Women's Movement and Nursing," *Nursing Forum*, 12:302–322, 1973.

Sadler, Alfred M., Blair L. Sadler, and Ann A. Bless, *The Physician's Assistant Today and Tomorrow*, New Haven: Yale University Press, 1972.

Schlotfeldt, Rozella M., "A Mandate for Nurses and Physicians," *American Journal of Nursing*, 65:102–105, 1965.

Schlotfeldt, Rozella M., "On the Professional Status of Nursing," *Nursing Forum*, 8:16–31, 1974.

Shetland, Margaret L., "An Approach to Role Expansion—The Elaborate Network," *American Journal of Public Health*, 61:1959–1964, 1971.

Shortell, Stephen M., "Occupational Prestige Differences Within Medical and Allied Health Professions," *Social Science and Medicine*, 8:1–9, 1974.

Silver, Henry K., and Patricia McAtee, "Health Care Practice: An Expanded Profession of Nursing for Men and Women," *American Journal of Nursing*, 72:78–80, 1972.

Smoyak, Shirley, "Co-equal Status for Nurses and Physicians," *American Medical News*, February 11, 1972, Chicago: American Medical Association.

Stein, Leonard. "The Doctor-Nurse Game," *Archives of General Psychiatry*, 16:669–702, 1967.

Sullivan, Judith A., "A Comparison of Manifest Needs Between Nurses and Physicians in Primary Care," *Nursing Research*, in press.

Wilson, Victoria, "An Analysis of Femininity in Nursing," *American Behavioral Scientist*, 15:213–220, 1971.

5 Women Leaders

MODERN-DAY HEROINES OR SOCIETAL DEVIANTS?

Connie N. Vance

Leaders reflect the values, strengths, and weaknesses of their groups and, indeed, those of the larger society. And therein lies a particular challenge for the leader who is a woman and a nurse. For the larger society and the sub-groups of society do not expect and value leadership behavior in women. Socialization and discrimination are still powerful forces affecting women and nurses (98 percent women) who try to exert strong leadership. In my research with identified leaders in nursing, these two factors emerged as continuing barriers to their full-fledged status as recognized leaders in the larger society.

Let us briefly analyze socialization and discrimination, specifically as they determine expectations and values about women as leaders.

SOCIALIZATION AND IDENTITY

Socialization is the process by which we develop an identity and expectations within that identity. These include sex-role expectations, and personal and professional expectations: what we should aspire to be, how we should or should not behave, what we come to value and expect in our lives.

We are all familiar with the sex-role expectations and stereotypes of maleness and femaleness in our society. For example, maleness is equated with such terms as dominant, competitive, independent, aggressive, objective; while to be female is to be compliant, accepting, dependent, passive, emotional. Strong social pressures reinforce these stereotypes. Expectations associated with leadership are more compatible with the male stereotype than the female one. The code words of effective leadership—competent, risk-taking, forceful, decisive—suggest images of strength and dominance. And these simply don't fit most people's conceptions of a woman. Le Roux, who has studied sex-role stereotyping and leadership, states:

Stereotyping regarding what females are like has lessened our initial credibility in leadership roles because traditionally females have not been viewed as authoritative sources in American society. This has affected our ability to influence others because source credibility is an important component of the influence process [1].

Reprinted with permission by *Image*, Copyright © 1979.

Because of our present value system and its socialization effects, a woman, to be a "true woman," a successful woman, must accept herself as the Other. As de Beauvoir puts it:

With man there is no break between public and private life: the more he confirms his grasp on the world in action and in work, the more virile he seems to be: human and vital values are combined in him. Whereas woman's independent success is in contradiction with her femininity, since the "true woman" is required to make herself object, to be the Other [2].

As a result of socialization with its concomitant sex-role expectations and values, women are still encouraged to seek approval, affection, conciliation and to be "other directed." They do this to the extent that they are concerned that their femininity is incompatible with being ambitious, powerful, competent, and successful. Representatives of the cultural party line also reinforce these role expectations and values. These representatives may be parents, teachers, friends, spouses, and colleagues. Epstein, writing from her research on women as leaders, states:

Because women are not generally counted among the successful, all women are regarded as deficient. Thus, women outside as well as inside the professions and occupations are regarded as second-class citizens, as incompetents dependent on males to make the important decisions: as giggling magpies who will contaminate the decorum of the male luncheon clubs and bars: as persons who can't be trusted to be colleagues [3].

THE WOMAN LEADER AS DEVIANT

It is my thesis that the woman who attempts to break out of the expected mold—who does not conform to the commonly accepted cultural feminine ideals and images—is often regarded as a *deviant*. Since in our society, professional and leadership roles still typically fall within the male-assigned role, the woman who dares to be different—to be successful and exercise power in her own right—is a role-breaker, an outsider. She fits into at least one or perhaps all of the definitions of deviance as conceptualized by Becker: varying too widely from the norm; something or someone essentially pathological; a symptom of social disorganization, and a failure to obey group rules [4].

Researchers at the Educational Testing Service report that young women continue to have a difficult time assuming leadership roles because there are few women leaders to model themselves after and because society treats such females as deviants. Even if a woman does manage to achieve a professional or leadership position, she is viewed with less respect and credibility than her male counterpart and is subject to more extensive criticism by both her male and female peers [5]. These researchers found that to challenge young women to prepare for leadership roles is to ask them to accept and learn behaviors that the majority of society stills considers deviant. "It is not a legitimized activity: it is something that is questioned," one researcher says [6].

Since deviance involves a violation of culturally accepted rules, the offender is duly noted as "different" and is often stigmatized. Some "successful" deviants are also secretly feared and admired as well as esteemed for their extraordinary courage in the face of powerful cultural constraints. Punishment of the deviant may take the forms of subtle put-downs and ridicule to open hostility and ostracism.

Numerous real-life "war stories" document this response to the "deviant" woman leader. Two brief examples are illustrative: one, a subtle put-down; the other, a serious infraction.

The "MacNeil/Lehrer Report" on PBS presented a program a year ago on upgrading nursing education, using the New York State Nursing Association's 1985 Proposal as a model. A physician on the panel was addressed as "Doctor," while the nursing educator with a doctorate was addressed as "Miss."

A female financial executive in a large company gained rapid prominence and prestige in her field. When she inquired about a merit raise, which her male counterparts had all received, she was refused. Her superior explained that since her husband had a fine position, she didn't need a raise. The executive went to court, cited her superior's discriminatory action, and won her case.

DISCRIMINATION AND NURSES

Discriminatory attitudes and behavior affect our lives deeply as women and as nurses. Persons possessing undesirable societal characteristics (of race, religion, sex, lifestyle) are considered inferior. Goffman states that on this assumption there are many forms of discrimination exercised by society, through which such a person's life chances are effectively, if often unthinkingly, reduced [7]. Nurses, reflecting the second-class, inferior status of women in society, have, through the years, been exploited, degraded, and controlled by others considered more powerful and superior. Their work, for example, has often been virtually ignored in relation to the physician's; their ideas and contributions have often been trivialized. Ashley has written:

The lack of progress and accompanying low status (of nurses) may well have worked to reinforce the belief that women are naturally inferior and incapable of advancing to levels of competence achieved by predominantly male professions. Nursing's problems, rooted in the traditions of economic exploitation, inadequate education, and long-standing social discrimination, have plagued the profession for the greater part of its history [8].

This discrimination, in the tradition of the self-fulfilling prophecy, leads to a devalued self-concept and a concomitant self-devaluation of one's work and talents. It leads to a low self-esteem and the flagellant self-hatred that is so common in women and in nurses. In the face of so many cultural constraints, is it any wonder that nursing and its leaders have met with so much resistance and failure in their attempts to become autonomous, competent, self-directed professionals and in their attempts to upgrade nursing and to impact on the larger society? Unless she is quite outstanding in many respects, the nursing leader's professional "life chances" are greatly reduced through discrimination.

Those nurses—and there are many in our past and present—who have struggled against all odds to strengthen professional nursing's purpose, are indeed *heroines*. They continue to come fullface against the tea and sympathy images and sex-role expectations of handmaiden, mother surrogate, assistant to the physician, uneducated doer, passive angel-in-white. They struggle against living out the self-fulfilling prophecy of the devalued feminine role of submissiveness, powerlessness, and ineffectiveness. They are well acquainted with discrimination in its many forms.

My doctoral research concerned itself with the study of contemporary leaders in American nursing, whom I term "nurse-influentials" [9]. Seventy-one leaders (70 female and one male) were identified in this national survey. Many of them have given their lives—their energies and talents—to advancing nursing within the larger society. They provide some clues, however, as to the impediments they have encountered in their professional endeavors. When asked to list the major disadvantages to belonging to a predominantly female profession, such as nursing, their four most frequent responses were:

1. Sexual stereotyping
2. Discrimination of various forms (income, status, educational)
3. Self-image problems (subservience, low self-esteem and self-confidence, insecurity, passivity, lack of assertiveness)
4. Isolation from the male perspective

Clearly, to do one's work competently—to be an influential leader—in the face of such odds requires courage and a touch of the heroic. The nurse-influentials speak to this point. When asked what had been important to them in their careers and what characteristics would be required of future nursing leaders, they named courage and the willingness to take risks.

THE LEADERSHIP CHALLENGE

We in Sigma Theta Tau are challenged to be leaders in our profession. As the founders of Sigma Theta Tau threw out the challenge for strong leadership, so we are still called by Sr. Rosemary Donley, our President [10]; by the theme of the 1977–79 Biennium, "Leadership in Action"; and by our profession and the public. A particularly relevant statement for nursing at this particular moment in history is made by Howe. She says that women in the next decade should focus on building strong and effective leadership in those areas where they are currently numerically dominant—in nursing, education, and social work—rather than diluting their possible power base by urging that those most energetic and talented serve as additional tokens in non-traditional fields of study [11]. To focus women's energies on these professions would be to develop and change the most important service institutions in our society [12]. Then, too, the values of the larger society might be transformed to reflect more humanitarian and person-centered ideals

I suggest three broad areas that we engage in, individually and collectively, in order to become influential leaders in nursing and health care and agents of social change.

First, we must end our isolation from the mainstream of broad social and political activity and from the arenas of power and influence. Many of our early leaders saw themselves as "social reformers," in the broadest sense of the word. One of these, Lavinia Dock, urged nurses to think in terms of their "latent" and "unsuspected power" and the ways it could be used in an "intelligent and energetic manner" [13]. We need to listen anew to these words. We must be willing to give up our self-image and the public images of powerlessness and helplessness. We must not align ourselves with the cultural stereotypic feminine expectations. Rollo May speaks of "pseudoinnocence"—a naiveté about the realities of power and its use, in which a virtue is made of powerlessness, weakness, and helplessness [14]. Probably endemic among women and nurses, pseudoinnocence is a defense against admitting and confronting one's real power. It allows nurses to deny their strengths and responsibilities within the larger world and leads them, instead, to expend their energies on narrow internal struggles and issues.

NURSES: A POWERFUL FORCE

I contend that nurses are a powerful force. If we acknowledged and acted on this fact, if we stopped being pseudoinnocent, more of us could become influential leaders in larger social arenas. The word "power" comes from the Latin root, *posse*, meaning "to be able." To be powerful is to recognize one's potential for being able—being able to do one's work effectively, for example. Influence, from the Latin, *influens*, means "to flow in." Influence is a dynamic, felt force; it causes an effect, a change, an impact. As one theorist puts it, power is potential influence while influence is kinetic power [15]. To become influential as nurses we must believe in our power and have the will to transform this power into active influence.

We are being influential when we communicate our message effectively to the public—to health consumers, to legislators, to other professionals. We must write and speak to other persons and groups as well as to nurses. We must join with outside power sources—not to have our own power diluted or co-opted—but in order to change the focus and direction of this power. Joining power sources can take many forms—becoming voting members of policy and planning boards (organizational, community, professional, consumer, feminist, etc.); becoming knowledgeable political-legislative activists in nursing and health care issues; being willing to take visible and responsible leadership positions within and outside our profession; becoming institutional and social change agents, wherever we find ourselves. Some nurses are doing all of these things, but we need more who will assume active roles. Take stock of *your* contacts, resources, and interests; you will think of many possibilities. . . .

Second, I suggest that our involvement in and support of higher education in nursing are increasingly important in the socialization of influential leaders. The "emergent" leadership in the nursing profession will come from the ranks of master's and doctoral prepared people—those who have sharpened their intellectual skills; who are aware of their potentiality and that of their profession; who have carved out an autonomous identity; who possess a clear sense of self and their value to society and its people. Ninety-five percent of the nurse-influentials in my study held higher academic degrees (33 percent held master's degrees and 62 percent, doctorates). When asked about the most important attributes needed by future nursing leaders, the top items named were scholarship and intelligence. When we consider the fact that in 1975, 81 percent of all registered nurses in the United States held less than a baccalaureate degree, then we know much attention needs to be given to this important area. Energies and money should be poured into graduate education. The brightest minds, the qualified, and those with leadership potential should be sought out and encouraged to obtain graduate education.

Leadership skills *can* be learned. The environments of our schools, universities, and patient care institutions must be restructured so that our practitioners are encouraged to be creative—to use their intellects—to demonstrate and be rewarded for excellence—to take risks—to be courageous in making needed changes. All of these are critical elements of leadership. We must be committed to finding the support and means to educate future leaders—to see the importance of investing in their futures—to know that if *they* succeed, we will *all* succeed.

THE STRATEGY OF TEAMWORK

Third, I refer to one of the most precious lessons of the Women's Movement, and that is the lesson of community. Many of us know with certainty that we have helped and have been helped by each other. However, the literature states that since women have traditionally not played team sports, they have not learned to be good team players—have not learned how to develop collective strategies for winning—how to be trustworthy allies—to trust one's teammates [16, 17]. In our society, women have learned, for various reasons, to disaffiliate from each other, to distrust and see each other as competitors, to devalue female friendships, to go it alone.

As a women's profession, we who are nurses have been plagued by many of these attitudes. It is my belief, however, that many of these characteristics are quickly becoming obsolete. We are experiencing the power and the joy of helping each other, of sharing in mutual successes. As we become more self-determined and self-assured professionals, we are learning the necessity of bringing others with us. We are developing support systems and coalitions of like-minded colleagues who join together for mutual benefits. All of this has a far-reaching ripple effect and is marvelously infectious. We are already experiencing the satisfaction of recognizing and supporting promising young leaders. We are committing them and ourselves to their future growth and their contributions to our profession. In essence, we are saying, "You are our future, and we will help you."

The mentor system is an example. It is a system common in the older, more established professions—a sort of patron-protégé system, whereby those more experienced and further along in their careers serve as role models, teachers, promoters, supporters, and door-openers for the newer, less experienced people in the profession. They could be called "creators of competence" [18]. The mentor system in nursing can be an exciting, effective way to socialize young leaders. It can also be a direct challenge to the notion that women do not share and help each other. The effects of mentorship could demonstrate the power of our numbers—organized, educated, informed numbers—in reforming and changing present values and outmoded institutional structures.

MENTORSHIP: AN IMPORTANT CONCEPT

Again, citing my research, the nurse-influentials attested to the importance of mentorship and the support of others throughout their professional careers. Eighty-three percent reported having mentors, while 93 percent reported consciously being mentors to others. Seventy-nine percent of their mentors are female; 21 percent, male. They reported that their mentors helped them through (1) career promotion, door-opening, and creating opportunities; (2) professional career role-modeling; (3) intellectual and scholarly stimulation; and (4) inspiration. Seventy-seven percent of the influentials also reported that nursing colleagues were greatly supportive to them in their work, followed by non-nursing colleagues (60 percent). Of those married, 86 percent of their spouses were greatly supportive, another necessary support system for the married woman leader.

It is important to recognize that in our profession, we do not need to face the fear and loneliness of being the token female—we can befriend, share with, and confirm each other. And we cannot wait for this mentor relationship to be administratively created in our colleges, universities, and patient-care settings. As each of you experiences some consciousness-raising about the importance of such relationships, then hopefully you will become sensitive to the opportunities of helping, sharing, and bringing others less experienced along with you. More of us will see it as an investment in our future, in our profession, and in young lives. Howe reminds us that we have immense latent power in two areas: simple numerical strength and information sharing [19]. The mentor system, developed more widely in nursing, would greatly strengthen us through increasing our numbers of informed, articulate leaders. The personal and professional benefits of such a system are limitless.

PERSONAL HEROISM NEEDED

The path to exerting strong, influential leadership in nursing contains many barriers—some due to the outside social forces that have been discussed, some due to our negative self-concepts and self-imposed fears. There *will* be continued stereotyping and discrimination. There *will* be counterattacks and backlashes, once gains have been felt. In the midst of these forces, President Donley's words remind us that to be successful leaders will "require investment of personal time and energy, hard decisions about the use of resources, and the willingness to be what we say we are—the elite in nursing." We will also have to learn to live with being deviants and with the risks and discomforts that this involves. We will need to have the courage of our convictions and the competence to match that courage. As Nightingale said, "Influence gained is not by preaching but by what we are. . . . Be heroic in your everyday's work." Indeed, we will be the modern-day heroines.

If we are anxious about the difficult aspects of our work and its future demands, we will, at the same time, begin to savor the exhilaration and satisfaction that comes with the taste of success. As we come to be successful, powerful leaders, we will actively seek more success and relish rather than fear it. We will be uplifted and uplift others. We will build powerful coalitions for change and become a counter-culture with different value and reward systems. We will decide what we want to have happen and make it happen. We will be able to do our work as we envision it.

We should have great faith in our power to become an influential force for reform and change. Toffler expresses my sentiments about our future: "We have many kinds of future possibilities. The single, most important ethic is to realize that nothing is written on the wall. It is all in our power to shape. . . ."

REFERENCES

1. Le Roux, Rose S. "Sex-Role Stereotyping and Leadership." *Nursing Administration Quarterly* 1 (Fall 1976): 28.
2. de Beauvoir, Simone. *The Second Sex.* New York: Bantam Books, 1970, p. 246.
3. Epstein, Cynthia Fuchs. "Bringing Women In: Rewards, Punishments, and the Structure of Achievement." In *Women and Success; The Anatomy of Achievement.* Edited by Ruth B. Kundsin. New York: William Morrow and Company, Inc. 1974, p. 13.
4. Becker, Howard S. *Outsiders; Studies in the Sociology of Deviance.* New York: The Free Press, 1963, pp. 4–8.
5. Lockheed, Marlaine E., ed. *Research on Women's Acquisition of Professional and Leadership Roles.* Princeton, N. J.: Educational Testing Service, 1975, p. ii.
6. "Researchers Find Obstacles in the Way of Girls Assuming Leadership Roles." *Burlington (Vt.) Free Press,* 23 March 1978, p. 16B.
7. Goffman, Erving. *Stigma; Notes on the Management of Spoiled Identity.* Englewood Cliffs, N.J.: Prentice-Hall, Inc., 1963, p. 5.
8. Ashley, Jo Ann. *Hospitals, Paternalism, and the Role of the Nurse.* New York: Teachers College Press, 1976, p. 93.
9. Vance, Connie N. "A Group Profile of Contemporary Influentials in American Nursing." New York: Teachers College, Columbia University, 1977. (Unpublished doctoral dissertation).
10. "Vision for the future." *Reflections* 4 (January-February 1978): 1–2.
11. Howe, Florence, ed. *Women and the Power to Change.* The Carnegie Commission on Higher Education. New York: McGraw-Hill, 1975, p. 14.
12. Ibid., p. 169.
13. Ashley, *Hospitals, Paternalism, and the Role of the Nurse,* p. 105.

14. May, Rollo. *Power and Innocence: A Search for the Sources of Violence,* New York: Dell Publishing Company, 1972.
15. French, John, and Raven, Bertram H. "The Bases of Social Power." In *Studies in Social Power.* Edited by Dorwin Cartwright. Ann Arbor: University of Michigan Press, 1959, p. 152.
16. Hennig, Margaret, and Jardim, Anne. *The Managerial Woman.* Garden City, N.Y.: Anchor Press/Doubleday, 1977, pp. 22–26.
17. Goren, Suzanne. "Nursing's Impact on the Health Care System/77: Women in Power, Nurses in Power." Paper presented at the National League for Nursing Convention. Anaheim, California, 27 April 1977.
18. Epstein. "Bringing Woman In," pp. 17–18.
19. "New View of Women and Power." *New York Times*, 11 July 1975, p. 9.
20. "Vision for the Future," p. 1.

Questions to Part I

1. Look back at the socialization process you experienced during your nursing education. In what ways were you socialized into a subservient role? An assertive role?
2. Compare and contrast your sex role socialization process with that of your professional socialization process.
3. During your professional socialization, in what ways were you "rewarded" for conformity? Was deviancy rewarded?
4. In what ways are the media images of nursing similar to or different from nursing as it is practiced today?
5. If the public were surveyed today, what do you think their image of professional nursing would be? Would it be the same as delineated in the Hughes article?
6. Discuss the factors that enhance nursing's bid for increased status. How successful have we been since Dachelet's article was published in 1978? Are the factors that inhibit nursing's bid for increased status the same as Dachelet described in her article?
7. How many nurses do you know that fit Vance's definition of heroines/deviants? Describe their behaviors. How effective are they?
8. Was Florence Nightingale a modern-day heroine or a societal deviant? Discuss your reasons.
9. When was the last time you read or saw something positive about professional nursing? Was it truly representative of the profession?

II Leadership
THEORIES AND ATTRIBUTES

Leadership poses a dilemma for many practicing nurses. The need for vital nursing leadership has never been more urgent, yet many nurses do not perceive themselves as health professionals who use leadership behavior in every facet of their nursing care. A leader, that is, a person who uses leadership behavior, is always "somebody else" with more of "something else" that nurses would do "anything else" to avoid.

As a result, the leader mystique is enveloped in an aura of superhuman, charismatic qualities that most nurses perceive to be beyond their reach. Given the processes common to our sex role socialization and professional socialization, we respond predictably; we decide that leadership is not an appropriate professional role behavior and should be reserved for the special few who somehow are better suited. Our preoccupation with the leader mystique overshadows a more essential element of leadership, namely, the nurse's use of leadership.

The basis for understanding leadership behaviors lies in its theories and attributes. Theories of leadership guide us in the conduct of our practice in the arena best suited for the exercise of leadership—our day-to-day practice. They are frames of reference that serve several purposes in helping us become comfortable with our leadership ability. First, theories of leadership help us identify what leadership behaviors are presently operative in our interactions with patients and what behaviors we still need to develop. Second, they invite comparison of leadership styles and behaviors that are effectively used in patient care settings with those behaviors that may not be as effective. Finally, the process of identifying and analyzing our own repertoire of leadership theories and behaviors diminishes the mystique surrounding leadership and gives a clearer picture of the leadership capabilities each nurse can draw on in her professional practice.

At the same time, the attributes of leadership represent a core of beliefs so fundamental that they beg for recognition as a conscious and viable part of every professional nurse's exercise of nursing leadership. The belief that the attribute of followership is one of lesser worth belies its real function as an indispensable corollary to leadership. The belief that the attribute of self-esteem is unbecoming to nurses who have been socialized to think of self-esteem and egotism as equivalent terms, fails to acknowledge that self-esteem is an affirming activity initiated by one's self, for one's self. Each time nurses affirm themselves through their professional practice, they not only give definition to themselves, they prevent others from engaging in stereotypical definitions of what they ought to be. The attributes of followership and self-esteem touch on an even more basic attribute—our own values. In the final analysis, each of us must decide what values are inalienable to our professional practice. This is not a random task, for every nursing action we take, every skill we use, and every measure of relief we provide is a reflection of what we value. If we do not recognize these attributes, who will? If we do not believe in the worth of our practice, who will? If we do not use values as the basis of our nursing practice, what then? The readings in Part II offer some insights to these questions.

6 Theories of Leadership

Ann Marriner

NURSING IS NOT recognized for the leaders it produces. Rather, leadership—the ability to lead, guide, direct or show the way—is a quality often lacking in the nursing profession. The reasons are several. Nursing seems to attract people who rank low on self-esteem and initiative and higher on submissiveness and need for structure than people in other occupations. Schools of nursing have placed little emphasis on teaching leadership, and what education has been offered has often been taught in an apprenticeship manner. The autocratic leadership style, so widely prevalent in nursing, does not foster leadership in others. Instead, it contributes to an attitude that nurses are paid to follow orders rather than to think.

Most nurses are female and role conflicts are common. A woman must maintain heavy responsibilities in order to run a household, raise a family, and pursue a leadership role in nursing. Leadership is associated with aggressiveness, which traditionally has been considered a masculine characteristic, while passiveness was thought to be within woman's domain. When a nurse does accept a position of leadership, she may find it less than rewarding. More than likely, her primary reason for choosing a career in nursing was so that she could work directly with patients, but her new role blocks fulfillment of her initial goal. The high attrition rate in nursing is directly associated with these reasons. For many the frustrations over role conflicts and the stifling atmosphere of an autocratic system are too much to endure. Unwilling to tolerate the barriers to service and self-fulfillment, many potential nursing leaders leave the field.

The problem of role conflicts in an autocratic system can be reduced by a greater stress on leadership in nursing education and service. Theories of leadership are numerous. The following survey covers the alternatives, beginning with the oldest notion and advancing to ideas currently in vogue. By familiarizing herself with them, the nurse can select and adapt the most suitable approach for dealing with different situations. As a role model, the nursing leader can reduce the autocratic atmosphere and some of the role conflicts [1–4].

GREAT MAN THEORY

The great man theory argues that few people are born with the necessary characteristics to be great. They are well rounded and simultaneously display both instrumental and supportive leadership behavior. Instrumental activities include planning, organizing, and controlling the activities of subordinates to accomplish the organizational goals. Obtaining and allocating such resources as people, equipment, materials, funds, and space are particularly important. Supportive leadership is socially oriented and allows for participation and consul-

Reprinted with permission of Charles B. Slack, Inc., from *Nursing Leadership*, Volume 1, Number 3, December 1978.

tation from subordinates for decisions that affect them. People who use both instrumental and supportive leadership behaviors are considered "great men" and supposedly are effective leaders in any situation. Because of its premise that leaders are born and not made, many find this theory unattractive as it suggests that leadership cannot be developed [5].

CHARISMATIC THEORY

A person may be a leader because of charisma, but relatively little is known about this intangible characteristic. What constitutes charisma? Most agree that it is an inspirational quality which some people possess that makes others feel better in their presence. The charismatic leader inspires others by obtaining emotional commitment from followers and by arousing strong loyalty feelings and enthusiasm. Under charismatic leadership, one may overcome obstacles not thought possible. However, charisma is so elusive that some may sense it while others may not [6, 7].

TRAIT THEORY

Until the mid-1940s, the trait theory was the basis for most leadership research. Early work in this area maintained that traits are inherited, but later theories suggested that traits could be obtained through learning and experience. Researchers labeled the leadership traits as energy, drive, enthusiasm, ambition, aggressiveness, decisiveness, self-assurance, self-confidence, friendliness, affection, honesty, fairness, loyalty, dependability, technical mastery, and teaching skill. Asking themselves what were the traits leaders possessed, various researchers arrived at different conclusions, but some common leadership traits were identified.

1. Leaders need to be more intelligent than the group they lead. However, a highly intelligent person may not find leadership responsibilities challenging enough, may prefer to work with abstract ideas and research, and if too advanced, may have difficulty relating to the group.
2. Leaders must possess initiative, the ability to perceive and start actions not considered by others.
3. Creativity is an asset. Having originality, an ability to realize new solutions to problems, and ideas of new ways to be productive is helpful.
4. Emotional maturity—integrity, a sense of purpose and direction, persistency, dependability and objectivity—is another important trait. Mature leaders do what they say they will do and are consistent in their actions. They often work long hours, applying themselves intensely, and spread enthusiasm to followers. Energy, drive, and good health are necessary to endure the long hours, overcome the obstacles, and sustain continuous achievement. Self-assurance is self-confidence. Hopefully, the leader perceives himself as an effective problem solver who can successfully meet the situations which will confront him.
5. Communication skills are important. The leader needs to perceive the meaning of messages from others and to speak and write clearly.
6. Persuasion often is used by leaders to gain the consent of followers. The leader may make suggestions, supply supportive data, ask penetrating questions, make compromises, and request action in order to persuade others.
7. Leaders need to be perceptive to recognize their allies from their opponents and to place their subordinates in suitable positions.

8. Leaders frequently participate in social activities. They can socialize with all kinds of people and adapt to various groups. Approachable, friendly and helpful, they gain the confidence and loyalty of others in such a way that people are willing to cooperate.

Trait theory expanded knowledge about leadership, but it was not without its flaws. Few, if any, traits are identified in all trait theory research. They are not mutually exclusive and there is considerable overlap between categories or definitions of the characteristics. It is neither clear which traits are most important nor which traits are needed to acquire leadership and which to maintain it. Trait theory does not view personality as an integrated whole, does not deal with subordinates, and avoids environmental influences and situational factors [5, 6, 8–14].

SITUATIONAL THEORIES

Situational theories became popular during the 1950s. These theories suggest that the traits required of a leader differ according to varying situations. Among the variables which determine the effectiveness of leadership style are such factors as personality of the leader, performance requirements of the leader and followers, attitudes, needs, and expectations of the leader and followers, degree of interpersonal contact possible, time pressures, physical environment, organizational structure, nature of the organization, stage of organizational development, and influence of the leader outside of the group. A person may be a leader in one situation and a follower in another or a leader at one time and a follower at others. The type of leadership needed is dependent upon the situation [5, 9, 12, 14, 15].

CONTINGENCY THEORY

During the 1960s, Fred Fiedler introduced the contingency model of leadership effectiveness. He identified three important dimensions of a situation for his contingency model: (1) leader-member relations, (2) task structure, and (3) position power. The leader-member relations refer to the amount of confidence and loyalty followers have in their leader. The task structure is related to the number of correct solutions to a situation. Position power is dependent upon the amount of organizational support available to the leader. Given the critical condition, Fiedler argues that one can predict the most productive leadership style.

If task is structured but the leader is disliked and therefore needs to be diplomatic, or if the task is ambiguous and the leader is liked and therefore seeks cooperation of the workers, the considerate, accepting leadership style probably will be most productive. When a disliked leader faces ambiguous tasks, a directive style is most productive. The most productive leadership style is contingent upon the situational variables. Fiedler's contingency theory is a complex three-dimensional model which is not easy to understand nor is it conclusively supported by research [5, 10, 15, 17].

PATH-GOAL THEORY

Robert J. House derived the path-goal theory from expectancy theory. Expectancy theory argues that a person acts as he does because he expects his behavior to produce satisfactory results. In the path-goal relationship, the leader facilitates task accomplishment by minimizing obstructions to the goals and by rewarding followers for completing their tasks. The leader helps subordinates assess the needs, explores the alternatives and helps subordinates make the most beneficial decision, rewards personnel for task achievement, and provides additional opportunities for satisfying goal accomplishment.

House noted that studies done during the 1950s revealed that leaders who structured activities for subordinates generally had more productive work groups and got higher performance evaluations from superiors. Structure refers to planning, organizing, directing, and controlling through such activities as clarifying expectations of subordinates, scheduling work, making assignments, determining procedures, and setting standards. Structured activity can increase motivation by reducing role ambiguity and allowing for externally imposed controls. In contrast, considerate leaders had more satisfied workers. They created an atmosphere of friendliness, warmth and support by tending to the personal welfare of their subordinates. Leader consideration seems particularly important for routine jobs. People who do a variety of tasks may find their jobs more satisfying and have less need for social support.

House recognized that individual differences will affect the subordinates' perception of leader behavior. For instance, experienced subordinates may prefer a task-oriented style while less mature, less experienced and consequently less secure subordinates may prefer a considerate leader. Subordinates with a high need for achievement probably will prefer a task-oriented leader while people with a high need for affiliation would prefer a considerate leader. The path-goal theory introduced subordinates as a variable [4, 13, 18, 19].

LIFE CYCLE THEORY

The life cycle theory predicts the most appropriate leadership style from the level of maturity of the followers. Paul Hersey and Kenneth H. Blanchard illustrate this theory in a four quadrant model (Fig. 6-1). A horizontal continuum registers low emphasis on the accomplishment of tasks on the left side of the model to a high emphasis on task behavior on the right side. The vertical continuum depicts low emphasis on interpersonal relationships at the bottom of the model to a high emphasis on relationships at the top. The lower left quadrant, therefore, represents a *laissez-faire* type of leadership style with little concern for production or relationships. The lower right quadrant represents an autocratic leadership style with considerable concern for production but little concern for relationships. The upper right quadrant designates a high concern for both tasks and relationships. The left upper quadrant represents a leadership style that stresses relationships but shows little concern for tasks.

The maturity level of the group or individual is depicted on a continuum from high maturity on the left to low maturity on the right under the four quadrants. The maturity levels are superimposed on the quadrants with dashed lines. The best leadership style for given levels of maturity is shown by a curvilinear line in the four quadrants. To determine the most appropriate leadership style, one must assess the maturity level of the individual or group, plot it on the maturity continuum, and project a line at a right angle from that point until it intersects with the curvilinear line. The quadrant in which the intersection occurs depicts the most appropriate leadership style. With increased maturity, less structure and emotional support are needed. High task and low relationship style is considered best for below average maturity. The leadership styles in quadrants 2 and 3 are recommended for the average group or individual.

This model is consistent with Argyris's immaturity-maturity continuum which indicates that as a person matures, he progresses from a passive to an active state and from dependency to independence. With maturity he passes from a need for structure and little relation-

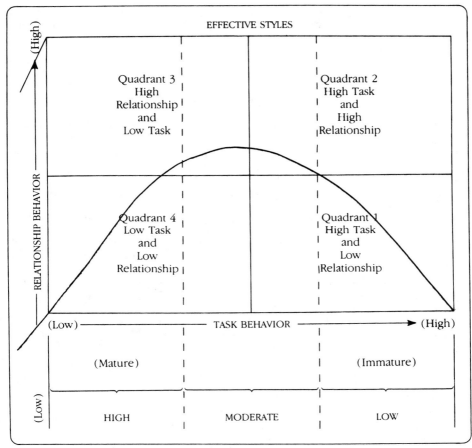

EFFECTIVE STYLES

Quadrant 3
High
Relationship
and
Low Task

Quadrant 2
High Task
and
High
Relationship

Quadrant 4
Low Task
and
Low
Relationship

Quadrant 1
High Task
and
Low
Relationship

RELATIONSHIP BEHAVIOR

(High)

(Low)

(Low) ——————— TASK BEHAVIOR ——————▶ (High)

(Mature)   (Immature)

HIGH   MODERATE   LOW

Figure 6-1. Life cycle theory of leadership. (Source: Paul Hersey, Kenneth H. Blanchard, and Elaine L. LaMonica: "A Situational Approach to Supervision: Leadership Theory and the Supervising Nurse." *Supervisor Nurse* 7 [May 1976], 20. Used with permission.)

ship through a decreasing need for structure and increasing need for relationship to little need for either. The progression is not always smooth. Stress may cause members of the group to regress, and the leader must adjust his behavior accordingly. The life cycle theory stresses the importance of the maturity level of the group and the leader needs to adapt leadership styles accordingly.

INTEGRATIVE LEADERSHIP MODEL

From a review of leadership theories, it is obvious that there is no one best leadership style. Leaders are rarely totally people- or task-oriented. Leader, followers, situation—all influence leadership effectiveness. Consequently, an integration of leadership theories seems appropriate. The leader needs to be aware of his own behavior and influence on others, individual differences of followers, group characteristics, motivation, task structures, environmental factors, and situational variables and adjust his leadership style accordingly. Leadership behavior needs to be adaptive.

REFERENCES

1. Diers D: Leadership problems and possibilities in nursing. *Am J Nurs* 72:1447–1448, August 1972.
2. Filley AC, House RJ: *Managerial Process and Organizational Behavior.* Glenview, Illinois, Scott, Foresman and Co, 1969.
3. Katz RL: Skills of an effective administrator. *Harvard Business Rev* 52:90–102, Sept-Oct 1974.
4. Kelly J: *Organizational Behavior.* Homewood, Illinois, Richard D. Irwin, 1974.
5. Fiedler FE, Chemers MM: *Leadership and Effective Management.* Glenview, Illinois, Scott Foresman and Co, 1974.
6. Kucha DH: The human relations approach to nursing administration. *Nurs Forum* 9:162–168, 1970.
7. Walsh M, Yura H: Super-vision. *Supervisor Nurse* 2:18–26, March 1971.
8. Claus KE, Bailey JT: *Power and Influence in Health Care: A New Approach to Leadership.* St. Louis, CV Mosby Co, 1977.
9. Dale E: *Management: Theory and Practice.* New York, McGraw-Hill Book Co, 1969.
10. Donnelly JH Jr, Gibson JL, Ivancevich JM: *Fundamentals of Management Functions, Behavior, Models.* Austin, Texas, Business Publications, Inc, 1971.
11. Freeman RB: Leadership in nursing. *Nurs World* 132:8–11, April 1958.
12. Hagen E, Wolff L: *Nursing Leadership Behavior in General Hospitals.* New York, Institute of Research and Service in Nursing Education, Teachers College, Columbia University, 1961.
13. House RJ: A path goal theory of leader effectiveness. *Administrative Science Quarterly* 16:321–338, 1971.
14. O'Donovan TR, Deegan AX: The scientific approach to supervisor behavior. *Supervisor Nurse* 3:39–43, 45, 47, November 1972.
15. Fiedler FE, Chemers MM, Mahar L: *Improving Leadership Effectiveness: The Leader Match Concept.* New York, John Wiley & Sons, Inc, 1976.
16. Fiedler FE: The effects of leadership training and experience: A contingency model interpretation. *Administrative Science Quarterly* 17:453–470, 1972.
17. Fiedler FE: Engineer the job to fit the manager. *Harvard Business Rev* 43:115–122, Sept-Oct, 1965.
18. Evans MG: The effects of supervisory behavior on the path-goal relationship. *Organizational Behavior and Human Performance* 5:277–298, 1970.
19. Hampton DR: *Contemporary Management.* New York, McGraw-Hill Book Co, 1977.

BIBLIOGRAPHY

Borgatta EF, Bales RF, Couch AS: Some findings relevant to the great man theory of leadership. *Am Sociological Rev* 19:755–759, 1954.
Christman LB: Nursing leadership—Style and substance. *Am J Nurs* 67:2091-2093, October 1967.
Cutler MJ: Nursing leadership and management: An historical perspective. *Nurs Administration Quarterly* 1:7–19, Fall 1976.
Flippo EB: *Management: A Behavioral Apporach.* Boston, Allyn and Bacon, 1970.

Haimann T, Scott WG: *Management in the Modern Organization.* Boston, Houghton Mifflin Co, 1974.

Hersey P, Blanchard KH: *Management of Organizational Behavior: Utilizing Human Resources.* Englewood Cliffs, New Jersey, Prentice-Hall, Inc, 1977.

Hersey P, Blanchard KH, LaMonica EL: A situational approach to supervision: Leadership theory and the supervising nurse. *Supervisor Nurse* 7:17–20, 22, May 1976.

Iafolla MAC: The dilemma of women leaders. *Nurs Forum* 4:54–67, 1965.

Leininger M: The leadership crisis in nursing: A critical problem and challenge. *J Nurs Administration* 4:28–34, March–April 1974.

McBride A: Leadership: Problems and possibilities in nursing. *Am J Nurs* 72:1445–1456, August 1972.

McFarland D: *Management Principles and Practices.* New York, Macmillan Publishing Co, Inc, 1974.

Merton RK: The social nature of leadership. *Am J Nurs* 69:2614–2618, December 1969.

Schurr MC: A comparative study of leadership in industry and the nursing profession. *Int Nurs Rev* 16:16–30, 115–132.

Sisk HL: *Management and Organization.* Cincinnati, South-Western Publishing Co, 1973.

White HC: Perceptions of leadership styles by nurses in supervisory positions. *J Nurs Administration* 1:44–51, March–April 1971.

White HC: Some perceived behavior and attitudes of hospital employees under effective and ineffective supervisors. *J Nurs Administration* 1:49–54, January–February 1971.

Yura H, Ozimek D, Walsh MB: *Nursing Leadership, Theory and Process.* New York, Appleton-Century-Crofts, 1976.

7 Nursing Leadership Process

Helen Yura, Dorothy Ozimek, and Mary B. Walsh

LEADERSHIP MAY OCCUR within the formal organization, and the situation is all the better if leadership is a companion process to administration, management, and supervision. However, leadership belongs to formal and informal organizations and is not bound by organizational boundaries. It can occur whenever, wherever, and with whomever there is need for goal setting and influence toward goal achievement by a person who is a leader and a person who is led.

With this in mind we have attempted to define leadership, designate the nursing leadership process, delineate specific behaviors inherent in the process, and determine the dimensions of the process.

The theoretical formulations about leadership provide a useful framework for thinking about, analyzing, synthesizing, and researching leadership further. Theoretical formulations in and of themselves have little value, however, unless they are put into action. In other words, the theories need to be operationalized for testing purposes and need to be applied to or serve as the basis for direct action.

The theoretical developments and the collective research related to leadership available at this time should give direction to the development of leadership for nursing and include a taxonomy of behaviors that would rightfully be labeled leadership behaviors; in addition, what is known about leadership, generally, should be applied to nursing specifically.

Thus the literature was searched for definitions of leadership. These were analyzed and other definitions were developed which seemed clearer and more appropriate to research development relating to leadership at the present time, and which were applicable to nursing.

For the purposes of this chapter, leadership is defined as the process of influencing the behavior of other persons in their efforts toward goal setting and achievement. *Nursing leadership is a process whereby a person who is a nurse effects the actions of others in goal determination and achievement.* This implies the defining and planning for nursing in an interactional setting. *Nursing* is an encounter with a client and his family in which the nurse observes, supports, communicates, ministers, and teaches. The nurse contributes to the maintenance of optimum health and provides care during illness until the client is able to assume responsibility for fulfillment of his own basic human needs; when necessary, she provides compassionate assistance for the dying.

Inherent in the operational definitions is a grasp of the direction of change and the ability to determine the direction and extent of change as well as to utilize the humane and moral

Excerpted from Chapter 3, *Nursing Leadership*. Reprinted by permission of Appleton-Century-Crofts, 1980. From *Nursing Leadership: Theory and Process* by Yura, Ozimek, and Walsh (2nd Edition), 1980.

means (communication, reward, punishment, coercion, etc.) that followers will accept as they pursue goal achievement. Failure to move or change means no goal achievement, no leadership, and no followership.

As our survey and analysis of the literature progressed, it was necessary to go beyond the definition of leadership and nursing leadership so that available knowledge would have meaning for nursing. Direct application of theory to practice was the goal. If the process of leadership could be determined—a process that would enhance goal setting and ensure goal achievement—a major step would be achieved toward the implementation of available knowledge related to leadership. This process, when identified and developed, could be learned as are all other processes needed for the practice of nursing—i.e., the nursing process, the research process, by teaching–learning process.

Available material in the literature on leadership and nursing leaders, including theories, definitions, opinions, behavior designations, expectations, etc., were analyzed to determine if evidence of a process could be found. As the review continued, it became obvious that a few key words and phrases were dominant and that clusters of behaviors thought to be leadership behaviors were related to these key words and phrases. The consistency in the use of key words and phrases (such as interaction, influence, guiding, satisfying individual and group needs, decision-making related to goal determination and achievement, changing, communicating, and providing) supported the contention that a process could be developed. Four key words were extracted from the words and phrases used most frequently. Most other frequently cited words and phrases related to one or another of these terms and seemed to be a dimension of or to flow from them. Terms could thus be clustered and categorized.

The four key terms were *deciding, relating, influencing,* and *facilitating.* These terms were felt to be strategic in putting into operation the definitions of leadership and of nursing leadership given earlier. A review of these terms satisfied the authors that these four terms were inclusive enough, with sufficient differences between and among them, to be of value. The sequence of the four terms was considered logical and useful.

After the components of the process were identified, the authors asked a sample group of senior baccalaureate nursing students and first- and second-year master's nursing students to respond to questions about these components. Respondents were asked if they perceived deciding, relating, influencing, and facilitating as essential to the nursing leadership process, and to rate the four component terms in order of priority. The authors' identification and ordering of the process components were supported by the respondents. All respondents agreed with the selection of process components and most supported the proposed ordering. Respondents were almost evenly divided as to placing *deciding* and *relating* as first in importance. However, there was a clear distinction when responses were viewed in terms of ordering in the second place. *Relating* was clearly designated for second place, in contrast to *deciding.*

The nursing leadership process is a process by which determined goals are achieved through the four components of deciding, relating, influencing, and facilitating. Permeating all components is the act of communicating. Inherent in the nursing leadership process is evaluation.

Participants in the nursing leadership process are the leader and the follower(s). Variables internal and external to the leader and follower(s) have an impact on goal determination and achievement when utilized in a nursing situation. Diagrammatically, the nursing leadership process is envisioned as is demonstrated in Figure 7-1.

Change occurs from the point of goal determination to the point of goal achievement.

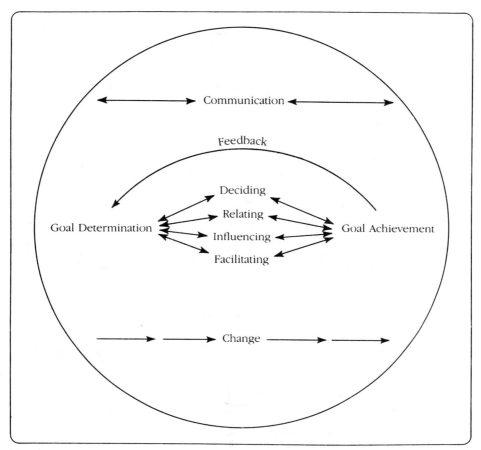

Figure 7-1. Nursing leadership process.

Feedback is needed to evaluate the realization of determined goals. Failure to meet the goals fully will reactivate the components of deciding, relating, influencing, and facilitating as demanded by the situation to fully achieve the determined goal(s) (Fig. 7-2).

Power is inherent in the leadership process, as is flexibility to manipulate components and subcomponents to achieve maximum effect. Power is given to the leader as long as followers sanction this. Power is increased if goal determination and achievement are accomplished in an effective manner. No one type of leadership style is viewed as appropriate to all of nursing. The variations encountered in nursing situations, with differences in follower participants as well as in the degree and number of crises and the amount of available decision-making time, demands a leadership style that is flexible even on a daily basis. Also superimposed upon the process are short-term, intermediate, and long-range goals in the nursing situation. This gives a multidimensional focus to utilization of the nursing leadership process. Change permeates the entire process from beginning to end. Change affects the partici-

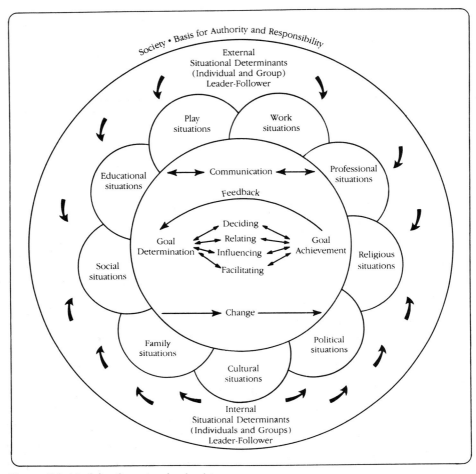

Figure 7-2. Models of nursing leadership process.

pants and the situation, for neither is the same once the process becomes operative. The acts associated with the nursing leadership process are always in the direction of goal achievement. Thus, if goal determination is legitimate, appropriate, realistic, and moral, and if the acts of deciding, relating, facilitating, and influencing are humane, are appropriate singly or in combination, are within the skill of the leader and are acceptable, expected, and viewed as helpful by the follower(s), then it can be said that goal achievement will occur and that the nursing leadership process is being effectively utilized.

The nursing leadership process is applicable with clients (well or ill), families, groups of clients or families, peers and colleagues and with special interest groups (consumer, health-related personnel and health professionals). The process is also applicable in the leader's immediate surroundings and with more distant groups—local, state, and national. It is possible to use the process despite a diversity of goals and even with diffuse goals that have a narrow and/or broad impact on those who are directly involved or who are touched or affected by goal achievemnt. An example of a broad impact would be the utilization of the nursing leadership process to achieve quality delivery of health and nursing service on a national level. Although the number of persons striving to achieve this goal is limited, the results of goal achievement will affect every citizen, alien resident, and visitor in the United States.

After the components of the nursing leadership process were identified, the human actions inherent in each were identified. These actions are called behaviors and their designation is termed a taxonomy of behaviors related to the nursing leadership process (p. 82). Permeating each of the four processes of deciding, relating, influencing, and facilitating is the act of communicating. Communication, however, is not viewed as a separate component because it cannot be separated from the four identified components. It is inherent throughout the process because the process components are only realized through communication. In the same way, evaluation (feedback) permeates each of the four components and is not separated out as a component in and of itself.

The style of nursing leadership will be determined by the behaviors demonstrated for each of the four components by the person who is the leader. Since the behaviors listed in the taxonomy indicate a large array of available behaviors, their precise utilization (and any additional behaviors, to be identified through practice and research) will depend on the leader's personality and knowledge, the followers' receptivity, and the variables in the setting. Thus no categorization of styles is deemed necessary or appropriate by the authors. The style emerges as the leader operationalizes the selection and combination of behaviors inherent in the use of the nursing leadership process with followers, in a particular setting, and appropriate to the goals to be achieved.

Leadership will be designated effective or ineffective according to the success with which determined goals are achieved. The level of success in leading must take into account nursing leadership behaviors inherent in deciding, relating, influencing, and facilitating.

To summarize, the dimensions of nursing leadership behavior can be illustrated diagrammatically in Figure 7-3.

The authors created premises related to the nursing leadership process and applied the components of the process for illustrative purposes, thus indicating the ease with which the process may be utilized. Each premise is accompanied by a myth that is refuted. The premises serve as guiding principles in implementing the process.

Premise 1: To use the nursing leadership process, the nurse must have knowledge and skill.
   Myth: A person is born to be a leader.

Factual knowledge from numerous disciplines is necessary if the nurse is to *inspire* the confidence and trust of her colleagues as well as the confidence of the clients for whom she is caring. She also must have sufficient knowledge to ensure her own self-confidence. She needs to be convinced of her ability to develop her own nursing care framework so that she can determine why an event is occurring and whether she can cope with it effectively.

The *decision-making* phase of the nursing leadership process requires a sound basis for making judgments, and this basis rests on the broad, inclusive knowledge and skills of the decider. When faced with more than one alternative in planning client care, the nurse must decide which is the best alternative or route to follow. The client, on a 1:1 caring plan, is involved with the nurse in the decision making. As the client asks questions and reveals problems he is facing, the nurse uses her knowledge and background experience to assist him and herself in making decisions about care. A wide range of assessment factors are

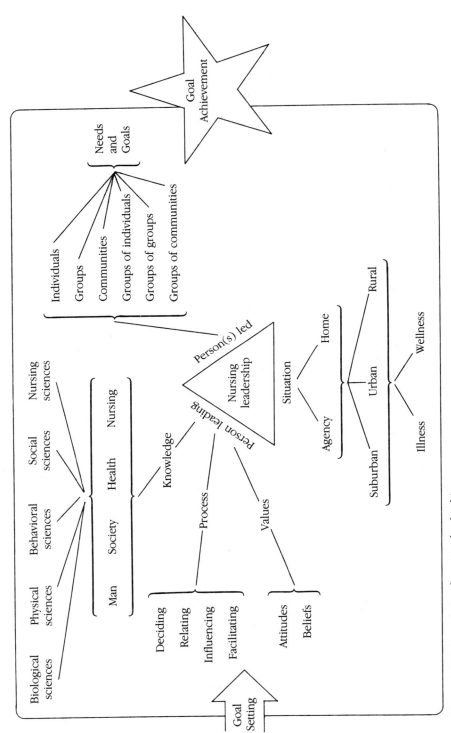

Figure 7-3. Dimensions of nursing leadership.

explored and various plans may be possible, each of which must be considered to determine the best route for the client at that time and in that situation. The nurse's knowledge will assist her in recalling scientific facts to guide decision making. For example, the diabetic client will require a much lower carbohydrate intake than he had with the high carbohydrate diet of his previous pattern. Or, a person who tends toward midmorning hypoglycemia should plan a carbohydrate-protein snack to ward off the untoward effects of such a metabolic incident.

When dealing with groups of nursing and health care personnel responsible for a group of hospitalized clients, the decision-making process becomes more complex. Not only does the nurse concern herself with the problems and needs of the client, his family, and significant others, but she also concerns herself with the problems and needs of members of the staff. Knowledge of human behavior becomes an important factor in dealing with groups of people, both clients and staff. An understanding of what to expect as well as how to deal with various behavior patterns, deciding what to do, and choosing one of several alternatives is crucial to effecting the nursing leadership process.

The knowledge acquired by the nurse provides her with a base from which she can determine the actual and potential problems of clients and the staff with whom she functions. Assessing these problems in light of her own abilities and strengths, she decides, sometimes alone, sometimes in collaboration with clients and/or staff, which is the best of several alternative routes to follow for the good of all.

Depending upon the persons involved in the situation and the problems identified, components of relating and influencing may change in priority or blend into components that are more difficult to separate precisely from each other than are other components of the nursing leadership process. One can argue that in order to influence, one must relate; and in order to relate, one must influence. Be that as it may, each component can be separately analyzed and then transposed from a higher to a lower position, or vice versa, as need be.

Relating to others requires an ample degree of charity (love), feeling, and value for one's fellow man. Trust and respect for another, be he client or co-worker, are essential elements in establishing a relationship that is productive of good effects. It is important that this kindness (charity), trust, and respect enter into and permeate all negotiations and encounters between individuals who relate to each other.

The nurse leader sees the client and treats him as a person who has abilities and rights, strengths and limitations, and who may be experiencing some temporary incapacity. In order to be of assistance to the client, the nurse communicates her respect for the client as an individual by word and manner. When the client senses such respect for his rights and feelings, he reciprocates, usually by extending the same degree of respect to the nurse.

The nurse leader, through her knowledge of human behavior, has established a sound basis for a good relationship by treating the client with respect.

In dealing with co-workers, whether peers, subordinates, or superiors, the same knowledge of human behavior applies. To function collaboratively for the benefit of clients and of staff, mutual trust and respect must permeate all endeavors. Through group efforts, the talents of each and all can be utilized so that the client benefits and the staff realizes satisfaction in worthwhile and productive efforts.

A sound knowledge of human behavior enables the nurse leader to provide a good, stable relationship between clients and personnel by establishing an atmosphere of mutual charity, trust, and respect for the abilities, strengths, and rights of each to the eventual benefit of the client and the satisfaction of personnel.

The knowledge necessary to carry out the *influencing* phase of the nursing leadership process should be constructive and broad. All of the knowledge used to make decisions and to relate to others is required for influencing. Positive influence is paramount so that the nurse leader is moving constructively and productively to benefit all. In her role of leader, the nurse may be able to exert influence because those who are following, whether client or staff, are doing so because of the nurse's role and not because of the directions or instructions she is giving. Knowledge about roles and status will help the nurse leader acquire insight into the client's and the staff's responses to her. The desirable effect of the nurse's leadership should be that the client sees her as a knowledgeable and capable health worker. Such knowledge proves to the client that the nurse can direct and guide him to achieve the health goal shared by both. Her role as leader is reinforced when the client sees the nurse as

Taxonomy of Behaviors Relating to Nursing Leadership Process (communicating and evaluating are inextricably incorporated in these components)

DECIDING		
analyzing	discovering strategies	perceiving
assigning	discriminating	planning
assuming	distinguishing	predicting
choosing	evaluating	probing
comparing	feeding back	responding
concentrating	formulating	revising
concluding	guiding	risk taking
data collecting	implementing	seeking
deducing	informing	selecting
delegating	inquiring	setting precedent
deliberating	judging	synthesizing
discerning	measuring	validating
disclosing	observing	

RELATING		
appreciating	effecting	recognizing
arbitrating	enhancing	reducing uncertainty
assisting	evaluating	resisting
attending	explaining	respecting
bargaining	feeding back	responding
behaving	gossiping	revealing
calming	greeting	sharing
comforting	ignoring	socializing
concealing	informing	speaking
conversing	interacting	supporting
conveying	(a) approaching	sustaining
cooperating	(b) initiating	touching
criticizing	(c) continuing	transacting
cutting off	(d) terminating	understanding
differentiating	(e) withdrawing	using self
dignifying	listening	valuing
directing	projecting	welcoming
discriminating	reacting	withholding

INFLUENCING

advancing	discharging	motivating
advocating	disciplining	neglecting
approving	disclosing	obligating
assenting	disguising	ordering
brainwashing	dissenting	pacifying
censoring	distinguishing	persuading
challenging	divulging	plotting
choosing	duping	politicizing
coercing	elevating	praising
comparing	evaluating	prodding
competing	feeding back	promoting
concealing	framing	proving
condemning	hiding	punishing
conditioning	identifying	reasoning
condoning	ignoring	rejecting
confronting	impressing	rewarding
controlling	indoctrinating	ruling
convincing	inducing	satisfying
credentialling	inspiring	separating
deceiving	internalizing	socializing
deferring	interpreting	subterfuging
demoting	legitimizing	suspending
detaining	managing	teaching
dictating	manipulating	tattling
directing	modifying	telling
disapproving	moralizing	threatening

FACILITATING

acquiring	dispersing	potentiating
altering	distributing	preserving
allocating	dividing	providing
arranging	enabling	publishing
authorizing	evaluating	recording
balancing	freeing	reimbursing
bargaining	getting	requesting
budgeting	giving	requisitioning
causing	involving	seeking
changing	modifying	showing
claiming	monitoring	starting
closing	negotiating	supervising
collecting	opening	surveying
creating	organizing	tending
demonstrating	paving	utilizing
directing	performing	

a person to respect not only because of her role but because of her knowledge and expertise in the health endeavors of both (client and nurse). The purpose of influencing, ultimately, is to establish plans of care and to set these plans in motion—to implement them. Through knowledge of resources, available personnel potential, and achievable goals, the nurse can influence the client to set reasonable goals and help him to seek resources and people who will be most beneficial to him.

Thus a wide range of constructive knowledge and skill is crucial to the nurse leader influencing the client in his search for reasonable goals and helpful resources and personnel.

To *facilitate* the entire operation, the nurse leader must know that all other phases of the process are completed satisfactorily or at least as fully as possible at the moment. Only if decisions have been made as to the best route(s) to follow, if relationships have been established, and if appropriate influences are felt, can the total process be facilitated. If, on reflection, it is determined that one or part of any component has been insufficiently explored and/or implemented, then facilitation is delayed until such components are completed.

Knowledge of what has been accomplished between and among nurse leaders and clients, as well as what the potential accomplishment is in terms of goals and desired ends, will assist the nurse leader in effecting changes and adjustments to enhance the situation. By knowing how to use the abilities of clients and personnel, the nurse leader can facilitate movement and can hopefully progress, by meeting the needs of clients, to a situation of stability and eventual total health.

The facilitation phase of the leadership process is effected when all other phases are moving well and constructively; the nurse leader acts as overseer and prime mover to ensure progress and stability to achieve a state of health for the client.

The extent of the impact of nursing leadership, the style and kind of leadership, and the effectiveness or ineffectiveness of leadership behaviors depend on specific utilization of the nursing leadership process and the number of persons participating. Degrees of complexity are determined by the quantity and quality of decisions; the method, kind, and quality of influence; the effectiveness of relating; the kind and amount of facilitation; the extent of goal determination; the amount of change needed to bring about goal achievement; the total number of individuals involved; and the number of communications needed among participants to achieve the goals set forth.

8 Followership

THE INDISPENSABLE COROLLARY TO LEADERSHIP

Dorothy F. Corona

IN A COUNTRY which places great value on leadership, "followership" is often overlooked. It is true there is a serious lack of leadership in our society but perhaps there is a more critical lack of the ability to follow with candor, intelligence and commitment.

To follow, according to Webster's Dictionary means "to come after, to pursue, to result from, to take as a model, to understand" [1]. There is nothing in this definition which implies lack of involvement, indifference, or apathy. Following has a connotation in the contemporary world of being unwilling to think, create or disagree, or incapable of thinking, creating, or disagreeing. It has often been confused with indecisiveness. It is viewed as an undesirable characteristic. One must look at following in the context of leading and the affected roles of both. Implicit in these roles are the values placed on them. Authority, communication, organizational structure, goals and behavioral characteristics inherent in these roles need consideration.

ROLE

Role theorists have identified that for every role there is a complementary role or a role which completes. If leadership is a desirable and necessary role in society then the role which completes it is equally desirable. That complementary role for leadership is followership.

AUTHORITY

A universal characteristic of society is that it seeks to organize itself. Organization may take many forms; however, all are designed to fix authority and accountability. Organization legitimates authority which in turn legitimates communication. Two of the several authority theories will be considered: Formal Authority Theory and Acceptance Theory can be described as *authority of position* and *authority of leadership* [2]. Formal authority theory or authority of position is related to that authority which is independent of the personal ability of the holder. Authority results from the position the individual holds in the organization. Authority of leadership exists when a person's skills are such that others will follow regardless of the formal position in the organizational structure. Barnard identified that authority

Reprinted with permission of Charles B. Slack, Inc. from *Nursing Leadership*, Volume 2, Number 2, June 1979.

results from the willingness of the workers to *accept* the authority of the person regardless of the position [3]. A person who possesses the authority of leadership is able to operationalize acceptance theory by inspiring and encouraging respect, thus creating a desire to follow.

The ideal organizational situation is to combine authority by position and by leadership. This type of leadership engenders confidence which makes following an inducement in itself [2]. In a society such as ours, based upon a constitutional republic, we are governed by a system of laws enunciated by designated leaders—lawmakers; the followers of the laws legitimate the leaders through the election process. Prior to the turmoil of the 1960s, hardly anyone either questioned the duly and lawfully elected leaders' right to lead or the followers' responsibility to follow. While authority to lead has been questioned from time immemorial, in the United States the "law" has been the standard authority and accepted by the overwhelming majority.

In modern times, and especially since the Nuremberg trials, the law holds each individual responsible for his or her individual actions regardless of the circumstances or forces surrounding those actions. Perhaps this brought about the phenomenon of "civil disobedience" or flaunting those laws an individual "felt" were unsupportable based on that person's moral conviction. Individuals perceived their values as more valid than law. What has been called an "individualistic society" came into focus. This type of society places more importance on the rights of individuals than on rights of an individual or group supported by law. There must be compromise between the "individualistic society" and the "pluralistic society" and it is this compromise which enlightened followers must make. To follow an individual who leads, requiring blind submission and absolute devotion, results in cultists, fanatics and demagogues. To follow a person who leads encouraging rationality, creativity, and discourse, exercises moral followership. Moral followership is dependent on moral leadership. James MacGregor Burns describes moral leadership as that "which tackles hard problems forthrightly, making hard decisions without regard for political expediency" [4]. Moral followership is, therefore, described as that which follows these decisions based on the good for the majority of mankind without undue regard for personal or individual gain.

MORAL LEADERSHIP

Moral leadership and consequently moral followership appears to be lacking in society. Traditional heritage and values are being forsaken to that which is most expedient for the individual. In nursing, the nurse's commitment to caring for others, the desire to alleviate suffering, the imperative to prevent illness for mankind has been compromised to delegate providing comfort to nonprofessionals, to preoccupation with operating gadgetry rather than working with patients and to concerning oneself only with the here and now in caring for the acutely ill. Nursing educators lack moral leadership when they are more interested in teaching the discipline than they are in teaching the learner. Nursing administrators exercise questionable leadership where they are more concerned with providing "bodies" and minimal credentials to staff a unit rather than concerning themselves with the characteristics and talents of those persons assigned to provide quality patient care.

Nurses are demonstrating a yearning for moral leadership to the extent that as followers they desire to be consulted when nursing decisions are made, to disagree when the facts are obscure, and to exhibit professional attitudes as consumer advocates.

FOLLOWERSHIP

Followership is imperative at this time. Enlightened followership provides strength and unity for the profession. It provides challenge of ideas. Growth doesn't take place without challenge, conflict and compromise. Worthy followers challenge a leader's ideas, then debate them and come to support them. In exercising followership, people close ranks against the outside marauders who seek to weaken or destroy by dividing.

No group, professional or otherwise, can be strong without unity. This is the key to nurse power. There are many schisms which divide professionals and especially professional nurses. On occasion, the ANA and the NLN are at loggerheads with each other, thus diminishing the effective leadership of both organizations. Hospital-educated baccalaureate and associate degree nurses have disdain for each other; nurses refuse to support the professional organization because they are told that the employing agency has greater interest in their welfare and the care of patients than their own professional colleagues. Nurses prefer to throw stones at the American Nurses' Association than to join and provide the challenge so essential to a viable leadership group.

Many nurses are cynical and divisive. They hold their leaders in contempt; they punish each other for not seeing things exactly as they see them. "Leadership doesn't prosper amid cynicism" [4]. Nursing needs support for those who speak for higher standards of nursing practice and education. Loyal followers are needed by those who articulate nursing's need for autonomy. Assertion that nursing is an essential service and that nurses are a great health manpower resource needs to be reinforced by every nurse. Nurse support will convince many that nursing is capable of accomplishing far more than that which is currently occurring. The value of nursing is not the "care and feeding" of the physician or unquestioned compliance with agency policy. It is rather serving patients/clients—to act on behalf of them and to support and sustain nurses who hold that commitment and are able to communicate it.

COMMUNICATION

The leader is predominantly occupied with the character of communication which induces acceptance by followers. Communication is authoritative when it promotes the effort or action of the group being led. Followers impute legitimate authority to communications from leaders provided they are consistent with the best interest of the organization or, in the case of a profession, those served and those doing the serving [2].

Communication is perceived through listening and, based on that listening, the message is interpreted. The decision to follow or not is predicated on the message heard. Followers may agree with the essentiality of the message even though they may not agree with each related issue. There are segments of professions where the message communicated is that after the professional is secure, the rest of society will be cared for. Nursing, at this point, is not in danger of this pitfall, however, the potential is there.

NURSING'S STRUGGLE

Nursing is vacillating; it is being swayed by many forces and the majority of its one million nurses ride the waves in a quasi-apathetic fashion. It is difficult to have gifted leadership and intelligent followers when there is no struggle. Nursing is in the throes of a struggle to become accepted as a contributor on the health care team, to the end that people's health needs will be better served. This is a real mission for nurses. But, for the vast number of practicing nurses, there is little which can be identified as pursuit of that goal.

Only as nurses become involved in the struggle and follow with determination, dedication and diligence, will nurses spawn the great leadership so desperately needed in this hour. Alfred North Whitehead made the observation that, while "advanced thinkers . . . are apt to be intolerant" [5], those who follow them can personify "genial orthodoxy." This puts followership in the position of change agent. Those followers can translate ideas into operations. They are the followers who complement the leaders. Whitehead calls these persons the "Apostles of Modern Tolerance" [5].

SKILLS OF FOLLOWERSHIP

Leadership and followership are relational concepts, inseparable, interdependent and influential only when interchange occurs [6]. Just as there are behaviors around which leadership is built, so there is a cluster of desirable skills which make one a useful and worthy follower. Followers should consolidate their efforts and present a modicum of unity. Nurses must appear as if they possess a common bond in serving humankind and, *indeed*, this commonality does exist. Loyalty is a characteristic essential to following, not a type of loyalty which is blind or acquiescent, but one which is built on respect and affection, if not for the leader, then surely for the cause [7]. The loyal follower is informed and supportive, and is willing to risk rational disagreement within the confines of the issue.

Nurses disagree poorly; rather than disagree, they frequently withdraw. Consequently, it has been easy to divide nurses. The art of confrontation and persuasion are foreign to many. Producing calculated conflict is repugnant to most nurses. Some nurses seem to fear the validity of their own intellect. No leader wants followers who won't challenge an idea. Challenge is how great ideas are honed. But to be productive, one must be cautious in criticizing. Continuous tearing down is not only destructive but demoralizing. Criticism demands positive reinforcement as well as negative comment. Proper challenging of that criticism is critical.

SUMMARY

In summary, the role leadership cannot be considered apart from the role followership. The fact of followership legitimates leadership and authority. Leadership and followership are interdependent roles. Accepted goals, communication, and appropriate organizational structure need to be clearly understood. Katz and Kahn have described some social patterns existing in which the group members are relatively unaffected by the interventions of their leaders [8]. These groups dissolve in impotence and anarchy. This won't happen to nursing if nurses are thoughtful, willing, articulate followers.

Effective followers use the recognized organizational structure to be heard. Follower does not imply legalism defined by rules and regulations where every "jot and tittle" receives equal emphasis. One uses judgment concerning rules and policies. If there are irrelevancies, ignore them and move on to the things which make a difference. Applicable, at this point, is a principle of Zen: "Put all energy and effort into what one does at the time one does it" [9].

The list shown in Figure 8-1 encapsulates some of the characteristics of the leader and the corollary behaviors manifesting desirable qualities of the followers. One can really see that all nurses are both leaders and followers from the listing.

LEADERS	FOLLOWERS
Studies and creates new ideas.	Tests new ideas.
Makes decisions.	Challenges where indicated.
Assigns appropriate responsibilities.	Knows when to accept responsibility and carries it out.
Creates an environment of trust resulting in freedom.	Uses freedom responsibility.
Takes risks.	Risks following.
Is reliable.	Is trustworthy and respectful.
Is loyal to followers.	Is loyal to leaders.
Is self-confident.	Knows oneself.
Assumes leadership position.	Follows when appropriate; uses the organizational structure.

Figure 8-1. Traits of leaders and followers.

If leadership is a commodity in short supply and great demand, leadership must be articulated with a vast number of willing followers. The quality of this followership is crucial. Michael Korda has concisely expressed it thus: "No matter how small the task, we have to teach ourselves that it matters" [9]. Followership is as indispensable as leadership in building momentum as a profession matures. For nursing, the hour is now.

REFERENCES

1. *Webster's New World Dictionary of the American Language.* New York, The World Publishing Co, 1973, p 27.
2. Hampton DR, Summer CE, Weber RA: *Organizational Behavior and the Practice of Management.* Glenview, Illinois, Scott Foresman and Co, 1973, pp 490–491.
3. Barnard CI: *The Functions of the Executive.* Cambridge, Massachusetts, Harvard University Press, 1938.
4. Burns JM: U.S. must be purposeful, not vagrant and uncontrolled. *U.S. News and World Report,* November 27, 1978, pp 63–64.
5. Whitehead AN: *Adventures of Ideas.* New York, Macmillan Publishing Co, 1956, p 57.
6. Blau P: *The Organization of Academic Work.* New York, John Wiley and Sons, Inc, 1973, p 188.
7. Stogdill R: *Handbook of Leadership.* New York, Free Press, 1974.
8. Katz D, Kahn RL: *The Social Psychology of Organizations.* New York, John Wiley and Sons, Inc, 1966, p 301.
9. Korda M: *Power! How to Get It, How to Use It.* New York, Random House, 1975, p. 259.

9 The Politics of Self-Esteem

Nancy P. Greenleaf

INTRODUCTION

This article examines the interrelationships between politics and self-esteem. Politics here means competition between groups or individuals for power and leadership. The overall focus is on nursing, a sex-segregated occupation [1, 2]; therefore, the self-esteem of women in nursing is of particular interest. Can we learn something about the power relationships within the health care industry by focusing on the self-esteem of the women who make up so large a segment of that industry?

Self-esteem is a reflexive term meaning that the object perceived and the perceiver are the same person [3]. It results from an evaluation of the self by the self. When the self-evaluation has positive results a person is said to have high self-esteem, or as Rosenberg suggests, might be known as an egophile [4]. Conversely, if the self-evaluation is negative, the person is said to have low self-esteem, to be an egophobe.

Power is of interest to two categories of people; those who have it and those who don't. Janeway says the ability to act is a liberating or enabling power and the ability to dominate is limiting or controlling power [5]. Oppressed people are concerned with becoming liberated, gaining control over the conditions of their lives. Dominant groups are concerned with maintaining their power and control over others.

When we speak of power struggles we refer to conflicts between individuals or groups for controlling power. We refer to the contenders in the conflict as "power holders" and "power seekers." If the contenders are of equal strength to begin with it is misleading to think of either as powerless. But groups or individuals do not always begin on equal footing; power relationships between dominant and subordinate groups differ from struggles between contenders of equal strength. Dominant groups, for instance, control resources and access to them such as money, media attention and consequent public opinion. Contrast the time and space allotted to press coverage of medical vs. nursing news, or the amount of federal money earmarked for medical research vs. nursing research.

Another powerful yet poorly understood resource of dominant groups is their greater opportunity to define the situation, themselves, and the other group [6]. The extent to which the oppressed group accepts the definitions put forth by the group in power has a great deal to do with their continuing acceptance of subjugation. We understand, for instance, that when medicine is defined as encompassing all health care, any challenge to nursing to define its own uniqueness is a futile effort.

The conflict between groups seeking liberating power and groups seeking to maintain

Reprinted by permission from "The Politics of Self-Esteem" by Nancy Greenleaf, *Nursing Digest*, Inc., Volume 6, Number 3, 1978.

controlling power is a complex process. Strategies to strengthen the position of the group seeking liberation become the focal point of the struggle.

One objective of this article is to examine the development of women's work as it emerged from work in the home. It is important to understand the commonalities of all women's occupations and not simply define nursing's situation as unique. The second objective is to gain a better understanding of self-evaluation and self-esteem, underscoring the significance of self-defined values and standards. The assumption throughout is that women in our society are in subordinate positions to men and that perpetuation of this inequality rests on both the dominant group's ability to define situations and individuals, and the subordinate group's acceptance of those definitions.

A model linking self-esteem and enabling power is proposed demonstrating the relationship of the two concepts and suggesting strategies to equalize the power relationships between dominant and subordinate groups.

THE POLITICAL ECONOMY OF WOMEN'S WORK

The term "women's work" is closely related to housework. Women's work is housework and housework is women's work. It is the work associated with the role "housewife" [7]. Work has been defined in various ways but most commonly has meant energy expended in the production of goods and services which in turn have value in the market place [8]. Housework, performed in the privacy of the home, does not have an historical claim to market place value. Because of this, the work of the housewife has not been perceived as work by sociologists [9]. Work is perceived as wage labor and takes place outside of the home. The term "working mother" clearly illustrates this for if housework meant work the term would be redundant. A "working mother" refers to a woman with children who works outside the home.

Galbraith speaks of the "convenient social virtue" as the ideology that gets people to do whatever it is that needs doing to benefit the economy [10]. In our modern industrial economy it is essential that someone manage the consumption within the household. The job is ". . . to select, transport, prepare, repair, maintain, clean, service, store, protect, and otherwise perform tasks associated with the consumption of goods" [11]. While single people do this for themselves, the majority of people live in families where housewives perform this service for the family. The value of their services has been estimated at roughly 25 percent of the GNP [12]. It is clear that if a man marries his housekeeper he saves money. He also reduces the national income [13].

It is important to keep in mind the relationship of housework to the economy when considering work done by women outside the home. Although 46 percent of women are in the labor force [14], most women who work outside the home are concentrated in sex-segregated occupations or professions [15]. (As of 1969, one-half of all women workers were employed in only 21 occupations, whereas one-half of all male workers were more broadly distributed in over 65 occupations [16]). Furthermore, many of these "female" occupations developed in part as an extension of the housewife role.

Before the industrial revolution, people produced at home most of what they needed to sustain themselves. All families did not produce all goods; there was trading between them, but the actual manufacturing of the goods took place in the home. Everyone old enough to work did so and the labor was divided between men and women. The men worked the land, planted and harvested the crops, hunted and tended the animals. The women prepared and preserved the food, spun the wool, flax, or cotton into thread, wove the cloth and made the clothing. The women also minded the children and taught them their ABCs and nursed the sick. The men provided the link with the larger community, trading surplus produce and goods manufactured by the women and participating in the political activity of the community. Laws defined married women as possessions of their husbands. Married women did not own property, make contracts, or vote.

As industrialization progressed the division of labor between men and women was maintained. One of the first industries to move out of homes and into factories was textile manufacturing. A descriptive analysis of nineteenth-century industrialization notes that:

Women were quickly drawn into textile work for a number of reasons; first, because it had been women's work before it was mechanized; second, because women could be hired more cheaply than men; third, because there was a shortage of male labor; and fourth, because there was opposition to enterprise which would draw the male population away from farming. [17]

The prevailing attitudes that everyone should work and thus be saved from the sin of idleness, a carryover from Puritan ideology, supported the move of women into the factories. However, as demographic changes due to immigration took place, and more men were available to fill jobs, attitudes toward women working outside the home also changed. By the 1840s ". . . The genteel lady of fashion had become a model of American femininity and the definition of 'women's proper sphere' seemed narrower and more confined than ever" [18]. Galbraith's concept of "the convenient social virtue" seems to have been operating long before he coined the phrase. Because male workers were more plentiful, it was more convenient for women to stay at home.

The development of other women-dominated occupations shows commonalities of women workers and women's work. In discussing the feminization of elementary school teaching in the nineteenth century, Oppenheimer notes that (1) women provided a cheap and relatively plentiful supply of labor, (2) there were few nonmanual occupations open to women, and (3) it is an occupation that requires a fairly high level of education [19]. Men with a comparable level of education could get other jobs with better earnings. It is also noteworthy that elementary school teaching may be seen as an extension of the housewife role of minding and teaching young children. Likewise, as public libraries multiplied in the latter part of the nineteenth century a need was created for well-educated librarians to work in them. Like public education, the libraries were tax supported, therefore the need was for inexpensive librarians. Libraries offered not only books and research services but a pleasing, welcoming atmosphere such as a genteel hostess might provide. Well-educated women were recruited from the upper classes and they perceived themselves and their jobs as a level above school teaching [20].

The situation was similar with nursing. Reverby points out,

Hospitals in America quickly saw the advantage of training nurses. Student nurses could be used to fill the hospitals' nursing needs; and better still, they didn't have to be paid beyond room and board. Between 1880 and 1900 the hospital nursing schools in the U.S. grew from 15 schools with 323 students to 432 schools with 11,000 students. Since cheap student labor provided the bulk of nursing care, hospitals did not hire their students after graduation [21]. Like other female occupations, nursing's roots lie in the housewife's role as caretaker of the sick family member.

All female occupations are valued. None is well paid relative to men's occupations [22]. In all cases we see a relationship between recruitment of women workers already or easily trained by virtue of doing housework, and low cost to the employer.

There are other important consequences of a sex-segregated labor market. One is that equal pay for equal work becomes meaningless [23]. When there are only a few men in an occupation they quickly rise to take the higher level jobs [24, 25]. People must be in the same job category to bargain for equal pay. Second, the socialization of women to be temporary workers affects their ability to gain control over the occupation. Young girls are brought up believing that they will become wives and mothers and while it is all right for them to work, they must fit marriage and child rearing into career plans. The modern mother is made to feel responsible for the emotional health and social adjustment of the children [26]. This is a powerful message which keeps women from making the same kind of career commitment that men do. The resultant moving in and out of the labor force creates an elasticity of supply and a relatively large labor reserve which means that workers are always replaceable. (In 1972, 1,127,657 RNs held licenses. Of the number, 778,470 or 69 percent reported holding employment in nursing [27].) It is perpetually an employers' market, for as Caplow points out, "it is almost impossible for a women's occupation to be effectively monopolized by the incumbents" [28]. Third, when women do work, often out of necessity, they find they still have the housework to do when they return home [29]. This fact inhibits full-time career commitment.

SELF-ESTEEM: THEORETICAL BACKGROUND

How are nurses' self-estimates related to the fact that they are women in a sex-segregated occupation? What is self-esteem?

Answers to these questions are found in social psychology. Much of the research on self-esteem is theoretically based on symbolic interactionism which in turn rests on the work of William James, George Herbert Mead and C. H. Cooley [30].

James, a pragmatic philosopher, developed the I/me dichotomy in which the total self is divided into the self as knower—the I, and the self as known—the ME [31]. It became difficult for James to differentiate between ME and MINE.

We feel and act about certain things that are ours very much as we feel and act about ourselves. Our fame, our children, the work of our hands may be as dear to us as our bodies are, and arouse the same feelings and acts of reprisals if attacked.

He extended the concept of ME by asserting that "a man's ME is the sum total of all he CAN call his." James's list of what a man might call his included his body, psychic powers, clothes, house, wife, children, ancestors, and friends. Though one may argue that for simplicity he left out a comparable list for women, the prevailing ideology of the day held that women did belong to their husbands and fathers. A better argument for the generality of James's statement is that he also listed friends as possessions. One can assume that autonomy was not lost because of friendship. James's derivations came out of the experience of men, an inference easily made from the context of his examples.

For better understanding he divided the ME into three parts:

Its constituents
The feelings and emotions they arouse (self-appreciation)
The acts which they prompt (self-seeking and self-preservation)

The constituents, each with attending feelings and acts were further divided into:

1. The material ME, including the body, family, near and dear material possessions such as home and hearth, life's work, and whatever would provoke intense grief if lost;

2. The social ME, which is manifested in the recognition one receives from others. Lack of such recognition was a horrible fate; as James says, "no more fiendish punishment could be devised, were such a thing physically possible, than that one would be turned loose in society and remain absolutely unnoticed by all the members thereof." He further states that a man has as many social selves as there are individuals and groups whose opinions he values. These social selves sound very similar to the social roles we speak of today. James emphasized what he called "club opinion" as one of the strongest forces in life. Like a code of honor, "club opinion" held that a thief must not steal from other thieves although he may steal from anyone else, or a gambler must pay his gambling debts although he may ignore other debts. (Another interesting example he gives is that you must not lie in general but you can lie as much as you want about your relations with a lady. Whether one may lie to protect the honor of the lady or at the expense of it is not clear.)

3. The spiritual ME, including all states of consciousness such as thinking, feeling, deciding, and desiring. Some states are more central or intimate than others, e.g., the will is more central than the intellect. These more central portions of the spiritual ME form the core or nucleus of the self as we know it.

According to James, self-examination (the I knowing the ME) leaves us with a sense of what we could be (pretensions or aspirations) and an evaluation of what we are (successes). Thus:

$$\text{Self-esteem} = \frac{\text{success}}{\text{pretensions}}$$

"The fraction may be increased as well by decreasing the denominator as by increasing the numerator." He points out the relationship of self-feeling to power; ". . . neither threats nor pleading can move a man unless they touch some one of his potential or actual selves." To influence another, one must first discover that person's strongest principle of self-regard and place one's threats or pleas accordingly.

C. H. Cooley, a sociologist, does not deal explicitly with self-esteem, but talks of self-feeling as an aspect of the "looking-glass self." He postulates that an individual's self-concept is determined by his perceptions of other people's attitudes toward him. He delineates the self idea thus:

a. *the imagination of our appearance to the other person*
b. *imagination of the other's judgment of that appearance*
c. *self-feeling [32].*

To have high self-esteem we need to imagine that others, when they perceive us, see what is really there and that it is all right in their opinion.

G. H. Mead was a philosopher with an interest in understanding social processes [33]. James dichotomized the individual into the I and the ME but his definitions differed. Mead indicates that the form of the self is the ME which develops by internalizing the attitudes of others in the group. He refers to the ME as "conventional" or as the "institutionalized individual [34]." "The I reacts to the self (ME) which arises through the taking of the attitudes of others." At least some of these attitudes which the ME incorporates are those expressed by others toward the individual as object. Therefore the individual develops self-attitudes consistent with those expressed toward him by significant others in his world [35].

The significant understanding is that self-feelings and attitudes, be they good or bad, originate outside of the self and come to belong to the individual through a process of internalization. According to symbolic interactionism, society is a precondition for the development of the self [36]. Self-esteem, then, results from taking on others' esteem of us.

Another provocative way of looking at self-esteem is from a developmental point of view. What are the major sources of self-esteem as the individual progresses through the life cycle? Belaief discusses this using Piaget's cognitive development scheme as a basis for two models of equality [37].

The first model, "social equality of opportunity" is derived from the juvenile stage where self-esteem is based on performance. Parental love is perceived as scarce and therefore one must compete for it (the esteem of significant other). This experience of self-esteem is never final; one is always in danger of losing it. Because of this constant danger, the individual experiences anxiety and others (peers) are placed in the position of rivals.

She calls the second model of equality "human equality." This type has two developmental derivations, one in infancy where the parents' sheer joy in the child's existence is experienced and the other during preadolescence when the person experiences a joy in the very existence of peers. In either case the esteem of significant other is not perceived as scarce or measured by some performance standard. Preadolescence doesn't rule out performance as much as it alters the relationship with peers, diminishing competition and sharing esteem. "I'm great and so are you."

Belaief suggests that society is fixated at the juvenile stage of development, perceiving the esteem of others as a scarce resource which depends on performance and superiority. She would like to see society move toward the second model where esteem is based more on sharing and one person's high doesn't somehow necessitate another person's low.

THE NATURE OF MAN IN THE NATURE OF WOMEN

In dealing with social science theories, we often assume that the "nature of man" is a universal term that includes women. As has been noted in James's case, this assumption is not necessarily true. Gould points out that many philosophers' views regarding universal human nature are contradicted by their views of concrete individuality in the case of women and that their statements regarding women are ideological in the sense of both reflecting and supporting the oppression of women. Thus, Gould notes that in Hegel's Philosophy of Right, the sphere of the family (woman's sphere) is specifically excluded from the domain of right, i.e., from the public sphere of civil society and the state. Kant holds that rationality is the dominant human characteristic and male, while beauty or aesthetic sensibility is a subordinate characteristic, and female. Gould argues that ". . . it is not because male nature is rational that men become rulers, but it is because men rule that rationality is assigned as a male trait" [38].

As we examine the universality of the philosophical assumptions underlying social science theory, further questions arise about the applicability of these theories to inquiries about women. How have feminist thinkers dealt with the self-esteem construct as it relates to women?

WOMEN AND SELF-ESTEEM

Virginia Woolf, writer and illuminator of women's condition, stated simply that women have not become great and famous or achieved as men have because they have received little privacy and less support, financial or otherwise. Men, on the other hand, have fared better because: "women have served all these centuries as looking-glasses possessing the magic and delicious power of reflecting the figure of man at twice its natural size" [39]. We don't know if Virginia Woolf was aware of Cooley's "looking-glass self," but the implication is hard to pass by.

Psychoanalyst Karen Horney exposed a major flaw in psychoanalytical thinking about the nature of women. She points out that the psychology of women has, like all science, been developed from a man's point of view. To illustrate, in the parallel phrases she makes the comparison of the psychoanalytic picture of feminine development and the typical ideas that a little boy has of a little girl (Table 9-1) [40].

When viewed from a symbolic interactionist perspective Horney's parallel phrases help explain why there are still clinicians trained in psychoanalytic methods who defend their ideas on the basis of clinical findings. It is indeed conceivable that women, defined as inferior by others, might come to define themselves that way.

Miller recently addressed this problem.

Women have always had to come up with a basis for worthiness that is different from that which the dominant (male) culture bestows. They have effected enough of a creative internal transformation of values to allow themselves to believe that caring for people and participating in others' development is enhancing to self-esteem. . . . This does not mean they are therefore recognized and rewarded for their value system. Quite pointedly, they are not; they are made to feel that they are of little worth—"I am only a housewife and mother." [41]

("I am only a nurse" echoes in my mind.) Miller attempts to derive a more accurate understanding of women's psychology as it arises from women's life experiences rather than as perceived by men.

Relating social psychology to the earlier discussion on power, we can see that both the situation in which we work and the characteristics by which we know ourselves have indeed been defined by others. Furthermore, we can see that it is functional for the present economic system for women (nurses) to believe in their inferiority, particularly in the work place. We can also see more clearly that reflections from the looking-glass need not be limited to perceptions defined by dominant groups. We can resist their definitions and define ourselves and our work. There has always been a segment of nursing to do so. We must recognize them, credit them, and continue their work.

LIBERATION AND SELF-ESTEEM

Recent interest in self-esteem has quickened in two arenas, education and politics. Both are rooted in the philosophical notion of democracy based on equality.

John Dewey employed the principles of William James's philosophy in his progressive movement in education. The trend for evaluation in education has been away from measuring objective behavior against outside standards toward developing subjective measures based on individual goal setting and self-evaluation. Also, interest in the causes of failure in school has prompted inquiries into how teacher expectation affects performance and how

Table 9-1. Horney's Parallel Phrases

BOYS' IDEAS

Naive assumption that girls as well as boys possess a penis.
Realization of the absence of the penis (in girls).
Idea that girl is a castrated, mutilated boy.
Belief that girl has also suffered punishment that threatens him.
The girl is regarded as inferior.
The boy is unable to imagine how the girl can get over this loss or envy.
The boy dreads her envy.

PSYCHOANALYTIC IDEAS

For both sexes it is only the male genital that plays any part.
Sad discovery (for girls) of the absence of the penis.
Belief of the girl that she once possessed a penis and lost it.
Castration is conceived of as the infliction of punishment.
Girl regards self as inferior (penis envy).
Girl never gets over the sense of deficiency and inferiority and has constantly to master afresh her desire to be a man.
The girl desires throughout life to avenge herself on the man for possessing something she lacks.

poor self-concept and self-esteem become the basis for self-fulfilling prophecies of failure [42].

Related to this, but from a different perspective, is pressure from political groups contending for equal opportunity to participate fully in the economy. A striking example of a political group's grasp of the importance of self-esteem is the Black Power Movement's slogan "Black is Beautiful." Likewise, in the Women's Liberation Movement, the emphasis on assertiveness training has focused attention on the need for a positive self-image as a prerequisite for assertive behavior [43].

Bloom makes connections between self-esteem, anxiety, and assertive behavior. She notes circular behavior patterns where you do not assert yourself, you lose self-esteem, you become anxious and therefore do not assert yourself. Conversely, asserting yourself by making known your requests or refusals increases your self-esteem and reduces your anxiety which in turn frees you to assert yourself [44].

Smith implies the importance of self-esteem in the title of her assertiveness training workshops for nurses: "Presenting Ourselves Proudly" [45].

The turn of the century debate between Booker T. Washington and W. E. B. DuBois asked whether protesting injustice, when one could not individually right it, was self-respecting. Washington argued that it was not self-respecting if correcting the injustice was impossible and claimed, in fact, that such protest betrayed a weakness by relying on the sympathy of others. DuBois strongly disagreed. Denying that protest was an appeal for sympathy, he maintained that if a person failed to openly express his outrage at injustice, he would eventually lose self-respect. What to Washington was prudent, was appeasement to DuBois [46].

How often do we take our fate for granted, assuming that protest will serve no purpose? But self-respect is closely related to self-esteem and self-esteem is our power base. Self-esteem comes from honest and appreciative self-appraisal and refusal to accept a stereotyped definition from others. Dumas illustrates the difficulties faced by black women executives when they are pressured to conform to the "mammy" image and fulfill everyone else's needs for "warm and soothing interpersonal relationships." The myth of the all-giving black mammy who nursed us all puts an added burden on black women in their jobs. Dumas protests when she points out that

. . . whether she likes it or not, the black woman has come to represent a kind of person, a style of life, a set of attitudes and behaviors through which individuals and groups seek to fulfill their own socioemotional needs in organizations. It is not surprising, therefore, that black female leaders are actively sought out by those who perceive themselves in a vulnerable position, under considerable threat, or powerless to accomplish without the help of these leaders some highly significant personal or professional goal. People who are relatively secure and strong manage to keep black women at a comfortable distance from the base of any real power. Black women's competence for their positions is imagined to be a function of their persons. Consequently, intellectual and professional expertise is considered of secondary interest, if recognized at all. [47]

Dumas protests the special exploitation of the black woman leader. Understanding it and exposing it, she refuses to assume a queen bee role, co-opted by the system and perpetuating the exploitation of others.

THE POLITICS OF SELF-ESTEEM: A SYNTHESIS

Janeway's enabling power concerns energy [48]. The *American Heritage Dictionary* defines energy as vigor or power in action. Energy can be directed for positive or negative use, and has a relationship to our self-esteem.

We know from experience that when we feel good about ourselves we have the energy or enabling power to accomplish our tasks.

Self-esteem ⟶ energy

And we know that when we are skilled at doing something we experience self-confidence and pride.

Competence ⟶ confidence ⟶ self-esteem

On the other hand, there are times when we cannot see things clearly and cannot accomplish much. We're working hard but getting nowhere.

Confusion ⟶ consumes energy

At times we must take risks in order to achieve a goal. Taking risks means we will be vulnerable. Fear of failure may keep us from taking risks even when we know it would be self-respecting.

Fear ⟶ consumes energy

At other times we realize that others keep us from doing what we want, or getting what we need. A common response to anger which we often feel we cannot safely express.

Oppression ⟶ consumes energy

Suppressed anger becomes rage. When we understand the oppression and get in touch with the rage we find a source of energy of which we were not aware. The rage becomes outrage and we will no longer acquiesce to the oppression.

Focused anger ————————————➤ energy

If we understand self-esteem as our power base, then strategies derived from the above scheme will strengthen that base.

IMPLICATIONS FOR NURSING LEADERSHIP

Nursing is in a key position to lead a movement to restructure the health industry to serve the needs of the American people rather than the profit and power requirements of health employers. Some important trends affect nurses' potential for controlling nursing [49].

There is a significant increase of women in the labor force. In 1974, 46 percent of all women 16 years and over were working outside the home [50]. This is up from 31 percent in 1950 and 20 percent in 1900 [51]. Statistics show that many RNs still drop out of the labor force to have children, but they are returning to work in greater numbers when their children enter school. They are thus more likely to view work relations, the quality of patient care, and level of wages in a long-range perspective. As Cannings and Lazonick point out, "Permanent wage workers are more likely to reject the traditional ideology of female submissiveness to males which has been very functional for maintaining and manipulating the hierarchical order of the health industry" [52].

Clearly the consciousness of nurses is changing. Nurses are seeing their careers more as long-term commitments rather than something to fall back on. They are becoming more assertive in demanding input into policy decisions affecting health care. Increased awareness of past economic exploitation and oppression is leading to a sense of entitlement, a right to participate fully. Above all, nurses are understanding the politics of self-esteem.

REFERENCES

1. Caplow, T. *The Sociology of Work*. Minneapolis: University of Minnesota Press, 1954, p. 236.
2. Oppenheimer, V. K. *The Female Labor Force in the United States*. Westport, Conn.: Greenwood Press, 1976 (original, 1970).
3. Wells, L. E., and Marwell, G. *Self-esteem*. Beverly Hills: Sage Publications, 1976.
4. Rosenberg, M. *Society and the Adolescent Self-image*. Princeton: Princeton University Press, 1965.
5. Janeway, E. On the power of the weak. *Signs*, Autumn 1975, pp. 103–109.
6. Daly, M. *Beyond God the Father: Toward a Philosophy of Women's Liberation*. Boston: Beacon Press, 1973.
7. Oakley, A. *The Sociology of Housework*. New York: Random House, 1974.
8. Vroom, V. *Work and Motivation*. New York: Wiley, 1964.
9. Oakley, A. 1974.
10. Galbraith, J. K. *Economics and the Public Purpose*. Boston: Houghton Mifflin, 1973.
11. Galbraith, J. K. 1973, p. 33.
12. Galbraith, J. K. 1973.

13. Benston, M. The political economy of women's liberation. *Monthly Review*, 24(1):13–27, 1969.
14. Women's Bureau, U. S. Dept. of Labor. *1975 Handbook on Women Workers.* Washington: U. S. Government Printing Office, 1975.
15. Oppenheimer, V. K. 1970.
16. Hedges, J. N. Women at work; women workers and manpower demands in the 1970's. *Monthly Labor Rev.*, June, 1970, p. 20.
17. Baxandall, R., Gordon, L., and Reverby, S. (Eds.). *America's Working Women: A Documentary History—1600 to the Present.* New York: Random House, 1976, p. 41.
18. Lerner, G. The lady and the mill girl: changes in the status of women in the age of Jackson. *American Studies*, Spring, 1969, pp. 6–15.
19. Oppenheimer, V. K. 1976.
20. Garrison, D. The tender technicians: the feminization of public librarianship, 1876–1905. *J. Social History*, Winter, 1972–73, pp. 131–157.
21. Reverby, S. "Health is Women's Work," in R. Baxandall, L. Gordon, and S. Reverby (Eds.), *America's Working Women.* New York: Random House, 1976, p. 347.
22. Oppenheimer, V. K. 1970.
23. Caplow, T. 1954.
24. Garrison, D. 1972–73.
25. Grissum, M. and Spengler, C. *Womenpower and Healthcare.* Boston: Little, Brown and Co., 1976.
26. Bowlby, J. *Attachment and loss: Vol. II, Separation.* New York: Basic Books, 1973.
27. *American Nurses Association. Facts About Nursing.* 1974–1975.
28. Caplow, T. 1954.
29. Hudson, M. "Diary of a Student-Mother-Housewife-Worker," in R. Baxandall, L. Gordon, and S. Reverby (Eds.), *America's Working Women.* New York: Random House, 1976.
30. Wells, L. E., and Marwell, G. 1976.
31. James, W. *Psychology* (the complete text of the classic one volume edition based on *Principles of psychology),* Greenwich, Conn.: Fawcett Publications, 1963 (original 1890), p. 166, p. 167, p. 168, p. 175.
32. Cooley, C. H. *Human nature and the Social Order.* New York: Charles Scribner's Sons, 1902.
33. Skidmore, W. *Theoretical Thinking in Sociology.* Cambridge: Cambridge University Press, 1975.
34. Mead, G. H. *Mead on Social Psychology.* A. Strauss (Ed.). Chicago: University of Chicago Press, 1934, pp. 238, 239.
35. Coopersmith, S. *The Antecedents of Self-esteem.* San Francisco: W. H. Freeman, 1967.
36. Mead, G. H. 1934.
37. Belaief, L. Self-esteem and human equality. *Philosophy and Phenomenological Research*, September, 1975, pp. 25–43.
38. Gould, C. "The Woman Question: Philosophy of Liberation and the Liberation of Philosophy," in C. Gould and M. Wartofsky (Eds.), *Women and Philosophy: Toward a Theory of Liberation.* G. P. Putnam's Sons, 1976, p. 22.
39. Woolf, V. *A Room of One's Own.* New York: Harcourt, Brace and World, 1929, p. 35.
40. Horney, K. "Flight from Woman Hood," in J. B. Miller (Ed.), *Psychoanalysis and Women.* Baltimore: Penguin Books, 1973 (orig. 1926), pp. 8–9.
41. Miller, J. B. *Toward a New Psychology of Women.* Boston: Beacon Press, 1976, p. 44.
42. Silberman, C. *Crises in the Classroom.* New York: Random House, 1970.
43. Adams, B. et al. *Woman, Assert Yourself.* New York: Harper and Row, 1974.
44. Bloom, L. et al. *The New Assertive Woman.* New York: Dell, 1975.
45. Smith, F. A. Personal Communication, October 20, 1977.
46. Boxill, B. Self-respect and protest. *Philosophy and Public Affairs,* Fall, 1976, pp. 58–69.

47. Dumas, R. "Black Women and Power" (Proceedings of the clinical conference), *Health coping in an unhealthy environment: nursing care needs of the black patient.* Mattapan, Mass.: New England Regional Black Nurses Association, 1976.
48. Janeway, E. 1975.
49. Cannings, K., and Lazonick, W. The development of the nursing labor force in the United States: a basic analysis. *Internat. J. Health Services*, 5(2): 186–216, 1975.
50. Women's Bureau 1975.
51. Baxandall, R. et al. 1976.
52. Cannings, K., and Lazonick, W. 1975.

10 Values: PART I

Jeanne Margaret McNally

WHAT IS the meaning of values? How are values formed? What do values do? What is the value of life and the value of health? This article is a combination of years of readings, workshops, discussions, and thoughts. Credit is given to all, known and unknown, who provided input.

WHAT IS A VALUE?

The term "values" is used frequently and in a variety of contexts. There often seems to be some implication that everything should be right and orderly, and problems should be resolved merely because the word "value" was used. Although not a new idea, the recent popularity of values and values education is a healthy sign that should be explored in nursing and nursing education. Values are beliefs that are important to us. A value also may be defined as an enduring belief that a specific mode of conduct or state of existence is personally or socially preferable.

A true value is characterized by the following criteria:

1. It is prized and cherished.
2. It is part of a pattern, *i.e.,* repeated.
3. A value is freely chosen from among alternatives only after due reflection.
4. A value is positively affirmed and acted upon.

Because these are demanding criteria, most people have very few values. People with very few values tend to be conforming, apathetic, inconsistent, and often very ambivalent. People with little internalization of values develop what is called *anomie*—a condition of extreme confusion leading to a psychological withdrawal from life characterized by intolerance for change, alienation from the external world, and loss of touch with self.

People who don't know what they want to do, where they want to go or who have no purpose in their lives suffer from anomie. Values may be expressed in a variety of ways, *e.g.,* that students are worried is an expression of values. The juvenile delinquent shares the values of his gang. The emotionally ill person values retreat from the world of reality more than the pains of everyday life. Everyone values something. Valuelessness, *per se*, is impossible.

Reprinted with permission from *Supervisor Nurse: The Journal for Nursing Leadership and Management*, May 1980.

VALUE SYSTEMS

Values are organized into systems according to a continuum of relative importance. A value system must provide meaning and practical guidance in a less-than-ideal world. We need values that give direction and purpose as we go about the real business of living. If the ideal is too far removed from reality, it will create frustration, guilt, and conflict. A realistic value system allows a certain degree of flexibility. Fundamental values remain relatively stable but they must be refined, extended, and adjusted to keep pace with change.

Values and value systems have specific functions. They serve as standards which lead us to take particular positions on social issues, and predispose us to favor one particular political or religious ideology over another. Moreover, they guide the presentation of ourselves to others and form a foundation for our evaluation of ourselves and others. They are central to the study of comparison processes and are employed to persuade and influence others. Our values help us determine which beliefs, attitudes, values, and actions of others are worth challenging, protecting, and agreeing about or worth trying to influence or change. Values help us rationalize (in the psychoanalytical sense) beliefs, attitudes, and actions that otherwise would be personally and socially unacceptable so that we will feel personally moral and competent—indispensable ingredients for the maintenance and enhancement of our self-esteem.

A value system consists of learned principles and rules which help one choose between alternatives, resolve conflicts, and make decisions. They therefore provide us with a general plan for conflict resolution and decision-making. Moreover, values serve as long-range goals which function to motivate. Values are both conceptual tools and weapons we employ to maintain and enhance our self-esteem. If value and motivation were suddenly removed from human life, there wouldn't be much left.

The content of certain values directly concerns modes of behavior and end states that are adjustment-oriented. These usually are concerned with compliance and getting along with others. People comply or obey for a variety of reasons. They may be afraid of the consequences; they may be seeking rewards; or they may feel an internal obligation. One way to get people to comply is to use threats or rewards or to put people in a highly managed or controlled situation that exerts subtle pressures by making refusal very difficult. It is very hard not to comply when a person feels compliance is expected.

Values fill ego-defensive needs. Feelings and actions that are personally and socially unacceptable readily may be recast by the process of rationalization and reaction formation into more acceptable terms. Social values represent ready-made concepts provided by our culture to ensure that such justification can proceed smoothly and effortlessly.

Values stimulate self-actualization. They involve a search for meaning and a need to understand. They provide for a better organization of perception and belief which provides clarity and consistency to our lives.

Basically there are two kinds of values—a *terminal* value which may be personal and social or an *instrumental* value which may be moral and competent. Terminal values may be self-centered or society-centered, intrapersonal or interpersonal in focus. Examples of these are personal salvation and peace of mind, world peace and brotherhood. An increase of one social value leads to an increase in other social values. A decrease in personal values leads to a decrease in social values. Instrumental moral values refer to behavior mostly with interpersonal focus. Examples of these are honesty and a sense of loving. When violated, moral values arouse a feeling of guilt. Self-actualizing values have a personal rather than an interpersonal focus. All individuals strive for a feeling of increased worth. However, this goal never is reached. Given one success, one bit of self-enhancement, human beings always strive for more. The violation of self-actualizing values leads to a sense of shame about personal inadequacy.

VALUES CLARIFICATION

Values clarification theory is concerned with how values influence behavior. Theorists in the field do not define a value but accept values as representing something important in human existence. Values constitute the internal standards individuals apply to their behavior. Most importantly, values are learned—and they change. We learn values first from our parents, primarily through reward and punishment. We then add to these values by our association with peers, with teachers, and with society at large. We quickly learn the results of behavior which is considered good or bad by particular groups.

Since we see values growing from a person's experiences, we should expect that different experiences would give rise to different values, and that any one person's values would be modified as her experiences accumulate and change. As guides to behavior, values evolve and mature as experiences evolve and mature. Because values are a part of living, they operate in very complex circumstances and usually involve more than simple determinations of right and wrong, good and bad, true and false. The conditions in which values work typically involve conflicting demands—a weighing and balancing—and finally an action that reflects a multitude of factors. Thus values seldom function in a purely abstract form. Complicated judgments are involved and what really is valued is reflected in one's life as it actually is lived.

Assessing attitudes, interests, and values is difficult and imprecise. Some standardized tests identify self-perceived values, but there is not *assurance* that they will be acted upon when one is under stress. Although our values depend heavily upon our reality assumptions, they are distinct from fact or information in that they represent what ought to be rather than what is. Because they involve goals as well as standards, values also are related closely to our assumptions about possibility.

Every individual operates according to a system of values whether or not it is verbalized and consistently worked out. In selecting goals, in choosing modes of behavior, in resolving conflicts, one is influenced at every turn by personal perceptions of what is good and desirable. Although everyone's value system in some degree is unique, an individual's values usually are grounded in the core values of the culture.

OPERATIVE VALUES

A person's values have varying degrees of affective reinforcement and ego involvement. Most people who have studied value systems make a distinction between conceived and operative values. Conceived values are conceptions of the ideal. For the most part they are values which the culture teaches and the ones most likely talked about in discussion of morality or ethics. However, conceived values, even though held with a good deal of intellectual conviction, sometimes have very little practical value. Operative values are the criteria an individual actually uses in making choices. Values are operative when an individual selects one line of thought or action rather than another—insofar as this selection is influenced by generalized codes rather than by impulse.

People's real values, then, must be analyzed not only in terms of what they say but in terms of what they do in situations that involve an element of choice. The intensity of the value often can be measured by how much time and energy the individual is willing to expend in following it, and what satisfaction she is willing to forego in its behalf. Finally, value strength can be gauged subjectively by how much satisfaction or guilt the individual experiences when the person either is true to the value or violates it.

Sometimes a discrepancy between an individual's conceived and operative values indicate an alarming schism between the "idealized" and "real" self. *We tend to become what we do not want to say.*

It is rarely, if ever, possible to bring conceived and operative values into complete harmony. The man who places a high value on nonviolence usually will fight rather than be killed, and the man who values complete honesty may lie to protect a friend. The complexities of human nature and human society make Utopia an ideal against which to measure progress, rather than a goal that realistically can be reached.

To practice responsible self-direction, individuals must find meaning in their world and have criteria by which to choose and evaluate. If a person's values are vague and inconsistent, her behavior will be aimless and confused. Values are necessary for the stability and effectiveness of society, which cannot function unless its members agree on responsible behavior and share basic purposes.

Different social institutions can be conceptualized as specializing in the enhancement of different subsets of values. The effects of Christian institutions are reflected mainly as variations of salvation and forgiveness. The effects of political institutions are reflected mainly as variations in equality and freedom. Thus, a person's value system may be an end result, at least in part, of all the institutional forces or influences that have acted upon her.

The affluent and educated typically regard values reflecting safety and security needs as relatively unimportant, not so much because they are not valued, but because they are taken for granted. Taking such values for granted frees them to place greater emphasis on higher order values, for instance, love, competence and self-actualization.

In every society people strive for whatever they judge to be good and right. Thus motives and values are inseparable. Essentially, a value is a learned belief so thoroughly internalized that it colors the actions and thoughts of the individual and produces a strong emotional and intellectual response when anything runs counter to it.

LEARNING VALUES

Values are learned. Adults begin teaching values explicitly the day a child is born and reinforce them through a system of reward and punishment. In addition to the explicit values they learn, children also internalize many others that may or may not coincide with what adults are teaching them. In the teaching of values, actions speak louder than words— and prove more effective than all the lectures. Children first learn values from important adults, especially parents and later from school personnel and peers. Association with people of different values leads children to modify their values. The process of value modification or value reinforcement is a life-long process. An individual's values are not wholly dependent on others. Each child interprets the values expressed in the activities and speech of others. Some he may internalize, some ignore. Individuals internalize values as they have meaning for them, as they perceive them, and as they have the capacity to understand them. The result of this internalization is unique to the individual and seldom, if ever, precisely what adults think they are teaching.

Values find one form of expression in the judgments people make about themselves and others. Any statement incorporating the idea that something is good or bad is a value judgment. As they grow older, people tend to judge themselves in terms of relaxed values while they will judge others in terms of ideal values. Adolescents judge themselves harshly in terms of their ideal values . . . this makes adolescence extremely difficult.

Value judgments, an inevitable part of living, can be expressed in ways other than words. Opinions, advice, thinking, actions, are all replete with value judgments. A value is both a judgment and an emotional response, *e.g.,* anger or fear.

Values differ radically from society to society and among groups in society. The general values of a society are those to which the majority of the society at least pay lip service and will defend in time of crisis. For Americans, the values associated with democracy are general values. Freedom and equality with responsible citizenship are values about which most Americans will agree, although many do not give evidence of their agreement in their actions.

TESTING VALUES

The mark of a mature adult is the ability to test values and freely to accept or to reject them. However, we cannot constantly question our values or all the values of our culture. To do so jeopardizes our security and emotional health. Much of our values systems we must accept without testing. Among these values are, of course, biological, economic, esthetic, moral, and religious values.

Even the process of physical maturation requires some recentering of values. As one grows older, for example, the values of physical excellence and youthfulness must be reweighed against the values of creativity, self-understanding, and other satisfactions which more properly belong to maturity. The tendency in our culture to worship the external attributes of youth makes this reorientation of values very difficult for many people.

Marriage and family problems also necessitate recentering the value system, as do problems connected with one's life work. The college student deciding on a career, the middle-aged woman who realizes belatedly that she hates her good job and would find much greater satisfaction in another line of work, the older woman who is forced to retire but wants to continue—all these individuals face problems peculiar to their age and situation which require realistic and clearly defined values for their solution. Spiritual values, too, are subject to continual redefinition in extension. As the individual's knowledge and experience broaden, a realistic value system must remain flexible enough to grow.

Change becomes increasingly difficult with age. We do not like to admit that as we grow older our ability to absorb new ideas diminishes. As we grow older we have to make a constant effort to remain open to the new. Obviously, this does not mean to embrace the new just because it is new, for this tendency, too, may be a poorly disguised form of conformism. If we cannot remain open to the new, how will we encounter new things? How will we endure this world of rapid flux and of new things?

BIBLIOGRAPHY

Belok, Michael. *Approaches to Values in Education.* Dubuque: William C. Brown Company, 1966.

Englehardt, H. Tristram, and Daniel Callahan. *Knowledge Value and Belief.* The Hastings Center, Institute of Society, Ethics and the Life Sciences, 1977.

National Academy of Science. *Experiments and Research with Humans: Values in Conflict.* Academy Forum, 3rd of a series, Washington, D.C., 1975.

Raths, Louis E., Merrill Harmin, and Sidney B. Simon. *Values and Teaching.* Columbus, Ohio: Charles E. Merrill Publishing Company, 1966.

Ringness, Thomas. *The Affective Domain in Education.* Boston: Little, Brown and Company, 1975.

Simon, Sidney B., et al. *An Introduction to Values Clarification.* New York: J. C. Penney Company, 1972.

Simon, Sidney B., and Howard Kirschenbaum. *Readings in Value Clarification.* Minneapolis: Winston Press, Inc., 1973.

Simon, Sidney B., et al., *Values Clarification: A Handbook of Practical Strategies for Teachers and Students.* New York: Hart Publishing Company, Inc., 1972.

Sprinthall, Richard D., and Norman A. Sprinthall. *Educational Psychology: A Development Approach.* Reading, Massachusetts: Addison-Wesley Publishing Company, 1974.

11 Values: PART II

Jeanne Margaret McNally

TODAY'S RATE of change is too rapid to allow time for testing values by results. Technological changes create new situations which may strengthen and validate values, require adaptation of values, or make some values obsolete. Thus, there is a great need for properly informed health education and continuing education related to the developing technologies and their application to society. Because health professionals have a responsibility to provide leadership in these areas, we need active educational programs to enable us to determine a rational course of action. For nurses and other health professionals, these decisions may involve population control, genetic intervention, behavior modification, human experimentation, abortion, control or limitation of research, the right to live, and the right to die.

Developing and understanding our own value system provides us with a foundation for leadership, and prevents us from drifting aimlessly. Health planners, policy makers, and practitioners often prefer to deny their role in value of life decisions. Many times we ask "How much is a life worth?" or "What is the worth of a life?" If asked such a question, most people in the U.S. would answer that life is so valuable that its worth cannot be determined. In other words, life is priceless. However, Victor R. Fuchs asked the question differently: "Who Shall Live?" The value of life can be viewed from quite different perspectives. For example, what is the value of life in war? abortion? What is the value of the life of a drowning child? What is the value attached to the life of the terminally ill? Immediately, values seem relative.

When faced with such questions, our values are reality tested. Our personal value systems will direct our course of action. Therefore, the ability to distinguish among different types of values and value claims is very important. There are three kinds of value claims to which nurses are frequently exposed.

1. *Personal value claims* are reflected in such statements as: "I like . . . ," "I prefer . . . ," "It is important to me that . . . ."
2. *Market value claims* are manifest in the statements a person makes when trying to convey what a certain object is worth in the marketplace.
3. *Real value claims* assert that a certain thing is better (*i.e.,* of greater worth or merit) than other conceivable and available alternatives according to particular criteria, *i.e.,* money, energy, or time. People making such a claim are not referring to the common or even expert opinion of what a particular thing is worth—nor are they merely expressing a personal opinion. They are claiming that a certain idea is better than another idea because, all things considered, it outweighs its alternatives in terms of explicit and important criteria. Moral value claims represent a particular kind of real value claim. [1]

Reprinted with permission from *Supervisor Nurse: The Journal for Nursing Leadership and Management*, June 1980.

The literature in economics and health offer three major methods for placing value on life: foregone earnings, willingness to pay, and social valuations. These take on an added dimension when resource allocations are at stake.

Foregone Earnings—The critical assumption is that an individual's wages reflect the economic value of his work effort—his so-called "marginal value." This depends both on how much he produces and on the value of his work as determined by the consumers of the economy. Should society value young skilled workers more than old unskilled ones—and allocate health care resources accordingly? Should we deduct someone's consumption from his income to achieve a net figure for his contribution?

Willingness to Pay—This method places value on life according to what individuals will pay to preserve it. "Consumer valuations" look at the choices people make in the economy generally with regard to assuming risks to their own lives. How much are people willing to pay to avoid life or health changes and the probability of death? Those who use the willingness to pay method tend to conclude that those with higher incomes and more wealth have more valuable lives.

Social Valuations—This method relies on the value society has placed on life in other situations, *e.g.,* court settlements and compensation claims. In this case, life is worth what some judge, jury, or agency says it is. One also could take the cost of saving or rescuing a life as implicit social valuation.

If one relies on social and political processes to determine the value of life, it is quite possible that public policy will reflect the belief that those with more social, political, and economic power are the most valuable. To the extent that individuals attempt to use values, the economic models used to determine the value of life can have power to influence behavior. These models tell us how market prices are derived, but they do not necessarily reflect basic values. Although the models can tell us the consequences of various alternatives, no model can make choices for us. Given information about the relationships between technological means and ends, about human resources, and about the time and money required, sound economics can show us how to maximize values.

We always will be faced with our value system.

REFERENCES

1. Belock, Michael, et al. *Approaches to Values in Education.* Dubuque: W.C. Brown Company, 1966.
2. Engelhardt, H. T., and Daniel Callahan (eds.), *Knowledge, Value, and Belief.* Vol. II. "The Foundations of Ethics and Its Relationship to Science." New York: The Hastings Center, Institute of Society, Ethics, and the Life Sciences, 1977.
3. Fuchs, Victor R. *Who Shall Live?* New York: Basic Books, Inc., 1974.

Questions to Part II

1. What leadership theories do you see practiced/used most often?
2. Think about something you would like your peer group to do together. Present your proposal three times, each time using a different leadership style. What was the effect of each style on the group?
3. In what ways do you use your leadership behaviors to achieve a health care goal? Compare and contrast the behaviors you have identified with those cited by Yura, Ozimek, and Walsh.
4. In what situations are you most likely to be a follower?
5. In your opinion, why are nurses so hesitant to be perceived as leaders?
6. How many nationally known nurse leaders do you recognize by name? If you find that you don't know too many, what may be contributing to this? Is there a relationship between the nursing leaders that you recognized and their visibility in the media?
7. If Florence Nightingale were alive today, would she be able to work with Gloria Steinem or Bella Abzug in advancing the status of professional nursing? State your reasons.
8. What does this statement, "I am only a nurse," say to you?
9. With what other profession or occupation do you feel nursing has comparable worth? State your reasons.
10. You have been asked to stand before your peer group and state what you value about your profession. What would you say?
11. "Do as I say, not as I do." Discuss this statement in relation to your professional values.

III Contemporary Leadership Behaviors

The vitality of a profession—its life force—stems from ideas; ideas that capture the thought and imagination of its members, who, as its custodians, live and fight for them until they are ideas no longer—they are reality. All nurses are custodians of their profession, a profession whose life force will weaken and die if there are no ideas to revive it and no fervent custodians to restore its vigor and renew its power.

As custodians of our profession, we are responsible for its vitality and for using behaviors that give it life and set its course in the direction it must go if its vitality is to reach out and influence others. Vitality gives life to assertiveness, expressing our rights and beliefs directly without violating the rights and beliefs of others. Vitality is the energizing force of advocacy as we use it to protect the rights of patients. Vitality glows in the supportive relationships of mentors that are shared among co-workers interested in mutual growth and learning. Each time we recognize and use our inherent self-worth, we activate the vitality that power gives as we influence patients in realizing their health care goals. Vitality, however, is only a partially realized force; it waits to be mobilized in the political arena where the greater issues of health care delivery are determined and where we have yet to exert influence that will prevail. To succeed, we must gather up and harness our collective vitality and drive its force toward collective action. No longer a dormant force, that vitality will be the spark in facilitating needed changes in health care and in resolving the conflicts that are bound to occur in the face of that change. Then, nursing will be a profession to be reckoned with. We are the navigators of our profession's future, and that future will depend on the course we chart to ensure that our ideas become realities.

The leadership behaviors selected for Part III are "ideas that won't keep." Something must be done about them or the new cultural image we are trying to shape and the leadership attributes we are learning to value and use will be left to wither, where-upon the vitality of our profession will be sapped and become extinguished.

Section 1
Assertiveness

12 The Six "A's" of Assertiveness

Marilyn M. Rawnsley

WE ARE a culture of fads. With predictable frequency the media heralds the latest craze to sweep the nation. The fate of such fads is also predictable; usually they enjoy a brief life in the spotlight then fade into memory as they are rapidly replaced by the next craze. Occasionally there appears a hardier species of fashion—possibly a mutant—that demonstrates substance and resiliency and is incorporated as part of the norm. Current examples of trendiness include disco dancing and running-for-health. Will either or both survive? It's too soon to be sure. What we can be sure of is that by next year there will be another fad.

Perhaps endless innovations are a tribute to American ingenuity; perhaps it is entrepreneurism run amok trying to build a better mousetrap; perhaps it testifies to a group preoccupation with excitement and a tendency to equate stability with boredom. Or maybe we are in endless pursuit of that elusive happiness that we thought was the American dream. But whatever their genesis, the fads continue to be spawned.

Education is not immune to fashion; consider the open classroom, team teaching, and modern math. At the same time that it is responsible for transmitting cultural values, education itself is influenced by the forces of fashion resulting in a peculiar dilemma. Which trends should be taught? And by teaching them do we legitimize their existence?

Assertiveness training is a widespread popular phenomenon that displays some trendy characteristics. The question to be addressed by this paper is whether or not this fad has substance. That is, can a conceptual basis of assertiveness be identified so that hypotheses for research and principles for practice can be derived? Without conceptual clarity of the phenomena of assertiveness—and its sequela, assertiveness training—two major risks are inherent: (1) professional resources may be invested into promoting a self-limited fad, and (2) a potentially valuable behavioral concept may be obscured by the jargon and showmanship of "pop" psychology.

Since much of the assertiveness movement is aimed toward women, nursing provides a target population, and it is a relevant topic for our study. As a humanistic practice discipline, nursing is concerned with developing and enhancing the communication and human relations skills of its practitioners; as an academic discipline, nursing is charged with systematic inquiry into phenomena that affect its practitioners and their practice. Analysis of its conceptual foundations is one phase of systematic inquiry into assertiveness.

Are the differences between the descriptors, "assertive and aggressive," real or arbitrary? One source defines assertive as "confident, positive and dogmatic" [1], and lists the second definition of aggressive as "disposed to vigorous activity; assertive" [1]. A later reference

Reprinted with permission of Charles B. Slack, Inc., from the *Journal of Continuing Education in Nursing*, Volume 11, Number 1, November 1980.

equates assertive and aggressive as synonyms [2]. Therefore, the terms are related seman-
tically.

Moreover, it is generally known that Freud postulated the aggressive drive, along with the
libidinal drive, as the major wellsprings of psychic energy. In some instances, the aggressive
drives narrowly interpreted pejoratively as leading to hostile attack. But just as sexual energy
can be the source of creative thought and artistic passion, so can aggressive energy be the
source of constructive action and competitive achievement.

*The aggressive part of human nature is not only a safeguard against predatory attack. It is
also the basis of intellectual achievement, of the attainment of independence and even that
of proper pride which enables a man to hold his head high amongst his fellows. [3]*

It can be argued then, that both "assertive" and "aggressive" are adjectives that describe
direct action-oriented behavioral responses. However, it is the position of this paper that
although both of these direct action patterns are elicited under similar conditions, they
manifest characteristics that suggest a difference in behavioral content and process rather
than merely a difference in degree of intensity of response. A paradigm of the conceptual
relationships between those behavioral response patterns has been designed to illustrate
these differences and is shown in Figure 12-1.

One assumption underlying this paradigm is that given a precipitating event perceived as
disruptive to one's integrity or wholeness, a response pattern characteristic of the individual
is elicited. A second assumption is that anger is the mobilizing force that directs the individual response to such threatening situations. The final assumption is that assertiveness is
constructive aggression.

Explanation of the paradigm is warranted. This behavioral schematic outlines the responses, intervening variables, behavioral pathways, and possible outcomes of a real or
perceived conflict with authority. Authority is broadly interpreted to include not only legitimate power but also any person, organization, or referent group to whom an individual
consciously or unconsciously ascribes superior or powerful status.

When a conflict between an individual and such an authority arises (and the conflict itself
may be real or perceived) then anxiety is evoked. Under these conditions, anxiety triggers
anger that is the powerful systemic activator that mobilizes an initial protective response of
"fight" or "flight." Individual and environmental variables may intervene at varying points in
this response pathway and the direction towards fight or flight may be a function of the
effects of one or more of these variables.

Fight or flight responses indicate an attempt to resolve the conflict either by acting directly
on the perceived problem (fight) or by moving away from the difficulty (flight).

Each one of the potential pathways under the flight response represents an attempt to
reduce distress by avoiding direct action. The choice between passivity or passive-
aggressiveness may be a consequence of its interaction of ego-defense structure, attitude
beliefs, and previous reinforcement experience.

Clarifying differences between the behavioral options outlined under the fight response is
crucial to a conceptual understanding of assertiveness. Given that the protective response
movement is in the direction of acting upon the perceived problem, then why would an
individual choose to act aggressively rather than assertively? Again, ego-defense structure,
attitudes and belief, and previous experience are important, as are the environmental variables. We need research that employs an experimental design to study this question.

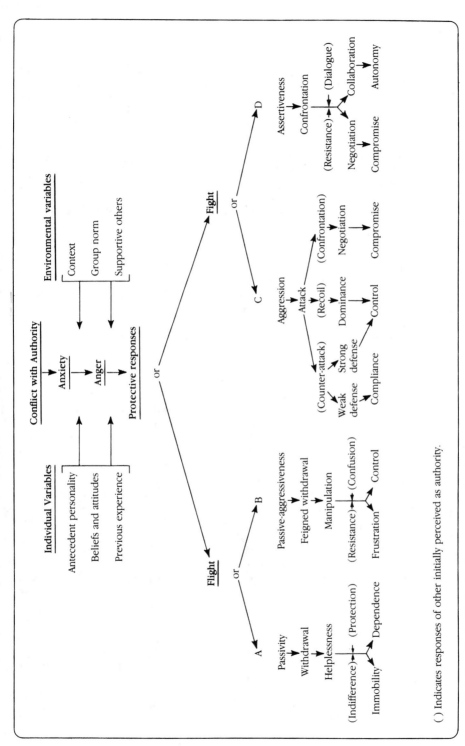

Figure 12-1. Paradigm of behavioral responses and pathways.

( ) Indicates responses of other initially perceived as authority.

119

But while we wait for this research there are speculations that can be made regarding the missing link in this conceptual chain and that missing link may be competence. On a professional level one cannot be assertive without the knowledge base and sound judgment that are essential to professional accountability. This is professional competence. Without competence one cannot be assertive; one can only withdraw, manipulate, or attack!

Therefore, if competence is essential to that constructive aggression called assertiveness, then nursing cannot rely on assertiveness training alone to help nurses achieve the professional autonomy they seek. Assertiveness training is based on principles of behavior modification and operates by shaping behavior through reinforcement of desired responses. But these behavior shaping techniques are situation specific in that they assume certain conditions or contexts. Generalization of effects is unlikely to occur if several variables are changed. Assertiveness training intervenes at the level of overt behavioral response and assumes that a change in behavior will modify antecedent variables such as personality structure and attitudes.

Can practicing new communications and human relations skills effect a lasting change in attitudes and beliefs, modify antecedent personality factors, and continue to operate despite opposing group norms in the absence of supportive others? That is the second question for empirical study. Meanwhile, the issue of competency as a prerequisite for assertiveness must be considered. It is quite likely that assertiveness training workshops for nurses that do not take into account the variable of competency will result in the aggressive behaviors outlined in the paradigm.

Several decades ago Eugene Bleuler postulated the four "A's" of schizophrenia—Autism, Ambivalence, Association, and Affect—in a pioneering attempt to describe that phenomenon [4]. In this paper five "A's" have been cited—Authority, Anxiety, Anger, constructive Aggression, and Accountability—as factors that relate to assertiveness and can influence whether or not the desired outcome—the sixth "A," Autonomy, will be achieved. By illustrating these concepts in a paradigm, it is hoped that clinicians may have access to another way of perceiving the responses of their clients, their colleagues, and themselves. It is further hoped that this paradigm can be helpful to nursing educators and administrators who must set priorities in allocating precious resources for continuing education in nursing. When use of educational resources are an issue, it could be argued that programs that address professional competence take precedence over assertiveness training workshops. Furthermore, it is implied that when assertiveness training is feasible, staff who demonstrate professional accountability may be the most appropriate participants.

Finally, it is hoped that this paradigm may stimulate research into the relationships it describes. Findings from empirical investigation of hypotheses derived from the paradigm may indicate to nursing effective ways to invest—not in a new fad, but in a new freedom.

REFERENCES

1. *Standard College Dictionary*. New York, Harcourt, Brace and World, Inc., 1963, pp 27, 87.
2. *Webster's Third New International Dictionary* (unabridged). Springfield, Massachusetts, G & C Merriam Co, Pub, 1968, pp 41, 131.
3. Storr A: *Human Aggression*, New York, Atheneum Pub, 1968, p iii.
4. Freedman A, Kaplan H, Sadock B: *Modern Synopsis of the Comprehensive Textbook of Psychiatry*. Baltimore, The Williams and Wilkins Co, 1972.

BIBLIOGRAPHY

Bach GR, Goldberg H: *Creative Aggression—The Art of Assertive Living.* New York, Avon Books, 1974.

Bloom LZ, Coburn K, Pearlman J: *The New Assertive Woman.* New York, Delacorte Press, 1975.

Curry JL: Assertiveness training for supervising nursing. *Supervisor Nurse* 9(9): 43–50, September 1978.

Fensterheim H, Baer J: *Don't Say Yes When You Want to Say No.* New York, Dell Pub Co, 1975.

Osborn S, Harris G: *Assertive Training for Women.* Springfield, Illinois, Charles C Thomas, 1975.

Phelps S, Austin N: *The Assertive Woman.* San Luis Obispo, California, Impact Pub, 1975.

Smith MJ: *When I Say No, I Feel Guilty.* New York, Bantam Books, 1975.

Taubman B: *How to Become an Assertive Woman.* New York, Pocket Books, 1976.

13 Assertiveness for Nursing

Stephanie Farley Pardue

ARE YOU UNWILLING to be an assertive nurse? The contemporary health care professional is expected to possess knowledge and skills far different from those required a decade ago. Today a nurse not only must demonstrate high level cognition in making complex health care decisions but also must present a "new image" to health care colleagues and consumers. This image should be that of an assertive, independent person.

Assertiveness is a behavior that can be learned. It is neither genetic nor the exclusive possession of extroverts. Assertiveness has been defined as "that type of interpersonal behavior which enables an individual to act in his own best interest, to stand up for himself without anxiety, and to exercise his rights without denying the rights of others" [1]. Analysis of this definition reveals no conflict with the role of a health care professional; yet, it does describe behavior that many nurses find difficult. Acting in one's own best interest, standing up for oneself without anxiety, and exercising one's own rights are contrary to traditional ideas that nurses have accepted about the nurturing, other-centered, self-denying characteristics of nursing. For many, assertiveness seems too self-centered or aggressive to accept.

After teaching an elective course in assertiveness for nursing students and conducting numerous assertiveness workshops, I noticed that common myths and misconceptions about personal and professional assertiveness follow characteristic patterns.

ASSERTIVENESS IS THE SAME THING AS AGGRESSIVENESS

This misconception seems to permeate almost all the groups who have participated in my assertiveness courses and workshops: nursing students, faculty members, administrators, and clinicians. In reality, assertive behavior maintains a balance between aggressive and passive behavior. It is the direct, honest, and appropriate expression of one's thoughts, feelings, opinions, and beliefs without undue anxiety and without infringing on the rights of others. Assertiveness includes making eye contact with others, smiling, initiating conversations, being able to say "no" in a matter-of-fact manner without feeling guilty, making requests of people, and asking for changes in behavior.

Aggressiveness is behavior that tends to dominate, humiliate, deprecate, or embarrass others for the purpose of winning—exerting power in an interpersonal situation. The aggressive person is usually insensitive to the needs and communications of others and is oriented primarily toward demonstrating one's own excellence [3]. Aggressiveness also might be expressed in passive-aggressive behavior. A nurse can exhibit aggressive tenden-

Reprinted with permission by *Supervisor Nurse: The Journal for Nursing Leadership and Management,* February 1980.

cies (in a passive way) by such means as waiting a prolonged time before answering the call light when she is irritated with a patient.

In addition to assertive and aggressive behavior, another behavior (non-assertive) is characterized by the inability to say "no" to requests, an unwillingness to express one's opinions or needs; nervousness and anxiety in conflict situations accompanied by a desire to avoid or suppress conflict at all costs; and timid nonverbal behavior [4].

The distinction among assertiveness, aggressiveness, and passivity (nonassertiveness) can be conceptualized more accurately as a behavioral continuum with an individual's responses fluctuating along the scale. For example, a nurse who demonstrates assertive behavior with respected colleagues may be nonassertive or passive with a saturnine physician. The tendency to alternate between assertive and other types of behavior is influenced by a variety of factors: the nurses's self-esteem; the perceived power distribution in the relationship; situational "triggers" such as fatigue or uncomfortable room temperature; and previous behavior patterns. Although assertiveness can be learned, it often is true that nurses tend to continue old patterns of behavior—even if they are dysfunctional. New behavior patterns are risky and anxiety-producing.

ASSERTIVENESS IS UNFEMININE

The myth obviously reflects the tenacity of inculcated socialization norms even though contemporary media and society present a changing role and image for men and women. The women's liberation movement has continued to alienate persons who perceive and describe advocates in pejorative terms such as hostile, macho, and power-hungry. Many female nurses express concern about maintaining their femininity while becoming assertive. Male nurses confuse their natural atavistic aggressiveness with assertiveness. Each nurse must clarify both a social and a personal definition of femininity and masculinity.

It is interesting to note that it is men who have defined femininity and normal female behavior in our society. Until recent years most psychiatrists, psychologists, and writers were male [5]. They defined women in terms of dependent relationships with men. A woman is expected to attract men; to see her primary role in life as a companion for a man and mother of his children. To be a woman is to be sensitive and nurturing, overly emotional, submissive, easily influenced, and fundamentally dullwitted [6–9]. Masculinity is defined as aggressive, independent, dominant, competitive, logical, not easily influenced, ambitious, and powerful. A man's major goal in life is to achieve success in a career [10, 11]. Traditionally women also have been expected to allow others to set goals for them rather than to initiate their own; to think of others before themselves; to avoid positive statements about themselves; and to be willing to help others without expecting financial reimbursement [12].

These same norms also carried over into nursing education. Often students are socialized into perceiving themselves as inferior to physicians. They are expected to give unquestioning care to patients or clients regardless of working conditions; to be independent in nursing knowledge and practice, but deferential to authority figures; to suppress true feelings in talking with patients or clients and co-workers; and to be oriented to procedure books and bureaucratic rule. In their attempts to be assertive, nurses must overcome distorting effects of sex role expectations and educational processes.

Assertiveness transcends the rigidity of archaic sex role constraints. Behavioral traits such as communicating openly and honestly, initiating needed changes, and saying no without feeling guilty are important for females as well as males. Assertiveness does not mean being pushy, obnoxious, insensitive, or devious. Removing the shackles of traditionally submissive, dishonest female communication is critical.

BECOMING ASSERTIVE WILL MAKE YOU SELF-CENTERED

Many nurses readily endorse the idea of assertiveness but express concern that they will become egotistic. Contrary to this expectation, the assertive person usually is much more cognizant of others' needs than is an aggressive or passive individual. If people previously have been unaware of their own needs, thoughts, and feelings, then it is likely that they will experience a transitional period of self-centeredness. This concentrated, self-assessment phase is a necessary step in becoming assertive. The nurse needs to determine who she perceives as more or less important than herself; her personal and professional "rights"; her own rationally defined "do's and don'ts"; and what she likes and dislikes about herself.

After completing this phase, the individual is ready to identify the behavioral changes necessary for mature human behavior. Many nurses have difficulty being assertive because they feel they are less important than physicians, or less important than clinical nurse specialists, or less important than the nurse with 10 years' experience. Self-deprecating comparative evaluations can paralyze the nurse with self-doubt. Realistically assessing one's own strengths and limitations is a necessary part of becoming assertive.

A review of one's personal and professional rights also may seem to be a self-centered reverie. In reality, it is an important re-orienting process. Herman states that the *Nurses' Bill of Rights* includes the right to be respected and listened to; to have and to state thoughts, feelings, and opinions; to question or to challenge; to understand job expectations and have them in writing; to say "no" without feeling guilty; to be an equal member of the health team; to ask for changes in the system; to have a reasonable work load; to make a mistake; to make decisions regarding health and nursing care; to initiate health teaching; to be a patient advocate or to teach patients to speak for themselves; and lastly, to have the right to change one's mind [13]. This *Nurses' Bill of Rights* incarnates the assertive nurse.

BECOMING ASSERTIVE MEANS THAT YOU WILL ALIENATE PEOPLE

It is a well-documented psychological principle that change in one part of a behavioral system will create stress in other parts of the system. If a nurse is caught in a "compassion trap," then it is likely that initial disequilibrium will occur when she exhibits her new assertive behavior. Adams describes a "compassion trap" as a problem exclusive to women who feel that they exist to serve others, believing that they must provide tenderness and compassion to all at all times [14]. The "compassion trap" dictates that a woman express herself only through meeting the needs of others: she must be compassionate to the exclusion of personal feelings. She often uses ego-distorting phrases such as "I feel so sorry for him that I must . . ." "They need me so much that I just can't . . ." "I'm the only one who really cares so I must . . . ." In reality, friends, loved ones, and co-workers have equal responsibilities in maintaining relationships and their own well-being.

Being caught in the "compassion trap" automatically obviates assertive behaviors. If an individual has formed a pattern of working or doing favors to avoid upsetting another person, tension will result when this individual starts asserting herself by assessing the rationality and fairness of requests. During this phase, the overly compassionate person might evidence resentment or a martyr-type self-image. Always suppressing one's own needs and desires eventually will lead to some type of uncontrolled expression. The individual could "blow up" in aggressive hostility or withdraw into a pathological state of depression. On the other hand being assertive permits honest exchange of thoughts and feelings and realistic give and take within relationships.

ONLY NURSING LEADERS NEED TO BE ASSERTIVE

This myth is often the most difficult to dispel. The importance of personal and professional assertiveness for *every* nurse cannot be overemphasized. The problems of high turnover rates and job dissatisfaction among nurses have been well documented. Longest states that attainment of goals through effective performance is an important factor in job satisfaction [15]. Herzberg, Mausner, and Snyderman indicate that the most potent job satisfiers are work characteristics that foster self-actualization and self-realization [16]. Hurka reports that job satisfaction of registered nurses is directly related to interpersonal relationships [17]. Other studies conclude that job satisfaction is enhanced in work environments which provide the opportunity for nurses to give high quality health care and to feel that their suggestions are heard and are considered important.

An assertive nurse is an individual who seeks opportunities to make needed changes in health care delivery; expresses her thoughts, feelings, and opinions about her work environment; and continually assesses the realities of job demands. She avoids falling into the "compassion trap" or martyr role and may experience greater job satisfaction because of her openness and honesty in interpersonal relations.

That patients/clients should have a much more active role in their health care maintenance and rehabilitation is recognized. The nonassertive nurse is likely to resent assertive patients/clients. However, the assertive nurse can serve as a role-model for health care consumers. In addition, a higher quality nursing care can be implemented only by assertive nurses.

CONCLUSIONS

Fostering assertiveness requires three steps: first, to help nurses to realize the importance of being assertive; second, to provide opportunities for nurses to learn assertive behavior techniques; and third, to support those striving toward assertiveness. The commitment to personal and professional assertiveness depends on the willingness of nurses to establish new behavior patterns and to perform honest self-assessments. Opportunities to learn assertive behavior techniques are available through reading materials, attendance at workshops or courses, and observation of assertive role models.

Providing support and encouraging others to maintain assertiveness are probably the greatest challenge experienced when establishing new behavior patterns. The negative feedback received when challenging traditional sex role and professional role prescriptions are continuous obstacles to assertive behavior. Ambivalent feelings also are experienced when establishing new behavior patterns. Without positive feedback from a variety of sources in the health care delivery system, the nurse will be tempted to regress to nonassertive or aggressive behavior patterns. It's an individual choice!

REFERENCES

1. Alberti, R. E., and M. L. Emmons. *Your Perfect Right: A Guide to Assertive Behavior.* Second Edition, Impact Publishers, San Luis Obispo, California, 1974.
2. Herman, Sonya J. *Becoming Assertive, A Guide for Nurses.* D. Van Nostrand Company, New York, 1978, pp. 17–20.
3. Osborn, Susan M., and Gloria G. Harris. *Assertive Training for Women.* Charles C Thomas, Publisher, Springfield, Illinois, 1975, pp. 25–30.
4. *Op. cit.,* Herman, p. 19.
5. Grissum, Marlene, and Carol Spengler, *Womanpower and Health Care.* Little, Brown, and Company, Boston, 1976, pp. 1–14.
6. Janeway, Elizabeth. *Man's World, Woman's Place: A Study in Social Mythology.* Dell Publishing, New York, 1971, p. 7.
7. Weisstein, Naomi. "Psychology Constructs the Female," *Woman in Sexist Society: Studies in Power and Powerlessness,* Gornick, Vivian, and Barbara Mason, editors. New York: Basic Books, Inc., 1971, p. 207.
8. Broverman, Inge K. "Sex Role Stereotypes and Clinical Judgments of Mental Health," *Assertive Training for Women,* Osborn, Susan M. and Gloria G. Harris, Springfield, Illinois: Charles C Thomas, Publisher, 1975, p. 9.
9. Wheelock, Alan. "The Tarnished Image," *Nursing Outlook,* 24 (8): 1976, pp. 509–510.
10. *Op. cit.,* Grissum and Spengler, pp. 1–14.
11. *Op. cit.,* Broverman, p. 9.
12. *Op. cit.,* Herman, p. 123.
13. Ibid., p. 27.
14. Adams, Margaret. "The Compassion Trap," *Women in Sexist Society: Studies in Power and Powerlessness,* Gornick, Vivian, and Barbara Mason, eds. New York: Basic Books, Inc., 1971.
15. Longest, Beaufort B. "Job Satisfaction for Registered Nurses in the Hospital Setting," *Journal of Nursing Administration,* (4) (Jan-June) 1974, pp. 46–52.
16. Herzberg, F. I., B. Mausner, and F. Snyderman, *The Motivation to Work.* New York: John Wiley and Sons, 1959.
17. Hurka, S. J. "Career Orientation of Registered Nurses Working in Hospitals," *Hospital Administration,* (26) 1972, pp. 17–19.

14 Am I My Brother's Keeper?

Gertrud B. Ujhely

"AM I my brother's keeper?" Cain asks of God in the biblical account of Cain and Abel. Implicit in this question is the theme of responsibility toward one's fellow man; in particular, responsibility toward the one who is weaker and demands protection, but at the same time arouses resentment and murderous rage in the stronger one. The theme has been a recurring moral question for mankind since the beginning of time—an archetypal theme, as Jung would call it. It is also a theme that is close to the hearts of health professionals, especially nurses.

To refresh your memory, as the account is written in the Old Testament, Cain and Abel were the first two children born of Adam and Eve after their banishment from paradise. When Cain and Abel each presented an offering to God, He accepted Abel's offering (that of the younger brother), but not the offering of Cain. Cain was hurt and angry, but God reprimanded him, saying, "Why are you angry and downcast? If you are well disposed, ought you not lift up your head? But if you are ill disposed, is not sin at the door like a crouching beast hungering for you which you must master?"

However, Cain did not listen to God. Instead, when he and Abel were in the open country, the Bible tells us that Cain "set upon his brother and killed him." When God asked Cain where his brother was, he answered: "I do not know. Am I my brother's keeper?" But God knew and cursed him: "Listen to the sound of your brother's blood, crying out to me from the ground. Now be accursed and driven from the ground that has opened its mouth to receive your brother's blood at your hands. When you till the ground it shall no longer yield you any of its produce. You shall be a fugitive and wanderer over the earth." Then Cain said to God: "My punishment is greater than I can bear . . . Why, whoever comes across me will kill me." And so God put a mark on Cain to prevent those who might "come across him" from striking him down.

Ginzberg [1956], in his study of legends surrounding biblical themes, enlarged on this cryptic episode in the Bible. According to Ginzberg, Cain was not really Adam's son, but the son of the serpent, who was Satan in disguise. Further, Cain did not make an actual sacrifice to God, but offered Him the leftovers of what he had taken for himself. This displeased God, and God chastised him. But Cain did not acknowledge his guilt, and instead insisted that he was treated unfairly by God. Also, Cain apparently coveted Abel's girl friend and, therefore, wanted to get rid of him. The brothers also fought over territorial rights. At one point when Abel had the upper hand, Cain asked for mercy, and Abel released him. When released, Cain killed his brother by hurling a large stone at him.

From *Perspectives of Psychiatric Care*, Volume 17, Number 5, 1979, pp. 204–210. Reprinted with permission from Nursing Publications, Inc., 194-B Kinderkamack, Park Ridge, New Jersey 07656.

Because he was the first murderer, Cain did not understand the concept of killing another, yet afterwards he tried to hide from his parents. But he had no way of hiding from God. According to legend, when confronted by God, Cain denied his guilt; he believed his action was God's responsibility since God had not accepted his offering. Since Cain had never seen a man killed, how could he know that the stones he threw at his brother would take his life? Besides, since Cain was the son of the satanic snake, he believed the responsibility for his evil nature lay with his "father," and not himself.

As we look at this sequence of events, we can distinguish three parts. In the first, Cain harbors negative emotions which he disowns, yet eventually acts out, because he is identified with them. He neither expresses his emotions, nor does he try to understand them. Instead, he broods until the emotions lead him to commit fratricide. Second, he does not assume responsibility for his act of murder. Yet, he is terrified of the consequences, for he is aware that he is vulnerable to retaliation by others. Third, God protects Cain from vengeful retaliation by placing the divine mark of protection on his forehead. He becomes a marked man in a paradoxical sense: he is marked as a sinner, yet the mark represents one of the letters of the holy name of God.

So much for the archetypal story. How does it relate to the question, "Am I my brother's keeper?" and what relevance does it have to nursing? To begin, Cain does not express negative feelings until he fails to receive positive feedback about himself. God looks upon Cain unfavorably because Cain's sacrifice had not been a genuine one; Cain was placing himself first, God second.

The question, "Am I my brother's keeper?" or, "Is it my fault if the patient does not follow his treatment plan?" arises when there is a divergence between the needs of self and the needs of others. As long as self and other operate in harmony, the question does not come up at all. When the patient conforms to his treatment plan, when I can respect the physician who orders medications, when I am able to have days off that I request, the question remains unformulated. "Am I my brother's keeper?" is asked when there is dissatisfaction with self and the world. Or, to put it another way, the question is posed when one becomes two, when unity or undivided harmony between myself and the other is jeopardized. The question arises when one's self-worth is put into question, and when a possibility exists that another who is younger and weaker may be perceived as more worthwhile than the self, the person of original power. These events have profoundly disturbing consequences.

For instance, the two-year-old with a new sibling often fears being displaced by one who is younger and weaker. All of us struggle to maintain our favored place at some point in our lives. If we lose the struggle, we experience profound rage; if we win, we are afraid of retaliation, knowing that we have hurt the other in *his* power needs. We may try to silence our fear by arrogance, or a swaggering attitude of self-righteousness, or be feigning ignorance of the consequences of our deed, but the fear is there. We fear not only blame and retaliation, but also being set apart, being ejected from the community, and losing oneness with our universe. No wonder we tend to be wary of conflict, and prefer to avoid it at all costs.

Consider the patient who does not cooperate with his treatment plan. How does his behavior affect you, the health professional? You might feel angry and threatened. You might fear the reaction of your superiors when you must account to them for the patient's behavior. Consider patients who blatantly question your authority. Or, how do you react when you are asked to submit to the authority of a physician who prescribes a medication of which you disapprove? What do you say when your nursing supervisor asks you to work a double shift when you are already exhausted from the tour of duty yet to be completed?

In all these examples, there is a question of how to assert individual rights and needs. Should you or should you not protect your own interests? One might say the experiences of present-day nurses are new variations on an archetypal theme, or new expressions of the eternal human dilemma depicted in the story of Cain and Abel.

No one can help feeling resentful when the original state of harmony with the other is shattered. Such unexpected events threaten our self-needs, and happen without being consciously willed, for they arise from inner or outer forces which are not under our control. However, we can control how we react. How we respond depends on the level of consciousness we have attained when the particular event occurs.

For instance, Cain was not able to confront his feelings of resentment and anger initially because he was too closely identified with the feelings. He perceived the source of his problems as originating in objects external to him, such as Abel, God, and even the snake who sired him. Cain assumed no personal responsibility, hence his actions focused on objects. Abel was weaker, so Cain eliminated him; his parents were stronger, so Cain tried to hide from them; Satan had operated in the past, so he blamed Satan. Cain tried to disclaim responsibility for his own deeds by asking, "Am I my brother's keeper?"

God had tried to help Cain acknowledge resentment and anger, but Cain was so identified with his subjective reaction, that he was unable to see the object in its own right. Cain wanted to reestablish the previous balance, to undo the refusal of his offering by eliminating the object which had caused a change in the balance (his younger brother). He wished to reestablish the position of only son with all its privileges—central focus and approval. As long as he needed to be preferred, the *only* one in power, the weaker one was life-threatening to him, and the source of the threat had to be eliminated.

Might this pattern also apply to our current nursing situation? We want to be in unquestioned control of the patient; we want the unquestioned good grace of the physician and our nursing supervisors. We want both control and approval for our service and/or sacrifice. When either or both of these desires are thwarted, our original state of harmony is threatened. Rage and a deep sense of anxiety at being cast out of the fold may ensue.

One way to respond to these painful experiences is to act, in a psychological sense, like Cain. Rather than experience the turmoil of our emotions as originating within ourselves, we view the pain as being caused by the weaker one (patient), or the stronger one (physician or the nursing hierarchy). We may plan how to get even with the patient, or dwell upon how unfairly we have been treated by the medical and nursing powers. We become threatened and isolated, believing ourselves to be the focus of hostility. We are alone, and we dread being alone, for seemingly even God has joined our pursuers.

It is small wonder, then, that we often cannot face either our inner feelings or the outer world, and that we try to disown all responsibility. We may attempt to cope by detaching ourselves. We do our day's work but are emotionally removed. If a patient does not want to cooperate with a treatment plan, so be it. If a physician prescribes a medication which is not appropriate, what concern is it of ours? If it appears that we might be asked to work another shift, we slip out the back door.

The price we pay for avoiding necessary conflicts is a sense of emptiness and a lack of meaning in our lives. If we refuse to shoulder our fair share of problems, we become dehumanized machines, cogs in the enormous wheel of the institution. Since emptiness, meaninglessness, and dehumanization deprive us of a sense of self, we may attempt to cover up the inner lack with an outer veneer of fancy uniforms, painted fingernails, and extraordinary coiffures. Also, we may attempt to compensate for the "nothingness" that lies inside by seeking exciting outer stimulation. Hence, we may choose to work on services where there is constant action—never a dull moment—yet never any time to engage in meaningful encounter with patient or staff.

The person who is alienated from the self in the belief that life must remain conflict free at all costs, is in a state of archaic consciousness. Persons who function on an archaic level of consciousness frequently come from families in which their own personhood was not valued. Often the parents were self-centered because of having been injured in their own personhoods. Such parents, consciously or unconsciously, tend to blame their own sufferings and disappointments on their children. In turn, the children accept the guilt projected on them, and view themselves as evil. Because it is unbearable to live with a poor self-concept, such a person is likely to disassociate the self from his/her feelings about the self, and to lead a shallow and superficial life. It becomes impossible to be close to others, including patients. Positive or negative input, particularly suffering on the part of the other would confront the person with overwhelming guilt and a negative self-identity. Instead, evil is perceived as existing on the outside in uncaring institutions and human beings. Evil objects must be used and exploited.

A second level of consciousness is also depicted in the account of Cain and Abel. We initially find that Cain possesses the legitimate and unquestioned power and status of a first-born son. Good feelings may become challenged when a younger sibling eclipses the older one as the focus of primary attention. When thus challenged, one option is to refocus attention on oneself by self-sacrifice. On this level, which Gebser [1972] calls the magical level of consciousness, two courses of action are open.

One, as described in the Cain and Abel story, is to eliminate the interfering object so that one's sense of specialness can be regained. Or, one may do exactly the opposite: instead of destroying the rival, one identifies with him.

And so, a nurse, acting out of this level of consciousness, may act in collusion with the patient's self-destructive efforts, since s/he "cannot bear to hurt his feelings." Nor does such a nurse confront the doctor, for s/he does not want to hurt the doctor's good feelings about her/himself. The nurse may comply with a course of treatment for a patient even if there is knowledge that the action is wrong. When faced with the inner furies of conscience, the nurse will try to evade the onslaught by becoming even more accommodating. To avoid causing those in nursing service additional aggravation, the nurse may work that extra shift, although exhausted. Of course, s/he is then prone to make errors which can cause grave consequences to patients, and for which the nurse will be held accountable.

Thus, the state of being one's brother's keeper, but not one's own, represents the opposite of Cain's mentality, yet is on the same magical level of consciousness. By such maneuvers, one can go through life under the illusion that one's omnipotence and central position are unchallenged. However, often such self-sacrificing acts can place others in a bad light, and hence may elicit reactions of retaliation. However painful, ostracism can be experienced as injustice by a person who views him/herself as an innocent victim who has sacrificed for a higher, selfless cause.

Gebser calls the third level of consciousness the mental level, in which you and I exist in our own right, and in which each of us has intrinsic value. I may experience your act as arousing conflict and pain, but I assume responsibility for my feelings, and am willing to explore the meaning of the act to me, and how it affects my relationship with you. I accord you the right to behave however you wish, but at the same time, I allow myself the prerogative to react subjectively (and to evaluate how I will respond in light of my reality and yours). In this state of consciousness, I perceive neither of us as having unlimited power, and I am realistically aware of the parameters of my own power.

When operating on the mental or ego level of consciousness, I can confront the patient who is not willing to cooperate with the treatment plan. I can tell the patient that while I am willing to help, her/his actions make it impossible for me to do so, and therefore, our relationship needs to be redefined. However, as a first step, I need to determine the cause and meaning of these actions. Perhaps the patient does not understand the treatment plan. Perhaps the patient would like to cooperate, but is unable to perform as requested. Or perhaps the patient does not want to be under my care because s/he does not like me, or believes s/he does not need care. It could also be that the patient expects me to "make her/him all better" without having to participate in the process.

Once I have determined the source of difficulty, I can more clearly define what my next move should be. If the treatment plan is unclear, I must provide instructions that are more easily understood. If the plan is too exacting, perhaps the patient and I can negotiate a scheme more in keeping with the patient's ability, or work together on upgrading the ability. Perhaps I should insist that the patient decide whether a particular treatment is desired, and if so, whether s/he wants it from me. If not, alternative treatments might be available from other therapists or nurses. The patient has the right to refuse my care. Conversely, I do not feel responsible for the choice; the patient is responsible for her/himself. However, I do accept responsibility for my own actions. In light of my overall goals, I may or may not wish to expend effort, time, and energy on someone who has so little use for them.

Similarly, I may be confronted with a physician's order that, in my professional judgment, is inappropriate. I can acknowledge the doctor's prerogative to prescribe, yet still insist that since I am accountable for my own practice, I cannot in good conscience give the patient what has been prescribed. The physician has the option to change the prescription or call for another nurse. I am not responsible for what the other nurse will do, nor am I responsible for the patient's medical management. However, I can alert the doctor's superiors. I might even alert the patient, for there is no need to cover up for the doctor when I am operating on this level of consciousness. Before I take such a decisive stand, however, I would endeavor to determine the doctor's rationale for giving the prescription.

Naturally, the possible consequences are endless in variety. What if the doctor persists and the patient comes to harm? What if he/she reports me to my nursing supervisors and I receive no support? What if I lose my job, and become excluded from the particular collective of peers with whom I work?

But the risks are worth taking. Asserting our own rights and needs, while according the other the same privilege, brings previously hidden information into the open, and helps evolve a form of consciousness which makes new approaches possible. Instead of the harmony of unity, we allow for the disharmony of duality, which eventually leads into a higher form of development. Of course, we often pay a price for our action, even if it is only being condemned by an irate physician whose omnipotence has been challenged. But, on the archaic level of consciousness, don't we pay the price of inner emptiness, stunted growth, and lack of relatedness to maintain the illusion of inner peace? And, on the magical level of consciousness, don't we pay the price of "killing" or self-sacrifice to maintain the illusion of power?

Actually, we have no choice of whether or not to pay a price. The only choice we have is what the price will be. It is not easy to attain or remain on the mental level of consciousness. To do so requires facing one's past and present suffering, as well as recognizing the feelings of anger and vindictiveness. It also requires facing one's sense of omnipotence, with the resulting fear of rejection and loss of power. It requires an ongoing assimilation of contradictory feelings and opposing values and needs. And it requires the ability to make decisions without any guarantee that one has taken the right stand. For, on this level, no universally right answers, attitudes, or actions exist.

Going back to the Cain and Abel story, we can gain some additional perspectives on the mental level of consciousness. God provided Cain with His mark of protection only when Cain acknowledged his guilt, fear, and sense of vulnerability; that is, when Cain was no longer identified with power and righteousness. All of us are apt to identify with universally valid moral law that we perceive as coming directly from God's mouth. Yet, God does not seem to appreciate our usurping His place, and rather views such behavior as hubris which must be punished. We are forced to acknowledge His superior power just when we are most self-righteous.

A true religious attitude does not become possible until we shoulder responsibility for our negative sentiments and acts. We have not caused the negative sentiments; rather, they arise in response to the actions of others, and as depicted in the Cain story, may even occur in response to God. Hence, we need not blame ourselves for having caused the sentiments, and for harboring them. Nevertheless, we have been given the responsibility to recognize that certain emotions originate within us, and to express our emotions so as to acknowledge the same right in others. When we assume our rightful responsibility in this manner, it seems to place us under divine protection, even if it does not always earn us the love of humankind.

How can a person on the mental level of consciousness recognize both the other and oneself, and at the same time remain aware of one's angry emotions? A person on the mental level of consciousness can maintain a sense of self-worth without feeling omnipotent. Such a person can recognize insults to his/her power without becoming annihilated by such insults. For this reason, there is no need for massive retaliation or self-sacrifice. (The hypothetical person may have always received recognition as a human being in his/her own right, while, at the same time, may have been taught to respect the rights of others.) The mental level of consciousness seems to result from a protracted process of dis-identification from the magical layer, and from injustices of the past. Thus, this person does not have to pit the entirety of him/herself against the other. On the contrary, s/he is aware of the higher power within the self and is willing to be its instrument, if the other is open to it. We might here paraphrase Fritz Perls: "I do my thing and you do yours."

To answer the question, "Am I my brother's keeper?" From the mental level of consciousness, we might say: I can only be my brother's keeper as long as his needs and mine coincide in terms of a third; a joint purpose that is congruent for both of us.

REFERENCES

Gebser, Jean, *Ursprung und Gegenwart,* Stuttgard: Deutsche Verlagsanstalt, 1966, Excerpted in *Main Currents of Modern Thought,* Vol. 29, No. 2 (November-December) 1972, pp. 80–88.

Ginzberg, Louis, *Legends of the Bible,* Philadelphia: Jewish Public Society, 1956, pp. 54–61.

The Jerusalem Bible, Genesis: Vol. 4, No. 1, New York: Doubleday, 1966, pp. 16–19.

Section 2
Advocacy

15 The Nurse as Advocate

A PHILOSOPHICAL FOUNDATION FOR NURSING

Leah L. Curtin

NURSES SEEM to be moving in the direction of the medical model with its emphasis on science, technology and cure. As individual nurses and as members of a profession we are seeking fundamental clarifications and asking radical questions. In partial reaction to this move toward the medical model we seem to be diverting to what is essentially a historical model of nursing with an emphasis on an intuitive approach. The answers that we reach, the direction that we choose will determine the future parameters of nursing.

Some sociologists have suggested that rather than developing as nursing professionals, professional nurses are evolving out of nursing! "Nursing will still be nursing, but it will be carried on by persons of other occupational affiliations [1, p. 528]. What then will nurses be doing while someone else is doing nursing?

According to some nursing leaders, nurses will be moving on to "meta-nursing [2]. Travelbee claims that "The role of the nurse must be transcended in order to relate as human being to human being [2, p. 49]. If the role of the nurse is viewed in such a manner, it is no wonder that nurses wish to move on to better things.

What is nursing? What is the role of the nurse? What is it that makes a nurse a nurse? Is it indeed the functions that we perform? How is it then that the director of nursing service, the administrator of a nursing home, the dean of a college of nursing, the primary care nurse, the operating room nurse, the public health nurse, the psychiatric nurse all claim to be nurses? We perform radically different functions and yet each of us claims the title "nurse." How can it be that those who, in the eyes of sociologists, have moved beyond nursing still consider themselves nurses? Could it be that rather than evolving out of nursing, these nurses are actualizing new possibilities within nursing?

Could it be that nursing *should not* be defined sociologically, but rather philosophically? Nursing can and should be distinguished by its philosophy of care and *not* by its care functions. Nurses themselves must formulate this philosophy and when they do, they transcend any particular function of nursing only to realize a more developed concept—a concept that embraces and unifies the experience of all nurses rather than denying or denigrating any of that experience [3].

NURSING—A MORAL ART

The end or purpose of nursing is the welfare of other human beings. This end is not a scientific end, but rather a moral end. That is, it involves the seeking of good and it involves

Reprinted from *Advances in Nursing Science*, by Leah L. Curtin by permission of Aspen Systems Corporation, © April 1979.

our relationship with other human beings. The science that we learn, the technological skills that we develop are both shaped and designed by that moral end—much as an artist uses a brush. Therefore, nursing is a moral art [4]. The wise and human application of our knowledge and skill is the moral art of nursing. Nursing science serves this art, and this art would not be possible without nursing science. This art is a moral art because it involves other human beings, our relationship with those human beings and the promotion of what we see mutually as "good"—health.

THE CONCEPT OF ADVOCACY

Anyone acquainted with the history of nursing is familiar with the various models proposed as models of nursing, such as the nurse as caretaker, the nurse as champion of the sick, the nurse as health educator, the nurse as physician assistant (extender, surrogate, etc.), the nurse as parent surrogate, and the nurse as healer. None of these seems adequate.

Perhaps the philosophical foundation and ideal of nursing is the nurse as *advocate*. The concept of advocacy implied here is not the concept implied in the patients' rights movement nor the legal concept of advocacy, but a far more fundamental advocacy founded upon the simplest and most basic of premises. This concept is not simply one more alternative to be added to the list of past and present concepts of nursing nor does it reject any of them—it embraces all of them. It is not structured rigidly so as to preclude alternatives, rather it involves the basic nature and purpose of the nurse-patient relationship. It is proposed as a very simple foundation upon which the nurse and patient in any given encounter can freely determine the form that relationship is to have, i.e., child and parent, client and counselor, friend and friend, colleague and colleague and so forth through the range of possibilities. This foundation is philosophically prior to any particular relationship and, in fact, enables that relationship to exist.

This proposed ideal of advocacy is based upon our common humanity, our common needs and our common human rights. We are human beings, our patients or clients are human beings, and it is this commonality that should form the basis of the relationship between us. It often seems that we have permitted traditionalism, elitism and more recently legalism to obscure this most basic of facts.

WHAT IT MEANS TO BE A HUMAN BEING

Even to begin to understand what the human relationship in the professional context means, we have to examine who we are and where we come from. We must approach these questions in the only way we know how, as individuals whose knowing begins with our senses. What we are examining are human beings, very special kinds of beings who exist in a visible ambience at a determinable point in time and space, beings who know and who know that they know, beings who laugh and cry—and sometimes know why.

Human beings cannot be fragmented. One of our deepest convictions, confirmed by all of our experience, is that each person is a unity [5]. I who think, I who know, I who feel, I who hope, I who fear, I who believe am one! As we grow and mature we come to realize that although we are separate and distinct from all other creatures and the world, we belong to them and with them because we have grown out of the growth of others, learned from their knowledge and benefited from their sufferings. Each person is an integrity, a unity, but a unity that is interrelated and interdependent.

Slowly and painfully, we have come to understand and demand our own dignity. We now know that freedom, respect and integrity are essential to our full development as persons. These concepts have crystallized in what we call human rights [6]. Although it has taken us a bit longer, we now realize that these rights belong to all persons—young and old, black, white, red and yellow; healthy and sick. The progress in this direction has not been smooth, nor is there anything to keep us from backsliding, but progress has been made [7].

Those concepts we call human rights derive essentially from human needs—*not* human wants, but real, fundamental human needs. Whether the right is physical (such as the right to bodily integrity) or intellectual (such as the right to learn), each is essential to our integrity—our unity—as persons.

HUMAN RIGHTS AND THE NURSE-PATIENT RELATIONSHIP

The relevance of this concept of human rights to the nurse-patient relationship is profound because the patient/client's human needs are magnified by disease. Moreover, the process of the disease itself renders the patient/client far more vulnerable to abuse. Furthermore, the disease process itself may well create new, fundamental needs, needs that must be addressed if the person is to maintain unity-integrity as a unique human being.

Nurses are in a unique position among health professionals to attend the patient/client as a unity because they are able to experience patients as human beings [3]. Not only do nurses attend patients when distress is immediate, but they attend them for sustained periods of time, often providing those intimate details of physical and emotional care that lead to a knowledge of this person as a distinct and unique human being. This knowledge is a precondition for the fundamental type of advocacy referred to here—not legal advocacy, not even health advocacy, but human advocacy.

The only way in which the *unique* human needs of patients or clients can be met is for nurses to attend them as unities. This requires not only an understanding of patients as human beings, but an understanding of each patient as a unique human being. Nurses must be sensitive to individuals and to their reactions to those needs created by illness that threaten the unity or integrity of the person.

Not only must nurses understand the specific physiological damage caused by disease processes, but they must also understand what illness does to the humanity of the sufferer. The wounds produced by illness stretch far beyond the person's physiological or even psychological limits and penetrate the existential depths of the person's being [8]. These very special wounds create very special needs—needs that must be met if we are to minister to the patient as a human being. These wounds must be addressed if we are to respect the human rights of patients/clients, if we are to accept human advocacy as the foundation of the nurse-patient relationship.

HOW DISEASE DAMAGES OUR HUMANITY
LOSS OF INDEPENDENCE

One of the very first things that illness does to human beings is to infringe upon their autonomy or independence as people. At the very least, individuals are required to go to another person, to place themselves before this person, to admit that they have a deficiency or a defect and to ask to have it alleviated. In effect, disease makes a petitioner out of an independent individual and threatens the person's self-image. The more personal or more threatening the disclosure is, the more difficult it is for a person to reveal the problem.

Ordinarily, when we meet with a threat we either fight or flee [9]. Yet we cannot flee from ourselves, nor can we fight that within ourselves which we cannot control. This is the ultimate threat, the threat that comes from within, and no matter how hard we try, we cannot have it alleviated without becoming a petitioner. The position of a petitioner is so repugnant to many that they will go to great lengths and take great risks to avoid it. If we are sensitive to this difficulty, the pain it imposes, the humiliation it brings, we can take some steps to alleviate it. So often it seems that health professionals (and nurses are no exception) are so caught up in their own business, their own knowledge and their own self-importance that they fail to consider this first humiliation of the patient or client. We must be willing to unravel the "medical mystique," to become more accessible and to remember that we too are human beings. It is only in doing so that we can begin to heal this first wound to the humanity, to assist individuals to overcome this first obstacle.

Loss of Freedom of Action

The second wound that impinges upon the humanity of the individual is the loss of freedom of action. The human being uses the body to transcend the body itself [10, pp. 28–29]. That is, unlike animals, we use our bodies for more than the fulfillment of physiological needs and instinctual drives. Human beings are bodily creatures, but they use their bodies to express their hopes, dreams, ideals and values. When we are ill we cannot command our bodies to do what we want them to do and thus in this sense our humanity is wounded, sometimes very seriously.

Insofar as possible we must assist the patient/client to communicate these essential aspects of their humanity. If they cannot do so, we must take steps to discover their value systems and then to respect them. The losses of freedom of action (verbal, locomotive, often intellectual) inflict another wound to the individual's humanity—and sometimes a very serious one!

Interference with Ability to Make Choices

In a third dimension our humanity is damaged by the interference of disease with our ability to make choices—not our right to make choices, but our ability to exercise that right. While there are many factors operant in decision making, it still remains that a decision to be truly valid, must be rational. This is a particularly sensitive area. Often professionals may consider only those decisions that agree with their own to be rational. This is not necessarily the case. However, we must be aware that pain, disability, trauma and drugs all becloud the ability to make choices as does the trauma caused by the loss of wholeness and the loss of ability to act.

Nevertheless, in all circumstances the right to consent rests within the individual. Under certain circumstances we may presume consent; in others we may obtain authorization to act; but the right always remains within the individual. If we are sensitive to this fact, we are far more likely to try to discover and act upon the patient's value system rather than our own or that of significant others. Because this situation has been greatly magnified by our increasing technological power to intervene in an individual's life, the responsibility to discover and respect the patient's value system has assumed vastly increased significance [11].

POWER OF HEALTH CARE PROFESSIONALS

A corollary of these factors, and perhaps one of the most devastating attacks on our person-hood, is that we are placed in the power of others. Many institutions in society exercise enormous power over us, but these powers have been recognized and surrounded with legal safeguards. It has been widely recognized, for example, that consent obtained under duress is not legally binding [12]. Few things in life are as coercive as the threat of suffering and death (in this instance imposed by illness). Yet what legal advocate, what laws of state, can protect us from these? Thus those persons whom we see as capable of relieving these threats can and do exercise enormous power over us. Not only do patients, generally speaking, lack the knowledge necessary to define the threat, but they also lack the ability to reduce the threat. Whether we as health professionals want it or not, we exercise enormous power over those whom we should serve. How do we use this power? What does this power mean in the light of human advocacy?

RESPONSIBILITIES OF HUMAN ADVOCACY

Information must be provided—at least enough to enable patients/clients to choose among options; but how and when patients/clients are told are at least as significant as what they are told. In the past (and often today), patients were uninformed largely because it was assumed that the health professionals, perhaps in concert with the families, knew what was best for the patients. Usually professionals do know what is best from the technical viewpoint, but it is doubtful that such knowledge extends into the realm of values.

Today, largely because of legal requirements, patients may be subjected to a tyranny of information. More as a hedge against malpractice than out of respect for human rights, patients are fed an enormous, disagreeable and indigestible lump of information—and all at one sitting. How much more patients would benefit from small amounts of information provided when they are ready for them and as they ask for them. If nurses and physicians worked collaboratively rather than jealously protecting territorial limits, the patient would greatly benefit. Because nurses have the opportunity to experience the patient as a unique human being and because they spend more time with the patient, nurses can more readily provide information as the patient requests it and when the patient is prepared for it.

Because individuals have been damaged by trauma or disease, and perhaps because they have been placed in the power of others, they have to a large extent *lost their freedom to define for themselves their own image of what it is they should be.* For example, there was a case of a 22-year-old male patient who was diagnosed as having primary cancer of the testes. He was a jockey, a husband and the father of two young sons. There was no evidence of metastasis. He was told of his diagnosis, the need for an orchiectomy and the effect this operation would have on his relationship with his wife. He and his wife discussed the situation and, considering the alternative, decided upon surgery. What he was not told, however, was at least as significant as what he was told. He was not told that he would lose his facial hair, develop breasts and develop a feminine speaking voice. How much did we impinge upon this person's identity? What did we do to his self-image? What image did he present to his sons? To his wife? What kind of comments did he have to endure at the race track? We do not know, but what we do know is that he committed suicide nine months after surgery.

So often by trying to do what we think is right by our value system, we trespass upon the authenticity of the person. Although in many cases our transgressions are not so great, in some cases they are profound. This man's decision might not have been any different if he had known all the facts, but the real question is whether or not the *individual rather than the professional* should make such value decisions. If we decide that a person cannot, how do we reach this conclusion? Can we not, should we not, ought we not assist the patient in decision making *AND YET RESPECT THE PATIENT'S DECISION* once it is made?

If these wounds are not addressed, and indeed if they are exacerbated, the most devastating of existential wounds develops. Insofar as patients' values are ignored, or replaced with others' values, patients cease to exist as unique human beings. Depersonalization may be partial or complete, but those individuals will die as the persons they were. If the depersonalization is complete, those individuals will not be able to create new values and goals in their life and they will lose a sense of meaning or purpose in their existence [13]. As the philosopher Nietzsche put it, "He who has the why to live can bear with almost any how" [14].

We must—as human advocates—assist patients to find meaning or purpose in their living or in their dying. This can mean whatever the patients want it to mean; it can range from enlisting religious aid to cracking irreverent jokes, from finding a new vocation to adjusting to the old one, from fighting the inevitable to the last breath to complete acceptance of death. Whatever patients define as their goal, it is their meaning and not ours, their values and not ours, and their living or dying and not ours.

Any application of human advocacy is subject to personal and situational interpretation by the practitioner. This is precisely why human advocacy can serve as a foundation upon which any practitioner in any given situation can develop the framework of the nurse–patient relationship according to the unique needs presented by that particular relationship.

According to Garver, violence is not so much a matter of force as it is a matter of violating persons physically, intellectually or psychologically [15]. Certainly not every limitation of a person's autonomy can be seen as an act of violence. To take this position would be to take the moral "punch" out of the notion of psychological violence. For example, one simply cannot equate a regulation limiting how loud patients may tune their television sets with the rendering of patients incompetent in various degrees by withholding information, thus interfering with their rational processes. The concept of psychological violence must be reserved to those cases in which grave or systematic harm is done to the person. The ability to distinguish those cases requires a sensitivity to the human needs created by illness and the unique manifestation of these needs in each patient, *NOT IN SERIOUS MATTERS ONLY,* but in the daily living experience of patients/clients.

Consider the daily living experience of an institutionalized patient. An individual comes into the patient's room to insert an I.V., and the patient does not even know about the I.V. or why it is being given. Another person comes in to administer a medication that the patient does not even know about or why it is being given. Still another person comes in to catheterize the patient, to administer an enema, to draw blood, to examine every part of the patient's body, to transport the patient here or there for this test or that, and the patient doesn't even know where they are going, what is being done or why it is being done.

Each individual violation may or may not amount to a serious infringement on the patient's autonomy, but collectively they constitute both physical and psychological violence. Note that the effect on the patient is systematic. Confusion, lack of knowledge, lack of explanation, the pervasive assumption that the patient's body belongs to the "professionals" to do with what they will—all lead to reduced possibilities for decision making. Such systematic violation leads to reduced possibilities for making decisions in other, perhaps critical, areas. Human beings are reduced to objects acted upon, in effect a wholesale reduction of autonomous decision making [16]. Patient and family are thus rapidly socialized into obedience patterns and nonconformity is swiftly punished in both subtle and not so subtle ways.

ESSENCE OF NURSING

Nurses can and do control the environment of the institution, and nurses can institute progressive and humanizing changes if they so desire. Explanations and working together with a patient are not extras that nurses may choose to do, they are the essence of nursing, the essence of the nurse–patient relationship. Obviously, in certain critical situations, there is no time for an in-depth discussion of values or even explanations. These circumstances, however, constitute only a minute portion of nurse–patient interactions and should not be used to negate patient rights in the majority of situations.

To claim that nurses can institute progressive change is not to ignore the many organizational and social barriers that nurses face. We can control our own actions. To be sure there are inflexible policies and insensitive orders from physicians, but the professional nurse has a great deal of latitude in the implementation of such policies and orders. Our ethical responsibility is not reduced by the actions of others, but in fact may be magnified by them [17]. Discretion and maturity are necessary components of the truly effective professional.

Nursing and the individual nurse are in very vital positions to help create a climate respectful of the human rights and needs of patients. No other profession and no other professional can exercise as great an influence over the environment of the institution (the environment of the patient) as do the nurse and nursing. If we, as a profession, work together to create an atmosphere that is open to and supportive of the individual's decision making, we may well perform our greatest service to patients/clients and their families.

In many instances nurses are not free to disclose certain information to patients/clients and their families. That is, they are not free unless they are willing to pay the price, a price that may well include loss of employment or even licensure. This situation is wrong because it violates both the patient's and the nurse's integrity [18]. Moreover, it constitutes a direct infringement of the nurse's right to practice nursing and interferes directly with the nurse–patient relationship [19]. This situation must, can and will be changed.

However, even the existence of such factors does not justify the daily violation of the patient in those matters that nurses do control. It is not an excuse for the psychological violence to which the person is subjected in the daily living experience as an institutionalized patient. The concept of human advocacy transcends even those situational problems created by physicians who knowingly withhold information from patients because it is based on the patient's humanity and the professional's humanity. This is certainly not a complex concept; rather it is so simplistic that it seems almost ludicrous to propose it. All patients—surgical patients, psychiatric patients, medical patients, pediatric patients, dying patients—are still living human beings with all that this implies. If we remember this—and remember too that we are also human beings—the concept of human advocacy is as natural as living and dying.

REFERENCES

1. Schulman, S. "Basic Functional Roles in Nursing: Mother Surrogate and Healer" in Jaco, E., ed. *Patients, Physicians and Illness* (Glencoe, Ill.: The Free Press 1958) pp. 528–537.

2. Travelbee, J. *Interpersonal Aspects of Nursing* (Philadelphia: F. A. Davis and Co. 1966).
3. Gadow, S. "Existential Advocacy: Philosophical Foundation for Nursing." Paper presented to the Four State Consortium on Nursing and the Humanities, Phase I Conference, "Nursing and the Humanities: A Public Dialogue," Farmingham, Connecticut, November 11, 1977.
4. Curtin, L. "Nursing Ethics: Theories and Pragmatics." *Nurs Forum* 17:1 (Spring 1978).
5. Chardin, P. de. *The Phenomenon of Man,* Wahl, B., trans. (New York: Harper & Row, Publishers 1959).
6. Dostoevski, F. "Notes from Underground" in *The Short Novels of Dostoevski,* Garnet, C., trans. (New York: Dial Press 1945) p. 149.
7. Dubos, R. *So Human an Animal* (New York: Charles Scribner and Sons 1968) p. 40.
8. Pellegrino, E. "A Humanistic Foundation for Medicine." Paper presented to the Second International Institute of Health Care, Ethics and Human Values, Mount St. Joseph College, Mount St. Joseph, Ohio, July 1976.
9. Gardiner, W. L. *Psychology: A Story of a Search* (Belmont, Calif.: Brooks/Cole Publishing Co. 1970).
10. Descartes, R. as quoted in Heidegger, M. *Existence and Being* (Chicago: Henry Regnery and Sons 1949) pp. 28–29.
11. McCormick, R. Lecture given to the Third International Institute for Health Care, Ethics and Human Values, Mount St. Joseph College, Mount St. Joseph, Ohio, July 1976.
12. Vinogradoff, P. *Collected Papers* vol. 2, ch. 20 (Oxford: Clarendon Press 1928).
13. Frankl, V. E. *Man's Search for Meaning: An Introduction to Logotherapy,* Lasche, I., trans. (New York: Pocket Books 1963) pp. 160–163.
14. Nietzsche, F. *The Birth of Tragedy and the Geneology of Morals.* Golffing, F., trans. (Garden City, N. Y.: Doubleday & Co. 1956) p. 299.
15. Garver, N. "What Violence Is." *The Nation* (June 1968) pp. 817–822.
16. Curtin, L. "Informed Consent: Information or Exploitation?" *Update on Ethics* 1:4.
17. American Nurses' Association. *Code for Nurses,* articles 1–3 (Kansas City, Mo.: ANA 1976).
18. Curtin, L. "Nursing Ethics: Theories and Pragmatics." *Nurs Forum* 17:1 (Spring 1978) pp. 4–11.
19. Curtin, L. "Nursing Practice—A Right and a Duty." *Nurs Ethics* 1:1 (Fall 1978) pp. 7–11.

16 The Nurse as Advocate

Mary F. Kohnke

MR. WOOD, a 48-year-old, 135-pound man, is lying in bed and moaning in pain. He is one day postcholecystectomy. One hour before the nurse had given him Demerol 75 mg. q4h, PRN. The medication had not been effective, according to the nurse's notes.

Mr. Wood's nurse pages the intern to request that the medication be changed. The intern refuses, as does the resident, saying that he has had enough medication for a man of his size. The nurse pursues the situation and contacts the attending physician to let him know what is happening. He comes to see Mr. Wood and changes the medication to morphine sulfate, 10 mg. IM. Mr. Wood experiences pain relief within 45 minutes after receiving the morphine.

Is the nurse's action an act of advocacy? My answer is no, this is not advocacy, it is just good nursing practice.

I believe that advocacy has been confused with legalities and ethics of nursing practice. We have to clearly differentiate between the three.

The classical definition of advocacy is "the act of defending or pleading" the case of another. In nursing at least, if not in law, I hesitantly offer a parallel definition: that advocacy is the act of informing and supporting a person so that he can make the best decisions possible for himself.

Thus, the act of advocacy or the actions of the advocate are two-fold. The *first* is to inform your clients or patient of what their rights are in a particular situation and then to make sure they have all the necessary information to make an informed decision. You as the nurse must first learn to gather the information before you can pass it on to your client. Then, you must, to the best of your ability, ensure that your clients know and understand the same information.

The information must be presented in a manner that allows the patient to hear what you are saying without imposing your own hidden feelings that may distort this information. In other words, the patient must not be put in the position of having to "psych out" the nurse.

People make decisions for all kinds of reasons, some of which have nothing to do with the immediacy of the situation facing them. The advocate must constantly be on guard not to feed into the unstated reasons that go into making a decision and thereby subtly support a decision that is not based on rational reasoning. For example, a person may make a decision that is contradictory to what he wants because he has a greater need to please others than himself. In the advocate role, your responsibility is to put your own opinion aside and clearly inform your clients of the consequence of their choices. If "A" is chosen, then "B" will follow.

Copyright © 1980, American Journal of Nursing Company. Reproduced with permission from the *American Journal of Nursing,* November, Volume 80, Number 11. This paper was originally presented to the Society for Advancement in Nursing, Inc. (SAIN), meeting in October 1979.

The *second* act of the advocate is to support clients in the decisions they make. Support may involve several actions or nonactions. One action is to actively reassure patients that it is their decision and they have the *right* to make it. They do not need to nor should they give in to pressures from others, be it family, friends, or health professionals. A second action may mean that you do not allow others to undermine your client's confidence in his own decision making. This may only be possible if you are in a position of authority to prevent others from harassing the client.

The decision a client makes is his own, even if, in your opinion, it is not the best decision for him. He has the right to make decisions freely and without pressure. This is advocacy in the finest sense of the word. It may be hard for us as professionals "who know best" to accept our clients' decisions, but it is necessary if we expect people to grow, and if we respect their right to make their own decisions. We can learn and grow not only from our right decisions, but from our mistakes as well.

Nonaction may be even more important than action, yet harder to do. Nonaction usually means keeping yourself from subtly undermining the patient's decision. It may also mean that you have to refuse the request of others, such as physicians, other nurses, or family members, who ask you to talk to the patient and convince him that he is wrong. This kind of refusal can have some disturbing repercussions for you if your colleagues or family members do not understand your responsibility to support your client's decision. For example, a physician may report a staff nurse to her superior if she does not "talk" his patient into signing a consent form for a procedure that he believes the patient should have.

The act of advocacy for those in the so-called helping professions is psychologically very difficult. It is almost in direct conflict with their image of themselves as the persons "who know best"—the experts who are paid to know and make decisions based on superior knowledge. We often see ourselves as the rescuers of mankind who are sick and need rescuing.

Rescuers often put themselves in the position of making decisions for others so that, in the end, they have to accept the responsibility for the decision. However, although we may be willing to make the decision, we are not equally willing to accept responsibility for having done so. Not only does making the decision for another rob that person of his responsibility and rights, it also places the professional in a very awkward position of being blamed if all does not come out well. Since most of us inherently know this, we then attempt to have clients make the decision we want them to make under the guise of their having done it themselves.

I believe that, in fact, we are only fooling ourselves if we believe that our clients do not know what is going on. This may be OK if all goes well, but too often, Murphy's law prevails (when it's possible for something to go wrong, it does). Then, when clients blame us, we act startled and surprised and ask, "How can you blame me?" Furthermore, we accuse them (openly or silently) of being ungrateful, never admitting for one minute that we got ourselves into the mess by our insistence of the "we know best" theme.

In the literature, this is often referred to as the games triangle or Karpman's triangle.* It is pictorially described as the rescuer-victim-persecutor triangle. An example of this is when teachers fall victim to the student who insists that the faculty adviser decide between two elective courses on the grounds that she knows best. Four weeks later, the student comes back and blames the adviser for "picking a lousy course. . . ." Another example is when the patient asks the nurse to explain to the family her desires because "they won't listen to me."

*Karpman, S. B. Script drama analysis. *Trans. Anal. Bull.* 7:39–43, Apr. 1968.

We can willingly accept the rescuer's role and, in fact, insist on it, or can be innocently put into it. The result is the same—whenever you make decisions for others or do for them what they should be doing, you automatically accept the responsibility for the results.

In the advocacy role, one should never get into this position. As your client's advocate, you must keep uppermost in your mind that clients must make their own choices freely. If not, this is not advocacy as I use the word; it is rescuing. The rescuer role has no place in the life of a professional, except when the client may be too young or in a coma, and thus is unable to make the decision.

The "we know best" attitude is something we have been taught as children because our parents practiced it with us and, in some cases, may even continue to do so when we are adults. This theme is reinforced in the school systems, and if one goes into the helping professions it is reinforced again, so that it becomes second nature.

Thus, to be an advocate, as a nurse, requires a reorientation and a constant guarding of self, so as not to slip into the "we know best" position. It also requires an element of faith: faith in human beings' ability to make their own decisions and, even more, in their right to do so.

CONSTRAINTS ON THE ADVOCATE

When discussing the constraints that can confront an advocate, there are two considerations that the nurse must remember. First, the patient's reluctance to make a decision, despite his desire to do so, will require extra care on the nurse's part in the informing and supporting processes.

Second, be very careful that you do not become triangled into the patient-family system. Knowledge of family theory and dynamics can be a great help. If you take sides with families, you may very well end up with them on one side and you on the outside.

These two areas may not be so much constraints from without as they are constraints from within. For example, one may see patients being manipulated by their families into making a decision they don't like. The nurse may want to intervene, only to find out that this is a lifetime game that they all play. Moreover, this pattern is one they want to continue despite the fact that, on the surface, they protest to the nurse.

The greatest area of constraint will be the institution. The major functions of advocacy are basically at odds with the culture of the hospital system. First, you inform. That, in itself, is a great sin because you will be labeled an "informer." By telling patients things that will make them ask questions, you get labeled a troublemaker. We give lip service to patients' rights. That's great until the patient begins demanding his rights. Then, watch out! If you are the instigator of this through information you gave, you are in trouble.

You may survive the first step, but if you then go so far as to support patients in their decisions, you have had it. For example, you have not only provided the information, but then you are told by the head nurse, the physician, or the administrator to go and convince patients that they are wrong. They *must* have the test or the operation or leave the hospital. If you refuse, you are, indeed, in a fix. You have, in effect, disobeyed a direct order from your superiors.

These are very real constraints. They are widely in operation today. I'm not trying to discourage you from ever being an advocate but only trying to alert you to the possible pitfalls.

There are ways in which pitfalls can be avoided. They involve being very knowledgeable about the system, the law, and how to handle yourself with the patient. If you use your knowledge wisely and do not get trapped in the emotional position of being a rescuer to the patient, it helps.

When your patient's rights are being infringed on, a wise word, well dropped, can make people retreat. If one says, "Well, Dr. Brown, I was only thinking of your interests. You know how sensitive people are these days and how quick they are to sue," this usually causes the person to at least stop and think. In other words, you must learn how to work within the system to the extent it is possible. People who have really been violating patients' rights will be very sensitive to this method.

One must be careful not to win battles and lose wars. Members of the health team must be educated to the dangers of the "we know best" rescuer's game. This you can do. You can show them the possible consequences of their behavior.

I suppose the bottom line of the advocate role can be summarized in the term *knowledge* or *to know*. Not to know is no sin, not to admit that one does not know is. The greatest sin or damage is committed under the umbrella of "We didn't know." But then, most of us may not want to know. We say, "What you don't know can't hurt you." However, I believe that it is precisely what you do not know that will hurt you the most. Ignorance is the greatest weapon of tyrants and the greatest defense of people who do not want to accept responsibility for themselves. When you are dealing with both, you have a dual problem.

The act of advocacy is, at its basic level, an act of loving and caring for others as you would love and care for yourself. In its true form, it is simplicity itself. However, the two-edged sword is that which is most simple is in fact complex, and that which seems most complex is most simple. The act of advocacy is just that—the most simple and the most complex.

Section 3
Mentoring

17 Mentorhood

A KEY TO NURSING LEADERSHIP

Margaret Smith Hamilton

ACCORDING TO Greek mythology, Ulysses, hero of "The Odyssey," left home to wage the battles of the Trojan War. Knowing he would be away for several years, he appointed Mentor, the trusted son of Alimus, to be the guardian of his household and tutor to his son. Hence the word mentor came to mean wise and faithful guardian and tutor.

Mentoring is an old and honorable way of assisting a neophyte in a profession. The arts place a high value on the mentor approach for training a novice. It has been a long accepted belief that aspiring professionals such as musicians and ballerinas learn best from an older accomplished professional—the expert. Some of the more established professions foster mentoring. The mentor-protégé concept has a deep, rich history for many men among the practices of medicine, law and business. Women have not been as fortunate in these professions. They have been equally deprived of mentoring in the predominately female professions. For many women and nurses their understanding of what a mentor is comes purely from what they have read or heard from others.

Nursing is a profession that has a demonstrated serious lack of talented mentors. The profession is depriving itself of a meaningful and resourceful way of promoting the growth and development of talented, creative, promising, young nurses. Nurses could gain tremendously from applying and mastering the concept of mentorhood in our practice. The purpose of this article is to take a comprehensive view of the matter and manner of mentoring, and to explore how it can facilitate and expedite the maturation of future nurse leaders. I am principally interested in focusing on the art of mentoring—what is a mentor; the understanding of the achievement of success and demonstrated leadership capacities that others have accomplished through such a relationship; how this mentor-protégé helping dyad operates; the impediments to establishing more mentorships that women and nurses have experienced; how it compares with nursing's panacea—the role model; and how leadership traits, encouraged through mentoring, can be cultivated in nurses through the development of mentors within the nursing profession. These are all areas of concern that need exploring if mentoring is to find a place in nursing and if nurses want to reap the rewards of this treasured tool of erudition and professional maturation.

THE ART OF MENTORING

What is a mentor? According to Webster's dictionary a mentor is ". . . a close, trusted, and experienced counselor or guide" [1]. The term mentor is used to describe a member of the

Reprinted with permission of Charles B. Slack, Inc., from *Nursing Leadership,* Volume 4, Number 1, March 1981.

mentor-protégé system. A mentor is the accomplished, more experienced professional who extends to a young, aspiring person, within the context of a one-to-one relationship, advice, teaching, sponsorship, guidance and assistance toward her establishment in her chosen profession.

In his ten-year comprehensive study on the developmental phases and tasks of adulthood in men, Levinson emphasizes the critical significance of mentors in the career advancement of men. He sees the mentoring relationship as a vital part of the developmental work of early and middle adulthood of men, and that the relationship is found most often in professional work settings. Defining mentoring not in terms of roles but in terms of the character of the relationship and the functions that it serves, he describes a mentor as a transitional figure, a mixture of good parent and good friend, who serves as a teacher, sponsor, and guide. The mentor possesses and represents the qualities that the younger professional someday hopes to acquire. An enhancer of professional skills and intellectual development, the mentor often facilitates and influences a novice's advancement within the profession. He can provide counsel and moral support during times of stress and encouragement during risk-taking endeavors. As a sponsor, he is an inviter, encourager, and welcomer into the adult world. He is the practical helper and guide as the young person struggles with the tasks, details, and challenges of his profession. With the hope that someday they may function as peers, a novice senses genuine concern from his mentor about his struggle to be successful. Most of all, Levinson found the mentor to be most crucial to his protégé in the supporting of and the facilitating toward the realization of a young man's dream [2].

Those who have described mentors for women call them a necessary part of the system of professional benefactorship, sponsorship, and protectorship [3]. They are advisors, supporters, and advocates who help define and promote the career of a neophyte. Epstein calls them "creators of competence" [4]. One woman executive describes a mentorship as having components of how a godfather and coach function. The godfather component is the protector who encourages the protégé, brings her along, and makes sure she is rewarded. The coach component is the intellectual component who helps to set a standard of professional performance and expectations, assists in accomplishing these goals and moving on to greater achievements [5]. Another describes how useful a mentor can be during that transitional process from student to working professional. She describes bright young women in busines; who are very competent at their work but somewhat naive about how the real world operates. She sees an important function of mentoring as explaining and pointing out the differences between the idealized world of academia and the harsh, real world of work. She offers pointers, suggestions, and criticism necessary for cultivating the kind of critical thinking it takes to succeed in the everyday operations of business [5]. Diamond, in discussing women leaders, describes a mentor as a person who believes in a protégé and helps the protégé to believe in herself and her ability to achieve her goals and evolve into a successful, autonomous professional with leadership qualities of her own [6].

Mentors are different things to different people. No two mentorships are the same. The dynamics and the intensity of the relationship varies. For some, a mentor comes along once in a lifetime, others never experience the opportunity. A few persons have the good fortune of having more than one mentor during their professional career. What they do share is a belief in the beginning professional. Theirs is a job of tutelage and guidance—tutelage in the ways of the world and guidance beyond the mere transferral of professional skills. Making learning an exhilarating experience for the protégé, and paving constructive avenues for creative energy are the ideal mentor's contribution to a novice. Whether they are actual architects of dreams or helpers in the execution of the protégé's dream, they somehow communicate the importance of dream making, career planning and strategy, and owning one's conception of career designing and putting it into perspective within their profession.

MENTORSHIPS: LEADERS AND SUCCESS

Many factors contribute to an individual's professional success. Not all successful persons can be classified as leaders. Leadership is a complex human quality that some say can be learned and others speculate about it as an innate human trait. But the attainment of success and the ability to function as a leader have been identified as results of a mentorship. Various correlations between mentoring and professional accomplishments have been established. The following is a look at some of those correlations.

It has been shown that achievement in business is very difficult without some mentoring along the way. Henning, in her study of 25 women corporate executives, found that they all had significant male, father-like figures who functioned as mentors and sponsors in their career development. They aided them, encouraged them, helped them believe in their capabilities, and protected them from others who were threatened by competent business women. Such a sponsor proved necessary for a woman who did not have family connections in business, if she was to make it to the top in any business corporation [7].

Another recent survey of top business executives showed that mentor relationships are fairly extensive in the business world among powerful executives [8]. The study found that executives who had a mentor moved into successful positions, earned more money at a younger age, were more likely to follow a personal career plan, were better educated and eventually sponsored protégés themselves. Compared to those who did not have a mentor, these persons demonstrated a higher level of satisfaction with their career progress and received greater pleasure from their work.

Roche, in a business survey of over 1,250 business executives, found that two-thirds had mentors during their first ten years of professional work. Few reported a mentor relationship during their education, stating they were more likely to seek out people in their chosen field of work rather than educators who lacked extensive experience in business. When asked to identify the factors that contributed to a good mentoring relationship in order of their importance, these persons listed a mentor's personal interest and open willingness, ability to share understanding and knowledge, counseling traits, knowledge of the organization and the people in it, the mentor's rank, respect from his peers, and his knowledge and use of power [8].

Estler identifies a mentorship as crucial in a woman's advancement to higher level managerial positions. She ranks mentoring, along with competency and compatibility as the three critical factors considered when screening women for promotions [9]. Reminding us that there are only a few women in educational administration holding positions of leadership, authority and power, Felton states the lack of mentors as one reason [4]. She states that women often lack the mentor who could be instrumental in their professional preparation and helpful in introducing them into the established networks that promote career advancement and success.

In an in-depth look at leadership, Zaleznik argues that the leadership personality is unique, differing fundamentally from a managerial personality [10]. A manager is a conservative, a regulator of the established, existing order of things, while a leader is driven to change and profoundly alters economic, political, and human relationships. A leader's talents are founded in two aspects of personal life history—development through socialization and, more importantly, development through personal mastery of the struggle for psychological and social change. It is in this struggle for personal mastery that many leaders get lost in themselves. The only certain way to interrupt such a preoccupation and self-absorption is to form a deep attachment to a strong teacher who understands and, by his ability to communicate, brings forth the potential of the gifted person [10]. Zaleznik believes that it is the one-to-one mentor relationship that accelerates and intensifies the young leader's development. It is this type of relationship that fosters in young people the ability to take a risk, to make a commitment to a professional philosophy, to freely share ideas and, in their interpersonal relationships, to be both intuitive to others' needs and empathetic of their situations [11].

More recently a mentor system in nursing has been recognized. After studying American nursing leaders and the influencing factors in their careers, Vance reported on the importance of mentorships in their lives. Out of 71 nursing leaders, 83 percent reported having mentors during their career development and 93 percent were consciously aware of being mentors to others. This group reported that mentors helped them by creating career opportunities, promotions, and opening doors; acting as professional role models; providing scholastic and intellectual stimulation; and being a source of inspiration [12].

THE MENTORING RELATIONSHIP

What is this mentoring relationship, when does it occur, why does it work, and how is it helpful? The mentoring relationship is a one-to-one relationship that focuses on the development of the protégé. Levinson called the relationship, ". . . a serious mutual non-sexual loving relationship . . . the most complex and developmentally important a man can have in early adulthood" [2]. A mixture of parent and peer, this transitional figure is usually 8 to 15 years older than his protégé [2]. This half generation split helps to avoid falling into a parental transference as well as identification as a peer.

Others define the relationship as "elitist" by its very nature [13]. Hierarchical, intense and exclusionary, the availability of mentoring has not been democratic. How one is chosen as mentor or protégé is often determined by such factors as gender, social class, and personality.

Roche found through his survey that the majority of mentor relationships started when the protégés were in their 20s and 30s. This usually occurred in the first five to ten years of their professional employment. The mentor's position when the relationship began was usually that of supervisor, department head, or company president [8]. This survey showed, as did Levinson's, that rarely did a man have a mentor after age 40. By that time the man had outgrown his mentor and was almost ready to be a mentor to someone else.

As in any relationship there are various dynamics at work during a mentorship. In an attempt to understand how it functions, the mentor-protégé relationship can be viewed as a helping dyad. A dyad is the simplest form of a social system. Social psychologists theorize about the social interaction of this helping relationship. Glidewell describes this socialization as a process that occurs on a one-to-one basis [14]. The helper in the dyad (a person of special power and status based on knowledge, skill, age, or magic) thoughtfully and precisely assists in bringing about new or changed behavior and alternative ways of functioning in the helpee. This can be accomplished by praise, rewards and, at times, punishment. A significant characteristic of a helping dyad is privileged communication. The person being helped is encouraged to expose his concerns and dilemmas in his interpersonal interactions. But he is also protected, by confidentiality, from high visibility, and therefore the societal consequences that would ordinarily accompany such exposure. It is this privileged communication that aids the helper in decision making and risk taking and reduces his rate of error and mistake making [14]. Such privileged communication is the basis of a mentorship.

What is inevitable in a helping dyad and why it remains only a temporary system is the potential shifting of the balance of power. In the beginning the novice is uncertain, hesitant, open to suggestions, and challenges little. As the relationship evolves and she gains a better sense of her professional self, style, commitment, and capacity for autonomous decision making, the relationship is more of a mutual give-and-take experience. It is at this point that the relationship usually terminates. The transition out of the relationship from helping dyad to colleagues varies. The men in Levinson's study report an abrupt, stormy parting of the ways that resulted in bad feelings on both sides [2]. Others see the termination as similar to leaving the safe nest of home [13]. Still others report the evolution into long-lasting friendships and peer relationships. Should the relationship not terminate, the protégé could be subservient to the point of exploitation or a prolonged relationship may increase the influence, control, and power of the protégé in ways that may be destructive and not helpful for either party.

A mentorship by its true nature is a nonsexual relationship. When and if a sexual relationship is formed within the same dyad it is often confusing and conflict laden for the young professional. There is potential deceiving of the self-confidence of the protégé engaged in a sexual alliance with her mentor. She can never be certain about what she achieved by her competencies and intellect and what she won by virtue of her sexual relationship [15]. As Sheehy points out, the protégé will have difficulty maintaining a healthy balance when her emotional, sexual, and professional need gratification all depend on one person [16].

Not to be underestimated in the work of mentoring are the benefits and rewards inherent for the mentor. The functioning of mentoring is growth-producing, and a mentor cannot help but continue in her own growth and expansion. One who is open and willing to share ideas will profit from such an interchange. Mentors can determine if they have been successful and influential when the behavior, decision making, and risk taking actions of the protégé seem to come naturally to him. Influencing is a two-way process and, as Yura reminds us, the actions of the person influenced may not always be directly observable to the influencer [17]. This is all part of the risk taking of the mentor—the one who engages in an influencing relationship. But mentors must take risks with people. Sometimes the emotional risks of working in a one-to-one relationship don't pay; however, as Zaleznik urges, it is that willingness to take those risks that is so crucial to the development of young leaders [10].

WOMEN: IMPEDIMENTS TO MENTORING

Mentorships are accruing recognition as an important relationship for women in their adult development. Only recently has a group of American women college presidents stated that a weak support system and lack of mentors for women have been the major obstacles for women in achieving their long-range professional goals [18]. Women in many fields have suffered from a lack of mentors. According to Daniels in *Working It Out,* a book about the lives and work of professional women, the sociology of most professions do not allow for the tutelage and support of a developmental significant mentor relationship. They lack that sponsorship of their work through regular professional contacts; objective and productive criticism; and the support of present research, studies, and projects on a daily give-and-take basis that would foster professionalism [19].

Why don't women and nurses have a rich history of mentorships? Several factors enter into it. The general socialization of women in America is geared toward belonging—

affiliative needs. The socialization of men has been toward competition—achievement needs. Since the purpose of mentoring is achievement, it is in direct conflict with traditional female goals. As Bardwick points out, there is a consistency of role expectations for boys and men that permeates our culture and society [20]. Because of this men receive support, assistance, and productive criticism from all walks of life and from all the contributors of the socialization process. How often have young boys heard from strangers, "That's a good job . . . son." Or the critical but useful reprimand, "I'd think twice before doing that . . . fellow." Females, on the other hand, don't receive this kind of social input. People have had different expectations for them or choose not to comment on their behavior out of fear of insulting them or hurting their feelings.

Another factor is the lack of emphasis on team sports and team involvement. The athlete-coach relationship recognized as so crucial to the development of boys, is only now being fostered in girls. Diamond discusses involvement in sports as a necessary pattern in the development of the competitive spirit and leadership abilities. She contrasts this with girls' play as seen as a cooperative interchange of play having no specific goals, no explicit end point, and therefore no designated winners or losers—more of a sharing, turntaking process [21]. This again points to the greater need for belonging—affiliation over that of success-achievement. Because women are socialized in this manner, they first try to please others by doing what is desired or expected of them before they do what they might want for themselves. Howe reminds us that this process leads to feelings of ineffectiveness and powerlessness [15]. A sure impediment to mentoring.

I believe, however, that what has been woman's largest obstacle to mentoring, as men know it, may well be our greatest advantage to mentoring as women know it. As Kjervik urges us, the affiliative needs of females, demonstrated in the skills of cooperation and collaboration, need not be considered weak but rather praised, acknowledged, and fostered [22]. Such a spirit of sisterhood and affiliation, when once tapped, could have tremendous potential for encouraging mentoring. What could be a more natural ingredient for successful mentoring? And that need not be in conflict with our achievement goals of independence, autonomy, creativity, and self-actualization.

There is a whole closet of devils that women are tackling now, as they emerge stronger and more determined than ever to accomplish what they want for themselves in life. Some research has shown that women have a disposition to become anxious over achieving success because they fear social rejection. They have feelings of being unfeminine due to success—viewing competition, intellectual achievement, independence and leadership as being in conflict with the concept of femininity [23].

We have learned from other generations, that premature choices, uninformed choices, and societal mandates of a woman's role have all contributed to a somewhat halfhearted commitment to a career or work. This leaves a woman with a work life that is not her first choice nor is it commensurate with her potential. Therefore her energies cannot be channeled into building and sustaining a positive sense of self [24]. It has been this dearth of strong and positive sense of self and lack of commitment to work that have prevented more mentoring for women and for nurses. To clarify the term commitment, I would like to say that a halfhearted commitment to a career is not the same as half-time work in a career. In nursing many part-time nurses have a full-time commitment to the profession and to their potential to be creative within it. On the other hand, many nurses in full-time work situations have little or no commitment to achievement, creativity, and self-expression.

Then there are the women who have been successful, but who for several reasons have not been able to mentor others. Levinson [2] states that there are fewer female mentors because women who survive in a working world dominated by men are usually too over-whelmed by the stresses and strains of making it. They are too "burnt out" to in turn offer or provide the opportunity of mentorship to younger women. When women who are accomplished today struggled up the ladder of success, there were no other women on the top to lend a hand. Becoming successful meant learning to survive as a woman in a man's world. The price of their success has been paid in a highly defended isolation [19]. Living with defended isolation within a profession has not been conducive to mentoring others. When older women have managed to become successful there seems to be a trend to be less than supportive to the young women beginning their own careers. Many women have learned to be successful in a painful, sacrificing way and in turn cannot help younger women in a mentor relationship. The notorious "queen bee syndrome" becomes their label. Queen bee behavior is for these women, a way of coping with the demands of being a contemporary professional whose history is one of being a traditional female.

There then comes along the reluctant mentor. The reluctant mentor is one who provides some guidance to a younger person but who because of personal limitations cannot be a true mentor. I believe that there are many reluctant mentors in the profession of nursing. These are the women who see the potential in others but don't know how to foster their creativity. Rigidity, discipline, high expectations, and the inability to create an atmosphere for sharing ideas are their trademarks. Being firm and demanding may encourage competition and achievement in the aggressive nurse, but could discourage the quieter, less aggressive one who may have less ego strength. The reluctant mentor may also be a product of the socialization process in nursing. She has not learned to be an aggressive decision maker, risk taker, and pioneer of ideas, so how can she foster these traits in others?

THE ROLE MODEL: NURSING'S PANACEA

Nursing uses the concept of role model frequently during the education and professional socialization of nurses. The profession has come to rely on the role model approach for demonstrating how a competent nurse should perform, defining the place of a clinical specialist, and as a source for emulation in interpersonal and interprofessional communications. When in doubt, look for a role model. It has come to mean all things to all nurses. It has become nursing's panacea for any lag in professional growth. In a broader sense, nurses have been encouraged to search for that illusive role model who exemplifies leadership or who has mastered the successful combination of career and family life.

The concept of role modeling comes from the knowledge base of role theory and has its roots in social psychology and the psychiatric concept of identification. Role theory has been an important way of providing a framework for studying the socialization process in nursing. It has been a way of transmitting to the beginning student the recognized way of performing as a nurse and the behavior required in a nurse's role. A role model is an individual whose demonstrated skills and techniques, personal organization of values, philosophical beliefs and attitudes, and overall style and behavior is viewed by another and contrasted with his own performance. The role model is observed and compared as a standard of excellence from which the individual can learn, imitate, identify with, and somehow magically incorporate into herself [25, 26].

How is a role model different from a mentor? The key difference is in the interaction between the two people involved. In mentoring there is a relationship. In the dynamics of role modeling there need not be a relationship. The model may never speak, be supportive of, or encouraging to the young professional. The role is one of passivity. Although some are and have been helpful it is not an inherent part of the process. The relationship is based on identification, the bulk of the work falling to the identifier.

Identification, prominent in theories of socialization, is a complicated psychological process whereby a person internalizes standards of another to become his own [27]. This is first seen in the child who internalizes his parents' morals and standards to become part of his own personality—the superego or conscience. They become so incorporated into the child's personality, that he grows up believing these traits and standards are his own. The established superego now functions, praises, criticizes himself and others using this personalized standard, now part of himself. Identification, a basic factor in character formation, is primarily a method of reducing tension. It is a way of reducing anxiety by identifying with the strength and achievements of the other person [28]. This psychological mechanism, an adjustive reaction necessary for children to develop, is for the most part constructive and positive. A person learns to employ this mechanism—to identify and imitate to reduce anxiety throughout his life. When a child experiences anxiety about how to be good, the easiest thing is to be like Mom, do what she says. When a nurse is anxious about how to perform, the easiest way out is to perform as the identified role model does. Mentoring is different. It doesn't reduce the fear or the anxiety through imitation. In the space of a one-to-one relationship it makes room for alternative ways and different behavior to be explored— ways that the mentor may or may not be employing but ways that are best and most creative, self-fulfilling, and self-actualizing for the protégé.

Role modeling according to Smoyak [29], "assumes that the imitator will achieve only the level of performance or skill which has been demonstrated. Other methods are needed to develop top notch performers." Others in the health field believe that role modeling is of limited effectiveness in helping women who are established in a profession to gain positions of leadership, power, and authority within that profession [13]. Since modeling fosters imitation rather than self-development, its place is early in one's career. It is helpful in making an initial professional commitment and as a key to a successful resolution of professional identity but is limited in its purpose after that. It is not helpful in moving up, making it, or becoming a successful leader within a profession.

Shapiro, Haseltine and Rowe, who have written about role models and mentors, note that it is misleading and hopeless to search for an ideal role model [13]. It should be discouraged because there will never be that perfect person with an exact combination of professional competence and ideology and personal life style that a student can emulate. Haseltine describes this concept of role modeling as a "sociological dinosaur," arguing that at best this concept is irrelevant and that by encouraging imitation and emulation it can inhibit and be destructive to a woman's advancement. So many factors complicate the modeling process: professional speciality and interests, personal style, professional philosophy, life style, marital status, and child care responsibilities. What might have worked in the past doesn't necessarily work now or is no longer relevant for today's woman. Circumstances are significantly different. For example, 20 years ago, new mothers were encouraged to be "modern" and bottle feed their babies, quit their jobs, stay home, and enjoy motherhood. Today, not only are women encouraged to continue with their jobs and work after giving birth, but they are also encouraged to breast feed their new babies through the first year of life. No two women work out the same plan for themselves. So if women depended on role models for this situation, they would get very discouraged.

Role models should be there to demonstrate to younger women how a woman in her profession functions, what is possible, and how she has handled some aspects of her life. Role modeling should be a way of looking over the goods without buying the product.

Through mentoring, a woman could be encouraged to construct her ideal role model, an intellectual abstraction, based on her own circumstances. It is this concept of an ideal model for her—a young woman's dream—that the mentor helps to realize.

MENTORING INTO LEADERS

The concept of mentorship in nursing has the potential to become an effective, exciting, and rewarding way of developing our future leaders. If mentoring is to find a home in nursing, we must understand our image of leadership and determine how its characteristics and traits can be cultivated through mentorships. A nursing leader must be competent, decisive, able to take risks, empathetic to others, capable of motivating others to be creative, and possess a good sense of her creative self. The amount of investment in self is a crucial component of leadership. Too little an investment or lack of confidence can lead to overdependence and diffusion of leadership. Too much or egotism can produce an autocrat or one not open to others' ideas [30]. It has been shown that through good mentoring a person can learn to achieve a healthy level of self-involvement.

Other qualities that have been associated with leadership are originality, capacity for intelligence, good judgment, achievement, emotional stability, initiative, responsibility, personal confidence and work confidence, adaptability, persistence, diligence, and a desire to excel [31].

Many professionals who had mentors during their careers believe they were significant catalysts in developing their leadership talents. One group of accomplished people who were mentored recognized the following personal characteristics as necessary ingredients for leadership: the ability to make decisions, motivation and the ability to motivate others, a high energy level, ability to complete assignments, and a willingness to work long hours. Others attribute the mentoring relationship to learning to take risks, believing in a professional ideology, accepting a philosophical commitment to sharing, learning to relate to people in an intuitive empathetic way, developing a creative approach to one's work, and intellectual stimulation and inspiration.

If mentoring has been shown to be helpful in the cultivation of young leaders, how can nursing incorporate this concept into the profession? Some ways to consider are: integration into our socialization process, improved professional self-esteem, and developed nursing networks.

Socialization: The socialization of the nursing profession begins during the basic educational nursing program. It is here that the student learns what constitutes professional nursing. Faculty, students, a broad academic education, and clinical experiences all contribute to the process. But this is only the beginning. The impact of all of this is felt when the student first enters the working world. The realities of how a nurse functions, the limits of her role, and how she is perceived by others are all brought home. It is this transition from academia to working reality that nurses have found difficult. Entering the working world as a clinical specialist after completing graduate school is another critical period in a nurse's socialization. Both of these times would be appropriate for nurse mentoring. A mentor could help with the transitional process by encouraging clinical growth and the application of graduate school theories in order to advance at an accelerated pace. Nursing faculty, nursing administrators, and nurse clinicians could all function in this capacity. Leininger discusses how she frequently has invited faculty and students to experience, attend or discuss with her conflict-laden, stressful, and complicated interprofessional interaction, and dynamics as an experience in learning the machinations of real life administration, leadership and political situations [32].

Another problem with this transitional period is what Stevens calls ignored role inculcation needs in nursing. This lack of role inculcation [33] (impressing upon the mind by frequent repetition) may lead to a failure to internalize the clinical role. She notes that students are often removed from the clinical practitioner and their interrelationships with the nurse clinical specialist. A new master's-prepared graduate in nursing is still naive and idealistic about the politics of any organization. She has the knowledge and potential for functioning as a clinical specialist but often has difficulty understanding the organizational machinations and the utilization of the consultative process and the managerial process. If not recognized and addressed, the anxieties and difficulties inherent in the functioning of an advanced practitioner and change agent will soon be externalized as the nursing profession's problems. What could be more beneficial at this time than a good mentor.

Some colleges and businesses have now started mentor programs, to help with this transitional process, whereby students and novices are assigned mentors. I don't believe that mentors can be assigned. The essence of mentoring is too dependent on the chemistry between the two people to be subjected to assignment. The best that nursing can do is to be aware of what mentoring is and aware of its value in our profession. Hopefully from this consciousness, future mentorships will evolve and develop as part of our extended clinical nursing socialization.

Self-Esteem: Mentoring has not been threaded through the development of young nurse professionals for many of the same reasons it hasn't been part of the socialization of women. Being a woman's profession it has been dealing with the same issues as a profession that women have as individuals. The dichotomous split of our achievement and affiliative needs and our failure to recognize this in nursing has contributed to our poor professional self-image. In diagnosing the difficulties of the nursing profession, Rawnsley identifies poor self-esteem in professional women as the reason for projection of personal insecurities and dissatisfactions upon nursing [34]. If we do not respect, enjoy, take pride in, and feel creative in our profession how can we communicate this to other younger professionals in a mentorship.

As a defense against our poor image many nurses have found their niche in the profession and usually stay there. An inherent problem in nursing is what Leininger identifies as "ethnocentrism." The belief that one's way of interactions, interpersonal communications, conceptual framework and socialization practices are better and more desirable than others are what constitutes ethnocentric behavior [32]. Historically this has been an issue for nursing. As a profession we tend to use this concept for security, protecting and maintaining one's status. How often do we see struggling over the best way to perform a certain technique or a strong push for adopting certain nursing philosophical beliefs? How can we mentor if we adhere to such a rigid, unbending, and barren state of mind?

A concentrated, organized design to improve nursing's self-esteem is desperately needed in the profession. Only through improved self-image could the concept of mentorship be widely implemented into nursing. One way is to deal with it as one would deal with the resistance to change. One of the most common methods in trying to overcome resistance to change is to educate people and communicate ideas to help them understand the need for the change and the logic behind it [35]. This could be accomplished in one-to-one discussions, group presentations and discussions, and nursing seminars on their ideas about mentoring. When fear, anxiety, and low self-esteem lie at the heart of the problem, it is the support and facilitation through the process of change that make new ideas and approaches possible.

Nursing Network: Mentoring cannot occur in a vacuum. Its effectiveness thrives on belonging to a larger, developed professional network. Many professionals have strong informal networks for information sharing, guidance, and intraprofessional protection. Nursing, as a group, needs to value such a network and encourage it on all levels. Lucie Young Kelly calls for a "good new nurse network" [36] that would promote nurses supporting nurses. Such a network could be a source of encouragement and support for the nurse who takes risks in her professional setting. Within this environment nurses could learn to trust, share, and depend on each other more often. It could be an atmosphere conducive to the development of nursing leaders through mentoring and peer support. With a focused recognition to the fertile territory or peer support, a strong nursing network could encourage peer relationships and peer groups that could share information, review work and provide feedback, explore issues and strategies, and assist each other in problem-solving techniques. A strong network would encourage mentorships that would help the nursing neophyte to move along in the profession quickly, work more independently, and develop a sense of colleagueship sooner. We would be moving toward a mechanism that would consolidate professional strength and heighten our awareness of our potential. Howe emphasizes that nursing, one of the most important service institutions in our society, should not commiserate over the fact that it is a predominately female profession but rather capitalize on our strength in numbers. She urges the development of a consciousness of "womanpower" [15], and calls for the significant task of establishing this as a knowledgeable power base for the profession. What better way to see this potential realized and to assure its perpetuation in the next generation than by an established mentor system in nursing. Learning, sharing, and enriching lives together would surely demonstrate the strength and high caliber of our profession. Might this not be the hidden, unrecognized, *sine qua non* of future leadership in nursing?

REFERENCES

1. *Webster's Third New International Dictionary.* Springfield, Massachusetts, G. C. Merriam Co., 1976, p. 1412.
2. Levinson, D. J., et al: *The Seasons of a Man's Life.* New York, Ballantine Books, 1978, pp. 98–99, 98, 147, 333–335.
3. Felton, G.: On women, networks, patronage and sponsorship. *Image* 10(3):59, October 1978.
4. Epstein, C. F.: Bringing women in: Rewards, punishments, and the structure of achievement, in Kundsin, R. B. (ed): *Women and Success: The Anatomy of Achievement.* New York, William Morrow and Co., Inc., 1974, p. 13.
5. Women finally get mentors of their own. *Business Week*, October 23, 1978, pp. 74, 79.
6. Diamond, H.: Patterns of leadership. *Image* 11(2):43, June 1979.
7. Hennig, M., Jardim, A.: *The Managerial Woman.* New York, Anchor Press/Doubleday, 1977.
8. Roche, G. R.: Much ado about mentors. *Harvard Business Review* 57(1):14–28, January/February 1979.
9. Estler, S., in: *Proceedings of the Conference on Women's Leadership and Authority in the Health Professions.* HEW Contract #HRA 230–76–0269, 1977, pp. 197–217.
10. Zaleznik, A.: Managers and leaders: Are they different? *Harvard Business Review* 55(3):73–75, May/June 1977.
11. Everyone who makes it has a mentor. *Harvard Business Review* 56(4):89, July/August 1978.
12. Vance, C. N.: Women leaders: Modern day heroines or societal deviants? *Image* 11(2):40–41, June 1979.

13. Shapiro, E. C., Haseltine, F. P., Rowe, M. P.: Moving up: Role models, mentors, and the "Patron System." *Sloan Management Review* 19(3):51–58, Spring 1978.
14. Glidewell, J. C.: A social psychology of mental health, in Golann, S. E., Eisdorfer, C.: *Handbook of Community Mental Health.* New York, Appleton-Century-Crofts, 1972, pp. 230–231.
15. Howe, F. (ed): *Women and the Power to Change.* New York, McGraw-Hill Co., 1975, pp. 28–29, 143, 169.
16. Sheehy, G.: *Passages.* New York, E. P. Dutton, 1976, p. 132.
17. Yura, H., Walsh, M.: Concepts and theories related to leadership. *Nurs Dimensions,* VII(2):86, Summer 1979.
18. Women's colleges: Issues for the 80's. *The New York Times,* CXXIX(44):B-12, November 19, 1979.
19. Daniels, P.: Birth of an amateur, in Ruddick, S., Daniels, P. (eds.): *Working It Out.* New York, Pantheon Books, 1977, p. 59.
20. Bardwick, J. M.: *Psychology of Women.* New York, Harper and Row, 1971, p. 140.
21. Diamond, H.: Patterns of leadership. *Image* 11(2):42–44, June 1979.
22. Kjervik, D. K.: Women, nursing, leadership. *Image* 11(2):35, June 1979.
23. Horner, M. S., Walsh, M.: Psychological barriers to success in women, in Kundsin, R. B. (ed): *Women and Success: The Anatomy of Achievement.* New York, William Morrow and Co., Inc., 1974, pp. 138–144.
24. Mogul, K. M.: Women in midlife: Decisions, rewards, and conflicts related to work and career. *Am. J. Psychiatry* 136(9):1142, September 1979.
25. Love, L. L.: The process of role change, in Carlson, C. E. (ed): *Behavioral Concepts and Nursing Intervention.* Philadelphia, J. B. Lippincott Co., 1970, p. 305.
26. Hardy, M. E., Conway, M.: *Role Theory.* New York, Appleton-Century-Crofts, 1978, pp. 140–141.
27. Nemiah, J. C.: *Foundations of Psychopathology.* New York, Oxford University Press, 1971, p. 159.
28. Shaffer, L. F., Shoben, E. J.: *The Psychology of Adjustment.* Boston, Houghton Mifflin Co., 1956, pp. 174–175.
29. Smoyak, S. A.: Teaching as coaching. *Nursing Outlook* 26(6):362, June 1978.
30. Zaleznik, A.: *Power and the Corporate Mind.* Boston, Houghton Mifflin Co., 1975, p. 205.
31. McNally, J. M.: Leadership—the needed component. *Nurs Leadership* 2(3):6–12, September 1979.
32. Leininger, M.: Territoriality, power and creative leadership in administrative nursing contexts. *Nurs Dimensions* VII(2):39, 40. Summer 1979.
33. Stevens, B. J.: *Nursing Theory.* Boston, Little, Brown and Co., 1979.
34. Rawnsley, M. M.: A nursing diagnosis . . . of nursing. *Nurs Leadership* 1(2):29–33, September 1978.
35. Kotter, J. P., Schlesinger, L. A.: Choosing strategies for change. *Harvard Business Review.* 57(2):106–114, March/April 1979.
36. Kelly, L. Y.: The good new nurse network. *Nurs Outlook* 26(1):71, January 1978.

18 Mentoring

AN ENCOUNTER OF THE LEADERSHIP KIND

Patricia Chehy Pilette

I believe in Man's possibility of believing in other.
I believe in my possibility of believing in other,
   the part of other I know,
   the part of other I have yet to know.
I believe in doubt—my doubt
   forcing me to question, to be restless
   to search and examine those things which shape me
   forcing me to be uncomfortable when I am stagnant.
I believe in relating, trusting, searching and reaching.
I believe in me and I trust your affirmation of me [1].

THE DEEPEST human need is not pleasure (Freud), or power (Adler), or even meaning (Frankl). Deeper than all of these is the need to believe in self and one's abilities. That is the deepest need. And next to it is the companion, ego-hunger for self-affirmation from another. Now and then we chance to stumble into a relationship that is job-focused, profession-focused but still available, assessable, and concerned with the affirmation of our being. We call this relationship *mentoring*.

I do not have an all-embracing definition of this special relationship. For its existential nature* defies the rigid specificity of a structured role description. I have, however, become quite mindful, through personal experiences of two seemingly essential elements of mentoring.

The first is elusive, yet obvious, and, by its very nature, the most basic element. I am referring to the *human-relatedness* factor—the human presence, the spirited meeting and engagement between mentor and "mentee." The term *encounter* comes closest to capturing the richness of this fundamental element.

The second factor and possibly the quintessence of mentoring is the element of *direction* that is intricately woven into the richly textured whole of the encounter. Anyone who has experienced mentoring is cognizant of this vital element. They know it both as a direction from within, a personal responsibility, and from without, as the gentle guidance or leadership of the mentor. This special leadership by the mentor aims directly toward the emergence of the "mentee's" personal and professional actualization. If one were to identify a primary principle of professional actualization, it would be that both kinds of direction are necessary means of growth, especially in the early stages of one's career.

*The concept insists on being derived from and placed in the service of experience.

Reprinted with permission of Charles B. Slack, Inc., from *Nursing Leadership,* Volume 3, Number 2, June 1981.

It must not be inferred, however, that growth cannot occur outside of or without a mentor's direction. Such inference would strip one of personal power. It is a necessary and helpful means of growth, but is not essential. That is, it is not intrinsic to the process of growth. It is useful to think of the mentor's leadership function as much like that of a midwife who brings the innate potentialities of the "mentee" into consciousness. The mentor facilitates this birthing process, yet is not the originator of it.

The concept of mentoring first began to prick my consciousness several years ago. I was working as a consultant to a small hospital's inservice department. The nursing director, through a supportive, nurturing relationship, insured for me much personal space in which to grow and test my abilities. That initial experience and subsequent ones constitute my awareness of the importance of a mentor in one's professional development. I want to share some of what I have learned from my personal analyses and research into the mentoring process. The intent of this essay is to put some flesh onto the bare bones of this process, to examine it as an encounter of the leadership kind.

EVOLUTION OF THE MENTORING ENCOUNTER

In mentoring, the interpersonal process is the critical vehicle for the growth-related meetings. This basic fact opens the door to an exploration of the unique, interactional stages which compose the "encounter." I identify four such stages within the encounter. The meaning of mentoring lies in the arrangement of these four stages, not as isolated but as related stages, building upon each other much like the girders of a steel superstructure join together to form a meaningful pattern. Each stage possesses its own particular qualities, challenges, and leadership style. The duration of each stage is individualized with the entire span of the relationship averaging two to ten years. A mentor is a skilled guide* throughout all of the four stages.

It would seem that in order to be truly helpful as a mentor, it is necessary to understand the basic stages of the process. They are the invitational, questioning, informational, and transitional stages.

Invitational: The first stage of the encounter derives its name from the basic theme it introduces—the invitation to try out one's thinking and test out one's dreams within the boundaries of a nurturing relationship. Personal and professional qualities of the mentor are essential ingredients in the creation of this fertile, relational environment. Personal qualities such as authenticity, responsive openness, and availability help reduce the "mentee's" resistance to change and/or learning. They allow the "mentee" to self-create within her own limits. Professionally, the mentor possesses the necessary characteristics of competency, accountability, and commitment but even more important is her† effluent humanism which enlivens these qualities. After dialoguing with one's mentor, it is not unusual to come away feeling intellectually, even sometimes physically, energized or renewed in a sense of well-being.

Of course, the "mentee" also possesses certain traits which invite a mentoring relationship. Some of these are a willingness to learn, goal-directedness, and a respectful trust in the mentor. "Achieving a mentor relationship . . . is like falling in love—you can't force it to

---

*In Greek mythology, Mentor was Odysseus's counselor. Athena assumed his form when she accompanied Telemachus, son of Odysseus, whom she guided in his search for his father.
†The majority of mentors in nursing are female [2].

happen, and it only works if the chemistry is right" [3]. Like any successful relationship, mentoring requires the qualities of free choice and compatibility to cement the relationship.

Central to the "right chemistry" is the notion of *vision*. For the "mentee" her vision usually takes form as a dream or career goal she desires to achieve. The mentor is someone who has fulfilled a similar dream or dreams and is willing to share the secrets to her achievement. Not only has she accomplished her goal, she has done so within nursing's parameters. And she continues to have fulfillment in and a romance with nursing; yet she is not blinded to its problems or deaf to its critique. She is a realist with a quixotic zeal for her work. She lives her vision; contrary to most of us who live by a model instead of a vision. When the model does not seem to work for us anymore, we abandon it and are left to search for another.

A mentor is a visionary in another sense in that she "sees in us potentials of which we ourselves are frequently unaware" [4]. She lures us away from the traditional and encourages us to "grasp our own gold ring." To be a visionary in this sense presupposes an uninterrupted attention to everything that happens in the other, to all she is not able to express, and to all the anticipated good that lies within. It is the very deepest form of affirmation, one whose roots rest in empathic responsiveness.

It becomes clear early on in this stage of the encounter's development, that a mentor is a leader who enkindles a pioneering spirit and elicits a great deal of admiration and respect. She exhibits a unique charismatic form of leadership that flows between the one-to-one relationship. Her motivational power emanates from the qualities within her that are nurturing and caring and that give evidence of her degree of wholeness. The effectiveness of this kind of leadership depends upon the relational integrity of the encounter. Such leadership is, therefore, more expansive than that of an apprenticeship and preceptorship wherein this quality is not demanded. The reason for which provides a further distinction between the concepts; mentoring is not caught up, as are the other two forms of leadership, with role conformity. It is not that mentoring rejects role-modeling, the inherent component of these concepts, but that it embraces and subsequently transcends it.

Questioning: This stage of the encounter's development is marked by the appearance of dissonance within the "mentee." For many, this is a period of vacillation, anxiety, and fear of being unable to meet the expectations and goals one has set for oneself. Self-doubt forces you to question, to be restless, which leads to a deeper self-discrimination and goal analysis.

The mentor in this stage of the encounter directs the clarification process. First, she seeks to help the "mentee" define her goals, to "tangibilitate" the intangibles. Her task is assistance in the ordering of priorities and determining a hierarchy of values. Under the mentor's supervision, the "mentee" projects herself into her future in order to transcend her present condition. This allows her to formulate a more realistic plan that will be effective in getting her from where she is now to where she wishes to go. Together, they manage her goals by defining the transitional steps of the process.

Clearly, the mentor functions as a footbridge in this stage, aiding the "mentee" to reach far beyond her initial, comfortable grasp. At this point, the "mentee" begins to "discover that the answers to her self-doubts lay within; and that potential for coping was there" [5]. The mentor frequently affirms this renewed sense of self-trust through the empowering endorsement "You can do it." It has been said that a mentor is a "creator of competence" [6] and rightly so, for theoretically her positive validation can lead to a perceptual reorganization of one's self-concept.

The need for a mentor is illustrated by this stage. Very simply, she affords the necessary perspective, or distance, to reflect upon one's professional situation. A space is created within the relationship for the "mentee" to analyze the war between the part of herself that finds change exhilarating and full of hope and the part of herself that fears disruption and loss. She then negotiates a treaty and plan between the two. Strengthened in her nadirs, she can appreciate the supportive, secure space of the encounter. She is then free to move on to the next stage.

Informational: "Whether we choose administration, clinical, or educational careers, somewhere we have to learn the ropes, sense the political climate, spot the behind-the-scenes action, gain insight into the field and have a sounding board for decisions" [7]. We have to test reality. And in order to do this effectively we need a certain amount of vital information. A mentor serves a Welcome Wagon function in this stage providing the necessary information and helping us establish an effective communication network. She bolsters our survival skills in our struggles to master new and recurrent stressful situations. She is the "nurse's" advocate, especially the neophyte who is enmeshed in such stressful issues as the defining of her professional boundary, redefining herself as a professional registered nurse, and learning and incorporating the institution's particular aspects of nursing. Much assimilation, accommodation, and reconceptualization is required from her. A nurse with a supportive mentor in the workplace will find herself less stressed, better able to demarcate her professional expertise, and functioning closer to her ideals.

In this stage of "learning the ropes" there are two components necessary for one's informational repertoire. The mentor is central to both. The first is to *learn the game plan of the institution.* Generally, this implies becoming familiar with written and unwritten workplace rules. Take, for example, the nurse whose goal it is to be a primary care practitioner. For her to learn the game plan she needs to know the type of government in the institution. Is it decentralized? How effective has the governing model been and what problems have been identified since its inception? She also needs to determine if the director of nursing services evidences a stern commitment to the primary concept, and if she is hampered in that commitment. Further, she needs to know what the nursing model is. If it is primary nursing, is it practiced throughout the hospital? Lastly, she must ascertain how long the concept has been implemented. Only a person traditional to the work environment, such as a mentor, can help the neophyte answer these questions from a reliable knowledge base.

Just as important are the myths that pervade the institution. For example, primary nursing may be espoused by the institution but in reality is far from being practiced successfully and completely. Another example of an institutional myth that might abound is the notion of the "merit" raise. Is it fact or fiction? Yet another is the atmosphere of the institution—is it humanistic and nurturing? Or is humanistic just an empty adjective when applied to the institutional value system?

The second critical aspect of learning the ropes is to learn who is the *power base* nearest you. This may not necessarily be the individual next to you in a line position. Also, the type of power that person holds is important. Is it a legitimate, decision-making or an evaluative power? Perhaps, it is neither. It may be a nonsanctioned, yet motivational power.

It is important to know the power holders and their sources so as to place one's trust appropriately. In this respect, a mentor is a "power guide" [7]. She helps you establish who will help or hinder your goal achievement. It is important to note that she, herself, is not usually directly involved in an evaluative capacity with the "mentee." She may, however, informally promote the "mentee" with those who are her superiors. A mentor is not intimidated by such promotion—for she does not "fear being eclipsed by the 'rising star' she has sponsored" [8].

Transitional: There is an adage that states "the greatest good we can do for others is not just to share our riches with them, but to reveal theirs to themselves."

Like a seed that has been planted, having been nurtured in previous stages, blooms into its full development, so it is with the emergence of a fuller sense of the richness of one's being in this final stage of mentoring. The transitional stage echoes the general increased self-assertion and assumption of more responsibility by the "mentee" for her own successful achievements. Self-reliance is a change congruent with and reflective of a change in belief or the reinforcement of one's belief system. This is a time of less dependence on the mentor, which may lead, as it commonly does, to termination of the mentoring relationship. Friendship is the most natural end of mentoring.

In the initial stages of the encounter process, the "mentee" possesses abundant energy and potential, but a relatively limited repertoire of leadership, survival, and awareness skills. A great deal of energy is used for their development. In the course of the encounter, the "mentee's" numerous personal and professional capabilities (cognitive, behavioral, and affective) are defined more clearly. Each meeting provides greater strength and growth for the next; every meeting provides the basis for a more mature individualization.

The cornerstone of this final stage is the "mentee's" autonomous self-governance, which is fostered "when someone believes in you and helps you believe in yourself, in your own ability to achieve what you set out to do" [9]. The "mentee" realizes and owns the resources that are hers alone.

NURSING NEEDS MORE MENTORS

Nursing's occupational landscape is littered with burned-out nurses—nurses who are stunted in their professional development. They don't feel part of a team, feel little or no support from nursing administration, rarely receive praise, feel no one cares about their welfare, and have little opportunity to grow. The lack of psychological and professional support in our institutions is a ripe condition for stress and stress-related phenomena such as "burn out." Nurses need affirmation. Until such a need is met, they will continue to burn out.

Nursing needs more advocates from within its own ranks to keep the excitement about nursing alive. There would no doubt be fewer burned-out nurses if mentoring was a vital part of our professional system. Yet, few workplaces encourage such a relationship. Granted, mentoring cannot be "forced" onto someone but the concept can be sanctioned within our institutions. It can be articulated, legitimated, and percolated down the hierarchial chain.

Mentoring, as part of the positive feedback system of an institution, could affirm nursing actions which are creative, innovative, or just plain right. Mentors could foster the dreams and visions that nurses have about nursing so that such dreams don't just end up being light and filled with airy expectations. They could also teach the basic tool of our profession—empathy—because mentoring requires a stepping outside of oneself, slipping into the other, and then exploring, as it were, this other from the inside out.

Nursing needs the person-centered leadership of mentoring. To me, it is an agent for the humanization of the whole of nursing's leadership process. It is so, because it draws from the source water of our humanness—affirmation. Excellence in nursing can be achieved through such affirmation.

In conclusion, to divide the mentoring process into a number of stages can seem arbitrary; however, if we recognize the mentoring relationship as a gradual process of growth through relatedness, we have the basis for such division. Each stage represents the challenges and qualities which ease change into place, beginning with the more external invitational stage and continuing to each successive stage of depth until the time when the "mentee's" inner guide suffices and the mentor is no longer necessary.

Nurses have far too long suffered from a lack of affirmation. Our Nightingale flame is flickering; mentoring can be the fuel we need.

Without either being concerned about it, they learned, without noticing they did, the mystery of professional survival: they received the spirit of affirmation [10].

ACKNOWLEDGMENT

An acknowledgment to Mary T. Chehy for her helpful review of the finished manuscript.

REFERENCES

1. Wise, J.: A creed. *New Day Album.* Fontaine House, Pastoral Arts Association of North America, 1970.
2. Vance, C.: Women leaders: Modern day heroines or societal deviants? *Image* 11:40, June 1979.
3. Williams, M.: *The New Executive Woman.* New York, New American Library, 1977, p. 207.
4. Schorr, T. M. (ed): The lost art of mentorship. *Am J Nurs* 78:1873, November 1978.
5. Schorr, T. M. (ed): Mentor remembered. *Am J Nurs* 79:65, January 1979.
6. Epstein, C. F.: Bringing women in: Rewards, punishments, and the structure of achievement, in Kundsin, R. B. (ed): *Women and Success.* New York, William Morrow and Co., Inc., 1974, p. 13.
7. Kelly, L. Y.: Power guide—the mentor relationship. *Nurs Outlook* 26:339, May 1978.
8. Pilette, P. C.: The mentor relationship, letter. *Nurs Outlook* 26:473, August 1978.
9. Diamond H.: Patterns of leadership. *Educational Horizons* 57:61, Winter 1978/1979.
10. Buber, M.: *Between Man and Man.* New York, Macmillan, 1965, p. 89.

BIBLIOGRAPHY

Dean, P.: Toward androgeny. *Image* 10(1):10, February 1978.
Henning, M., Jardim, A.: *The Managerial Woman.* New York, Doubleday Co., 1977.
Levinson, D.: *The Seasons of a Man's Life.* New York, Ballantine Books, 1978.
Page, C.: The ins (and outs) of office politics. *Boston Evening Globe,* September 12, 1978, p. 23.
Sheehy, G.: *Passages: Predictable Crises of Adult Life.* New York, E. P. Dutton and Co., 1976.
Shubin, S.: Burnout: The professional hazard you face in nursing. *Nursing 78* 8(7):22, July 1978.

Section 4
Power

19 The Promise of Power

Beatrice J. Kalisch

MOST NURSES TODAY are so preoccupied with their current professional lives that they generally give little thought to future conditions, for themselves or for their profession. Yet more than half of these nurses practicing in 1978 will probably still be active in nursing in the year 2003, and the face of nursing in that year will depend on the cumulation of decisions and events that take place between now and then. Consequently, an endeavor to scan the future and attempt to forecast the condition of American nursing just after the end of this century may offer helpful insights for directing progress.

LOOKING AHEAD AND LOOKING BACKWARD

Time is a three-fold present: the present as the person experiences it, the past as the person's current memory, and the future as the person's present expectation. Obviously forecasting is not and cannot be a purely objective exercise. The future does not exist; the forecaster must try to invent it. As she does so, her suppositions about what ought to happen are intertwined with assumptions about what will and what can happen. Existing or past trends do not always define the future, since a totally unexpected happening may create some new trend that is much more important than any now recognized. Would anyone in medicine, for instance, have predicted Pasteur's discovery of microbes twenty-five years before he detected them? Or physicists have predicted twenty-five years before Hiroshima that atomic fission would be achieved so soon? Yet these two developments are among the most significant occurrences of the past 150 years.

Without exceptionally powerful evidence pointing to a radical break between past and future, most forecasting is possible only through the projection into future time of social phenomena which can be shown to exist somewhere in the present or past. A good parallel exists between the practicing nurse and the nurse who attempts to forecast the future. Just as the practicing nurse has to take into account the past health history of her patient, so the nurse forecaster has to take into account the past development of her profession.

Progress in any field is not a function of mere chronology. The earlier is not necessarily the lesser, nor the latest always the best; "modern" does not always connote the highest form of development. In the history of nursing, just as in the lives of individual nurses, there are moments or periods of great achievement, such as the establishment of the first Nightingale schools in 1873; and there are also moments or periods of decline, such as the proliferation in the early 1900s of hundreds of very weak nurse training schools, which existed almost solely to supply student nurse labor to hospitals. At various times in the future, nurses may strive to regain lost ground and may gain inspiration from certain bygone practice standards,

Copyright © 1978, American Journal of Nursing Company. Reproduced with permission from *Nursing Outlook,* January, Volume 26, Number 1.

such as the individualized "one patient/one nurse" care which characterized early private duty nursing. Thus, in speaking of progress in nursing, the forecaster is concerned not so much with the calendar as with the ongoing march of nursing toward the realization of the profession's fundamental values and potential.

In considering nursing's progress up to 2003, we are probing the principles of critical evaluation of nursing—past, present, and future. But what does "progress" mean? The word, coming from the Latin verb *progredior,* means "going forward." Now all going with nurses, as with other beings, is *not* going forward. Some crustaceans, for instance, move backward; crabs usually crawl sideways and can proceed in any direction without really turning. In the crab's philosophy of life, the term progress, in the sense of moving forward, would be confusing; forward and back, outward and in—all would be one to the crab. Many nurses, unfortunately, identify progress with vigorous movement. If the going is ceaseless and energetic, it is judged to be progressive, as with the nurse who "never lets up," or the nursing practice setting in which "something's doing every minute."

The least reflection should serve to dismiss the correlation of progress with mere energetic activity, for the most vigorous movement may be the most futile or ruinous if it is misdirected. Energetic activity and development are, of course, the means through which progress in nursing may be achieved. But to judge progress, one must judge the consequences of change: Toward what values do specific nursing activities tend?

The idea of progress emphasizing personal or collective fulfillment can be stated simply as change for the better in nursing care. American nursing in 1978 is in such a period of flux and there are so many diverse forces at work that it is often difficult to tell if the profession is moving forward, backward, or sideways.

ESTABLISHING A RESOURCE AND POWER BASE

The critical challenge facing nursing over the next twenty-five years will be to acquire a solid resource and power base upon which to move the profession forward. Ever since the beginning of the profession the absence of such a base has been the most crucially limiting force in nursing's march toward achieving its potential, and economic developments in the years leading up to 2003 will not make it easy to achieve such a base. For, by 2003, the United States will have moved away from the values of growth, extravagance, and exploitation toward sufficiency, frugality, and stewardship. In short, the principle of conservation will replace gain as the prime motive of economic life.

Economist Kenneth Boulding uses the concept "spaceman economy" to describe the future consequences of scarcity [1]. According to him, since our overpopulated globe is beginning to resemble more and more a spaceship of finite dimensions, with neither mines nor sewers, our welfare depends not upon increasing the rate of consumption or the number of consumers—both of these are potentially fatal—but on the extent to which we can wring from a minimum of resources a maximum of richness and amenity. A good life will be possible, but "it will have to be combined with a curious parsimony"; in fact, "far from scarcity disappearing, it will be the most dominant aspect of the society; every grain of sand will have to be treasured, and the waste and profligacy of our own day will seem so horrible that our descendants will hardly be able to think about us" [2].

The health care industry, and specifically nursing, will feel the effects of this scarcity perhaps even more acutely than other components of society. Health services have always been scarce, even though the health care industry has been receiving an increasing share of the gross national product. And nursing services in particular have never been available in any great abundance—not even enough to meet society's basic nursing needs.

A static financial base will intensify these health care shortages and will force the industry to use its financial and manpower resources much more efficiently. The phenomenon of scarcity has momentous consequences, of which one of the most important is the utter inevitability of politics, defined as the art and science of government, and the need for government to distribute scarce resources in an orderly fashion. Assumptions about scarcity are absolutely central to future nursing practice, education, and research; and the relative scarcity or abundance of future health resources will have a substantial impact on the character of nursing standards.

Long before 2003, the nation will be forced by the current health care crisis to solve the disproportionate outlays for health services which take funds away from other parts of the economy. In 1978, health care costs will exceed $185 billion. By 2003, unless drastic changes take place, the annual figure will be in the vicinity of $1 trillion. Consequently, the questions about *who* gets *what, when, how,* and *why* in health care will be closely reexamined and answered anew during the next decade; by the year 2003, strict limits on the resources allotted to health care will undoubtedly be mandated.

The 1978 nurse is typically apolitical, largely because her socialization places political involvement outside the purview of professional nursing. The 2003 nurse, in contrast, will be operating within a health care system constrained by increasingly scarce resources, on the one hand, and burgeoning demands for quality nursing care, on the other. If nursing is to meet those demands, then nurses in 2003 will recognize the absolute necessity to become considerably involved in the political process. They will know that nursing must acquire and maintain a fair share of the financial base available to the health care industry, today dominated almost entirely by physicians or medically dominated institutions.

IMAGINATION AND POLITICAL AWARENESS

Nurses in 2003 will have at least two fundamental qualities which are generally underdeveloped in nurses today; creative imagination (the capacity for expressing their creative potential) and political awareness (in the wider sense of a determination to define the aims of the health care industry and to markedly influence the decision-making processes). They will have been prepared for such tasks through a broadened professional socialization directed toward the development of a full awareness of the complicated workings of the health care industry, knowledge of points of leverage in helping to shape the system, and a willingness to fight for principles in the face of competing forces which threaten to undermine or dilute quality nursing care. By 2003 a structural evolution will have occurred through the advance of socially committed nursing science, shedding light on decision-making mechanisms, defining individual and collective nursing projects, and transforming ideas, opinions, and attitudes into action.

While in 1978 many politicians are little aware of the so-called nurse vote but highly aware, for example, of the school teacher vote, in 2003 the vote of the nation's two million active nurses (double the number of active nurses in 1978) will constitute a potent force with which to contend. Like the National Education Association in 1978, which brings together the collective action and influence of teachers, the American Nurses' Association and the political arm of the organization, N-CAP, will be readily associated by the nation's policy makers with the advancement of health care. Several nurses will have been elected to

Congress, and perhaps one will have won office as a state governor. Many candidates for state, local, and national office will seek endorsement from district and state nursing groups. Nurses will routinely work for the election of candidates who espouse their views.

As nursing in 2003 will be closely associated with health consumerism, politicians will find that advocacy of quality patient care and protection of patients' interests are effective means of garnering votes. Many local and state nursing groups will form coalitions with health consumer groups to elect public officials who are concerned with the welfare of nursing and health care recipients. From hospitals to public health agencies, to colleges and universities, to planning groups and regulatory agencies, nurses in 2003 will sit as members of boards of directors, will occupy positions as top level administrators, and will wield considerable power as policy makers.

Despite the overwhelming historical evidence for the rapid mortality of all institutional structures, we tend to think of the particular set of health care institutions that we have inherited and grown accustomed to as eternal, immutable, and, above all, right. They are not. Through a lack of critical reevaluation, some health care institutions and practices may persist long after the conditions that made them viable and socially useful have vanished.

The United States, with its advanced technology, substantial financial resources, and highly developed acute care services, has the potential for the best health services in the world. That potential, however, is far from completely realized, since we lag behind many industrialized countries in caring for our citizens' health, as measured by vital health indices. More than two dozen other countries have a higher life expectancy for males, while about half this number rank above the United States in life expectancy for females. At least a dozen other countries have a lower infant mortality rate, and nearly a dozen have a lower maternal death rate. The same disparity is evident among population groups within the United States.

RESOLUTION OF THE HEALTH CARE CRISIS

Described as the "most rapidly growing *failing* United States industry" in 1978, health care faces a crisis of momentous proportions [3]. Millions of Americans now receive virtually no health care, and millions of others receive it only sporadically. Most health care is delivered at staggering financial costs and, in many cases, with unnecessary suffering. For millions of Americans—the poor and near poor who live in rural or inner city areas—the medical care system is not merely inadequate; it is almost nonexistent. On any measurable health index, the poor and racial minorities fare much worse than the rest of the population: higher mortality rates, greater incidence of major diseases, and lower availability of medical services.

It is clear that the United States cannot continue to tolerate this situation, wherein the availability of health services is too frequently determined by financial means or geographic location. Health care should be regarded not as a privilege, but as a basic human right for all citizens, and access to health care should be seen as a corollary to the right of life itself.

The present health care crisis, which will have to be resolved between now and 2003, comprises interacting problems that exacerbate each other through various kinds of threshold, multiple, and combined effects. Thus, the complexity of managing the combination of problems has grown faster than any particular problem itself. Such a labyrinth is already taxing nurses' cognitive skills and will continue to do so through 2003, since a premium will be placed on analyses and evaluations of various courses of action and independent judgments in developing the most effective means of implementing quality nursing care within the shifting health care complex.

Nursing input into current efforts to solve health care problems is notably lacking, despite the fact that about one out of every 200 Americans (or 1 million) is an active registered nurse. Delays, failures of planning, and a general incapacity on the part of nurses to deal effectively with even the current range of health care problems are all too visible today. Nursing's ability to cope with large scale complexity will improve substantially by 2003, however.

Undoubtedly, a system of national health care, embracing cradle-to-grave health insurance, will develop on an incremental basis, building on Medicare and Medicaid as they exist in 1978, moving next to maternal-child care and then to comprehensive population coverage. This system will closely adhere to the principles of cost effectiveness.

Greater use of the services of nurses will occur as they will provide primary care to large parts of the population. Emphasis will be placed on prevention, and the major locus for health care will be ambulatory settings, not hospitals; thus, nurses in 2003 will provide much more care on an ambulatory basis than they do today. Physicians will be employed on a salary basis to provide specialized medical services, mostly of an acute care nature. Some physicians will still carry on a lucrative private practice by catering to the wealthy few who choose not to receive health care underwritten by the government.

EXPANDED NURSING PRACTICE

The expanded scope of nursing practice in 1978 already encompasses certain functions that have been traditionally performed by physicians. Nurses practicing in this new role have generally recieved specialized preparation beyond their basic or graduate programs. By 2003, these "expanded" functions will have become an integral part of the nursing role and of nurse preparation programs. The increased responsibility will be generally viewed, as it is today by some nurses, as an opportunity for the nurse to enlarge the informational base that serves her as professional foundation for nursing assessments, diagnoses, and interventions.

Under a system of national health care, nurses will be considered cost effective by policy makers, not only because their salaries will be lower than physicians, but also because the preventive, wellness-oriented care that nurses offer can save millions of dollars in diseases prevented and can significantly upgrade the quality of life for millions of Americans. This type of care will be increasingly sought by consumers, in contrast to the biomedical model, which emphasizes the treatment of acute disease and explains disease solely in measurable biological terms. The biomedical model represents a rather recent view of illness—most people aren't aware that it is only about a century old—but it nevertheless forms the conceptual basis for most health care in America and has a tremendous impact on health policy.

Even though this model prevails, the word "health" is often used so imprecisely and inaccurately that it leads to misunderstanding and to false expectations. "Health center," "health examination," "health promotion," and "health insurance" are terms commonly misused today. In each instance, the activities encompassed by these designations are largely concerned with problems of disease. And the institutional frameworks within which nurses function today concentrate almost entirely on biomedical patient services and de-emphasize the supportive, preventive, and psychosocial tenets of nursing, which have been downplayed since they were espoused by Florence Nightingale.

TECHNOLOGICAL INFLUENCES

Biomedical technology is growing rapidly, but it will have become obvious by 2003 or before that medical technology cannot be improved indefinitely without encountering limits of scale beyond which further improvement is of no practical value. Some technologies in medicine are already near this point and the rest soon will be, for the expensive substitution of one ever more efficient form of technology for another simply cannot continue forever.

In effect, the better the existing technology is, the harder it is to improve upon. How much further will the current thrust in biomedical technology run? It can hardly continue indefinitely if the past is any guide. Trends at some point begin to reach a limit, and turn into the common S-shaped curve which has its kinetic analogue in the motion of a pendulum.

Although a condition of diminishing returns will prevail, some significant technological breakthroughs will continue. By 2003, transplants will have become very popular with the hundreds of thousands of debilitated people needing new limbs, hearts, lungs, and other organs. Spare-parts surgery will be limited only by cost, the number of surgical teams available, and the supply of spare parts.

At the same time, such surgery will give rise to difficult moral and legal problems that the nurse will be expected to help resolve. Which of the many patients in need should receive a new organ? Should there be an open market for kidneys? Or just a black market? Should an individual be free to decide whether his organs can be transplanted at death? Or should relatives be allowed to make money by selling his heart and lungs? Other new technologies by 2003 may include:

artificial hearts, perhaps as common as artificial limbs are today.
synthetic skin for burn injuries.
regeneration of bone and eventually of vital organs.
laboratory-synthesized whole blood substitute for emergency transfusions.
implantable brain-stimulation devices to control appetite, induce sleep, and relieve head-
aches.

Diminishing returns will clearly be seen, however, for the more scientific work that is done, the more likely it is that new theories will be corrections or refinements of previous ones, necessarily leaving most of the old structure of knowledge intact. Thus, new knowledge may not be translatable into new technology. By 2003, some additional advances will have been made against mental illnesss, arthritis, degenerative vascular disease, and some cancers; but the billions of biomedical research dollars will have yielded so few practical, cost-effective breakthroughs that biomedical, disease-oriented research will have given way to prevention as the major research and development focus.

Nurses will logically play a pivotal role in conducting this research. This is not to say that an ongoing program of biomedical research will not exist but rather that a far greater share of research resources will have to be allocated to preventive and psychosocial solutions.

THE NURSE HERSELF

The personal characteristics of the nurse will also undergo marked change. In 1978, the *majority* of nurses are still characterized as submissive, dependent, malleable, conforming, and "mild-mannered." By 2003, the *typical* nurse will be described as confident, independent, autonomous, and even assertive. Nurses will be regarded as health professionals in their own right, who are as valuable to society for their unique contributions as physicians are for theirs. Nurses will be much more willing to accept responsibility and accountability for their performance than they are today and will engage in independent practice as well as in cooperative decision-making with physicians and other health care providers.

Unfortunately, some physicians will still resist the nurse's egalitarian role on the health care team. The years between 1978 and 2003 will be characterized by some degree of conflict between physicians and nurses as health care roles are realigned. Government guidelines for health care providers will help in the resolution of differences. Nurses' involvement in institutional politics and their ability to tolerate the anxiety associated with confrontation will, of necessity, greatly increase.

A MAJOR CHALLENGE

We confront a major challenge during the next twenty-five years, and we should not deceive ourselves about the magnitude and duration of the task. No one nurse, no one development, no one invention can supply more than a small piece of the eventual solution; the final result will be a mosaic of mini-elements, some designed by nurses, others fashioned by the accidents of history. Progress in nursing has been and will continue to be a zig-zag. No sooner has one obstacle to professional fulfillment been removed (such as large scale exploitation of student nurse labor), than others have loomed up (such as access to third party payments). Any satisfaction that is gained will always release new needs so that the unending battle will have to be joined again and again.

Only by postulating goals and understanding why we select those goals rather than others can we assess the ways in which change in nursing interacts with change in society—whether the change be large scale, such as a radical revamping of the health care system, or small, such as a new nursing intervention for a particular type of patient. Of necessity, an assessment of our goals involves forecasting. We want to know just how the change will or will not fulfill our postulated goals, not only now but also into the future—for one, two, or even three generations. To do this requires some exercise of the imagination, some movement out of the quantifiable into the unknown.

REFERENCES

1. Boulding, K. E. The economics of the coming spaceship earth. In *Beyond Economics: Essays on Society, Religion and Ethics,* ed. by K. E. Boulding. Ann Arbor, University of Michigan Press, 1970, pp. 275–287.
2. Boulding, K. E. Is scarcity dead? *Public Interest* 5:36–44, 1966.
3. Califano, J. A. What is wrong with U.S. health care. *Congressional Rec.* 123:E4281–E4283, July 1, 1977.

20 Identification and Explanation of Strategies to Develop Power for Nursing

Nancy D. Sanford

EVERY NURSE appointed to a health systems agency board has some measure of power. The nurse may or may not attend board meetings, committee meetings, and briefing sessions, may or may not read the thick packets of information received regularly, may or may not seek input from other nurses, may or may not study in depth the controversial issues before the board, may or may not influence the HSA board and staff. Every nurse has this measure of power. It is not nearly enough.

Every nurse on an HSA board has the opportunity to study the strategies used by those who wish to maintain the "status quo" in the health care system. These strategies are well described by Berg [1]. They are as follows: (1) Emphasize the great American tradition by saying that any attempt to change the system is 10 miles down the road toward "socialized medicine." (2) Shift coalitions according to the issues. For example, if the issue is deleting obstetrical beds, seek out religious group coalitions. (3) Emphasize professional elitism. It is difficult for the non-professional or even the less powerful professional to counter charges that only physicians and administrators really understand the complexity of the system well enough to sift out what is good for society. At the same time, keep the language at a technical and statistical level so that all but the most courageous challengers are prevented from entering into the discussion. (4) Charge inadequate data to support change. HSA staff are so busy striving to interpret and comply with regulations that they really don't have time to collect data, and the data available are inadequate in most cases, so the charge is successful. (5) Threaten impending disaster if any hospital beds are denied funding. The public is easily alarmed by such threats. (6) Pack the audience with opponents of a proposed change.

The nurse on the HSA board can study these strategies and use them with equal skill in reverse, or plan to cut them off by careful preplanning. That is not nearly enough.

The nurse can even go beyond these strategies and use those employed by planners who do want change [2]. These include: (1) Focus on a few crucial issues. No person can obtain sufficient information on all health issues. The nurse must, as do effective legislators, select a specialty and gain a reputation for knowledge in that health planning area. (2) Attack one target area at a time. Once the target is established the nurse must stick to the game plan. The nurse must decide who counts and who does not count in regard to achieving the victory. (3) Use eminent good reason backed up with very good homework. HSA board members and staff are impressed with anyone who knows the facts and states them clearly and objectively. (4) Externalize the conflict by bringing in outside experts to give a different perspective on the issues causing conflict.

From *Power: Nursing's Challenge for Change,* American Nurses' Association, 1979, pp. 15–26. Reprinted with permission of American Nurses' Association.

The nurse can become quite skillful in using these strategies. It is still not nearly enough, if we are to develop power for nursing.

In October 1977, 24 nurses with varying degrees of involvement in California HSAs met together to determine how to get more power for nursing. This issue was so important that most of the nurses traveled at personal expense.

We determined some priorities. Our personal priority was to develop political ability, our professional priority was consumer advocacy, and our health care priority was comprehensive health care. We decided that we wanted to become involved as powerholders, not just participants. We felt that would be enough.

Over and over again, throughout the conference, we became aware that we had to learn more about the realities of politics, or more precisely, the realities of power.

There isn't much written about power. It is as if to write about the inner workings of power is to reveal too much. One of the few scholars willing to study power and then candidly write about it is Adolf Berle. He was an intimate advisor to Presidents Franklin Roosevelt, Kennedy, and Johnson. He has had close contact with many other powerful people as well. In his study of power, Berle discerned five natural laws of power [3]; they are (1) power invariably fills any vacuum in human organization, (2) power is invariably personal, (3) power is invariably based on a system of ideas or philosophy, (4) power is exercised through, and depends on, institutions, (5) power is invariably confronted with, and acts in the presence of, a field of responsibility.

Berle found these laws of power to be valid whether applied to the head of a family, the head of a business, or the head of government. The laws of power are just as relevant to the nurse who would be a powerholder on an HSA board as to a politician who would be president.

To identify and explain strategies to develop power in nursing it is necessary to study these laws in more detail.

POWER INVARIABLY FILLS ANY VACUUM IN HUMAN ORGANIZATION

Power fills a vacuum because humans desire peace and order. People are willing to give power and money to those who seem able to bring order out of disorder and chaos. In fact, powerholders sometimes deliberately create chaos (choosing wisely) so that they can then step in and exhibit excellent leadership qualities and win wide support.

Power fills a vacuum because a certain instinct for power resides within nearly everyone. Whenever a power vacuum exists, many people reach out to fill it. Eventually one person must defeat the others, or win them over by some promise of a share in the power, once obtained. The winner is one who really wants to be a powerholder. If the winner does not appear to have that desire, then we must look behind the scenes and determine who placed that person in the "apparent" powerholder role.

Power comes forth when assertive people, with an idea that matters, and a group capable of being organized come together. That person who can express the idea in such a way to mobilize the group and direct the efforts of the other assertive people is the powerholder. When power fills the vacuum, it becomes a reality and it has an impact on the community.

Nurses have a deep desire to fill the vacuum that exists in the field of health care planning. We have assertive nurses, we have over a million nurses capable of being organized, and we have an idea that matters. For example, we believe in comprehensive health care. We believe that every individual has a right to information about preventive and corrective health measures. We believe that people have a right to health services in which they have a voice in making decisions [4]. Surely most people would agree that a power vacuum exists within the health care system in regard to prevention and informed consent, because chaos, disorder, and neglect reign.

Before we move to assert our power, however, it would be wise to consider our history. Krause [5] relates how nurses have made six major attempts to fill a power vacuum in the field of health care: (1) We have attempted to gain autonomy by educating nurses in university settings but have found we still can't control our practice as do physicians in medical schools. We are still restrained by laws that say our practice must be performed under the general supervision of physicians. (2) We took on all the "dirty work" (and then passed it down to L.V.N.s, aides, orderlies, and others) and still found that although we had some people below us in the hierarchy, it did not move us up any. When nursing took on anesthesiology we made it seem attractive enough that the physicians stepped in and took it over, claiming the ultimate expertise. (3) We assumed the managerial position and said, "Our role is to manage what happens in the health care setting." That was OK until we made it attractive enough that both physicians and hospital administrators stepped in and claimed the ultimate authority. Even still, we made it attractive enough so that non-nurses have stepped in and claimed greater managerial skill. (4) We attempted the outside mover strategy and sought to serve the community through visiting nurse service and made it attractive enough so that hospitals stepped in and purchased nearly all of the nurses and their services. (5) We seized the technology and made ICUs and CCUs a successful reality, but hospitals own the technology and physicians dominate the hospitals. (6) We have sought power through unionization but we have made that so attractive that hospitals buy off the nurses with small salary and benefit increases rather than give up any control over patient care. And, we have made it so attractive that labor unions are stepping in to offer their services, and their price is looking good to the average nurse.

Krause and others believe that nurses can achieve power in spite of past failures [6, 7]. Nurses may find power in the HSA, because we are organized, because we do have an idea, and because we are respected by the community.

As we move forward, however, to fill the power vacuum in health care, whether it be by an idea about prevention, care of the aged, or something else, we must anticipate that when we make it attractive, others will attempt to wipe us out. We must anticipate that and be prepared to hold our own.

What if we replaced our "Year of the Nurse" billboards and signs with other signs reading, "Nine out of every ten patients in convalescent hospitals suffer from either bedsores, constipation, depression, incontinence, or perineal rash. It doesn't have to be that way. Ask a registered nurse how these problems can be eliminated through better health care planning."

What if, concurrently, we sent letters to all nurses, giving them a briefing on the issues and a model reply to offer the public?

In recent times all great powerholders have turned to the masses for support of their ideas [8]. The general public does not want their parents, or other loved ones, to suffer from bedsores, constipation, depression, incontinence, or perineal rash.

Then if need be, the next sign might read, "Guess who doesn't want to help eliminate bedsores, constipation, depression, incontinence, and perineal rash? We're getting lots of pressure from the nursing home industry, physicians, the drug industry, the hospital supplies industry, the paper supplies industry . . . Help us prevent illness! Call 555-2370."

Isn't it more than a little scary to confront that much power, that much money? Can we, could we, fill the vacuum? We have nurses in large numbers and we have ideas that matter. We have to identify those nurses who are powerful enough to organize us well enough to hold our own and more, against those who have always managed to keep us and our ideas subservient.

POWER IS INVARIABLY PERSONAL

Power is an attitude; it doesn't exist without a powerholder. No class of people, no minority group, no elite group, can achieve power or use it, without organization. Behind that organization is a person. Power is invariably personal.

Power comes when someone is vested with it, through appointment or election, by an institution, or when an individual brings power into existence, by developing an institution and thus becoming its leader.

Power, the ability to make others do as you wish, in an effort to obtain a goal, has only two limitations [9]; they are (1) extraneous fact (or everything else going on in the world) and (2) conscience or intellectual restraint (deciding what you cannot or what you will not do). How the nurse powerholder will react is invariably personal.

Nurses have a long and fine tradition of service to others. Our credibility is good and we are viewed as being concerned about patients and without a vested interest [10]. Thus, the public would likely place trust in the nurse powerholder.

Knowing that power is invariably personal, will nurses support one of their own in attaining power? Norris says:

While pettiness, put-downs, backbiting and sabotage among nurses are usually blamed on the nature of the interaction among women when they are thrown together, I personally believe that women are as loving and know as much about loving as men—if not more. I believe that their rage, destructiveness, jealousy and intolerance of others' success arises out of centuries of subjugation as women and more than a century of put-downs as nurses. . . . We need to restructure our behavior, hard though that is, so that we encourage, foster, indeed demand the movement of our nurse colleagues into status positions, power positions, prestige postions—where they are closer and closer to where the power is and where the real decisions are made. [11]

It seems to me we are ready to support the nurse who will reach out for power and grasp it. It seems to me we are ready to support the nurse who will, using subtlety, cleverness, and exquisite timing, grasp the power and hold on to it. The question is, will we recognize it when we see it?

In 1976, in Atlantic City, a debate raged on in the ANA House of Delegates about direct membership. A nurse stepped onto the mike platform and said with all the dignity she could muster, which is considerable, "Jo Elliott, Colorado." She then proceeded to explain in very clear and simple terms why the three-tiered membership structure was important. I'm sure that many delegates did not know of the power she once held and still held, but they did know she was a powerful woman. The vast auditorium was hushed, and then applause exploded. Had the vote been taken at that time, the issue of direct membership would have been soundly defeated. However, a delegate who didn't know a thing about timing, but did know that she had been standing at the mike a long time, chose to say her speech too. The moment was lost. Debate raged again and a compromise was later made.

Power is an attitude, timing is a gift; both are essential for effective leadership. We can teach a nurse content; we are rarely successful at teaching timing. Will we recognize it when we see it?

Why didn't organized nursing recognize Anne Zimmerman's charisma, timing, and political skill 20 years ago? Why didn't we put her in the ANA presidency then—and fill every publication we owned with her picture and her quotes—and then why didn't we place her in the House of Representatives or Senate (if she had been willing)?

POWER IS INVARIABLY BASED ON A SYSTEM OF IDEAS OR PHILOSOPHY

Without an idea, an institution cannot be created nor can it continue, *and* without an institution, power cannot be generated or expanded. Furthermore, the idea must be one that attracts followers, gains their loyalty, and brings forth their time and energy.

We have an idea, a national policy for health care [12]. Will it turn anyone on? I believe, for example, that prevention and care of the aged are timely ideas. Is that enough? Do enough nurses care? Do enough people care?

The major reason we have inadequate care for the poor, the aged, the minorities, and the rural population is because that isn't where the money is [13]. A recent political cartoon [14] tells where the money is—the money is in cancer and heart disease. More about that later.

If we are to enter the power arena of health care, we have to know where the money is and where the power is (and they will be found together). Let us consider that for a moment.

Ginzberg [15] tells us that since the government is now the source of more than 2 of every 5 dollars expended for health care, the health industry is, and will remain, in the political arena. We have to consider what that means if we are to enter into that arena. Nobody talks about it directly. It means that for any significant health care issue, the politicians count votes. And they don't just count heads. They also take into account who will most likely protest a change and actively organize against it. From experience they know that those who stand to lose are much more likely to organize than those who stand to gain [16].

Consider next Dahl's report in *Who Governs?* [17] of how a cancer agency funded anticancer drug development to fight existing cancer but was unwilling to fund basic research to find out the cause of cancer, research that might *not* bring profit to a corporation, but that might *prevent* the development of cancer in the first place, totally eliminating it as a source of profit.

What if we did find a cure for cancer, for heart disease, for the common cold? Consider the economic complications for our society. Consider how many people would be out of work. Consider how many nurses would be out of work. Are we ready to deal with that? I believe we may be, if given the facts. I believe that more than any other health care group, because we have seen so much pain and suffering, vomit, bile, sweat, sputum, and despair, that we MIGHT be willing to make a financial sacrifice to prevent illness.

We must not go naively into the political arena of the health care industry. In 1976 we spend $638 per person, or a total of $139 billion, on health and its many facets [18]. Where the money is, the power is, and powerholders don't give it up easily.

During my term on an HSA board I learned that the idea of Public Law 93-641 is to improve the level of health, encourage a healthful living environment, and provide for the availability and accessibility of high quality services at reasonable cost for all residents.

A logical, thinking nurse would anticipate, therefore, that money, time, and energy would be devoted to finding out (in each community) who isn't getting care, what kind of care they need, and what is quality care anyway? I received and read many pages of material, but very little of it had to do with these basic issues. I ponder over why, out of all the health planning issues, CAT scanners and kidney dialysis machines capture so much print? Our society is not likely to turn away from newer technology. In the meantime, people continue to need availability and accessibility of high quality services at reasonable cost. I feel "had" sometimes.

I bring up these hot issues because the nurse on an HSA board cannot hope to achieve power if he or she does not have some insight into the subtleties of power and economics.

Ginzberg says, "The health care system cannot be significantly modified by *any* single change, even one so sweeping as national health insurance" [19]. I'm not so sure. If the people had advocates, who really let them know what is happening, then might the people say, "I'm mad as hell, and I'm not going to take it anymore." Is our idea, our vision of the way it ought to be, strong enough?

POWER IS EXERCISED THROUGH AND DEPENDS ON INSTITUTIONS

The powerholder must either work through an existing institution or build a new one. There is no other way to exercise power beyond one's own personal space.

The powerholder must give considerable time and loving care to the institution *because* an institution does not support a powerholder unless it gets something back in return.

The powerholder must constantly remind the institution that he or she fulfills a need no other could fill as well. Whenever the powerholder falters, someone else is ready to fill that vacuum. The powerholder must either squash the opponent (hopefully with cleverness, good humor, and grace) or be squashed.

The powerholder must delegate power if it is to be expanded, and each portion of delegated power must enhance the power of the powerholder. When it does not, the powerholder must resolve the problem or else falter, and then withstand the next challenger.

As you can see, that is a lot of work for the would-be nurse powerholder on an HSA board, for she or he must please two institutions, the HSA and organized nursing. That takes time (and timing), political skill, and tremendous desire.

Whether we like to face it or not, the nurse must know who to talk to, how to talk to them, and who to call upon to speak for them at the appropriate time. If power is invariably personal, and if power is through and depends upon institutions, then we must teach nurses how to mobilize the institutions.

Barritt says that if nurses are to be effective powerholders in HSAs, we must prepare them better. We need to teach them about humanity and the nature of the profession. We have to design curriculums that provide knowledge of economics, political science, urban and rural planning, and health economics, and they must share classes with other health professionals [20].

The president of a great university, who by nature of his position places other men in presidential positions, always gives them one bit of advice, to read Machiavelli's *The Prince* at least once a year [21]. I wish someone had given me that advice. We don't talk much about Machiavelli in class or in the nursing literature. Perhaps it is as Max Lerner says:

May I venture a guess as to the reason why we still shudder slightly at Machiavelli's name? It is our recognition that the realities he described are realities. . . . Let us be clear about one thing: ideals and ethics are important in politics as norms, but they are scarcely effective as techniques. The successful statesman is an artist, concerned with the nuances of public mood, the approximations of operative motives, with the guesswork as to the tactics of his opponents, and with back-breaking work in unifying his own side by compromise and concession [22].

In order to make the rules better, you have to know what the rules are; in order to modify the rules to your advantage, you have to know what the rules are; in order to win the contest, you have to know what the rules are. Society has been all too willing to protect women from the harsh realities of the rules of power. Physicians, hospital administrators, and college presidents have been all too willing to protect nurses from the harsh realities of the rules of power.

Some nurses do learn the rules of power, modify the rules, and win with the rules. Some use the power more graciously and more humanely than others. So it has always been.

Our society wants certain things and is willing to accept the rules of power to get them. There isn't any trend to change that, but some groups want greater participation [23]. Nursing is such a group.

POWER IS INVARIABLY CONFRONTED WITH AND ACTS IN THE PRESENCE OF A FIELD OF RESPONSIBILITY

A recognition of the field of responsibility, and the organization of a communication system within that field, with the powerholder, is what leads to a democratic power base. When any significant group of people is not included in the communication system, tension builds up.

The powerholder must enter the field of responsibility and through persuasion, argument, example, favor, or force attempt to maintain power. This power is very personal. The positive or negative reactions of the people in the field of responsibility have a potent effect upon the powerholder.

Berle [24] tells how President Woodrow Wilson mastered the power position of presidency of the United States, but couldn't handle the senior power position in the world, at the Paris Peace Conference. He says Wilson's illness, like Roosevelt's, was the result of unendurable strain that made them particularly vulnerable to disease. He further states that in 1933 he saw a number of rather obscure men suddenly thrust into power. The results were more devastating than most people know. Some of these men survived, others never recovered. The opinion of those in the field of responsibility has great potency.

The powerholder must strive to appear calm, cool, informed, and capable at all times. And this is the fact, no matter how much we may want to deny it.

The powerholder must make contact with the intellectuals in the field; in our case, nursing. This communication will enhance the powerholder's resources. The nurse on the HSA board will sometimes have to make a decision on the lesser of two evils. At such a time it is comforting to have some intellectual advice.

I believe the ANA commissions would be willing to connect the appropriate nursing intellectuals with the HSA nurse, if asked, and if the need was clearly stated. For such a liaison to work, however, the nurse powerholder must be very sure of her or his own sphere of knowledge.

Power is invariably confronted with and acts in the presence of a field of responsibility. That is a full-time job in itself. The only significant channel of communication within nursing is through ANA and its component parts. And then we are faced with the problem that only two in ten belong, and few of those read the information sent out. Most nurses know, however, that even if they do not belong, ANA speaks for them and fights for them. In fact, our communication system may work better than we think.

In the fall of 1977 it looked as if nursing might obtain a measure of power. Representative Martha Keys introduced a bill providing for the inclusion of registered nurses in policymaking PSRO groups. The federal government promised to back the bill. At the hearing on H. R. 3167, however, the HEW representative withdrew his active and specific support. Quite obviously someone counted votes and decided that both Representative Keys and ANA were less powerful than their opponents.

I read about this blatant putdown in the November issue of the *American Journal of Nursing*. The very next day I was one of only two HSA board members willing to spend a morning meeting with a representative of the federal government who wanted to know how we were progressing and how the government could help us. After a while I said, "The health care industry seems unwilling to change and we have heard reports that certain groups of physicians have spent large amounts of money to have consultants assist them in developing strategies to wipe out the effectiveness, if any there be, of PSROs and HSAs. How can we trust anyone? He replied, "You've got a problem, but you can count on us, that is why we passed this law." I then said, "I understand Dr. Goran promised to support a bill to include nurses in PSROs and then pulled out at the last moment." This man nearly fell apart, as they say, and then he said, "How did you know about that?" He then went on to say that he had been involved and that he felt "really rotten" about it. Now, I know that when I receive my *AJN* it is not brand new news, but this representative of the federal government was totally surprised anyone in California would know about what happened in Washington during the hearing on H.R. 3167. What if we used the power of our press to carry out one good idea? The time is right. They don't think we are paying attention, and it is for sure they pay very little attention to us.

The rules of power are becoming clear. If we are to share the power of the HSA we must: (1) Fill a power vacuum. (2) Place powerful people in the powerful positions. (3) Further develop and promote our idea of comprehensive health care. (4) Exercise our power, our ideas, through our institutions of organized nursing, all of them. (5) Expand and enhance the communication within our field of responsibility, nursing.

I suggest we start by asking all of our families, friends, employees, colleagues, and students to say, when admitted to any health care facility, "I prefer my care to be given by a member of the American Nurses' Association." When asked why, they will reply, "Because I understand they believe in prevention."

REFERENCES

1. Berg, Robert L. "Movers" and "Statics" Refine Political Strategies in HSAs, *Hospital Progress* (September 1977), 68–69.
2. *Ibid.*, 67–68.
3. Berle, Adolf A. *Power*. New York: Harcourt, Brace & World, Inc., 1969, 37–134.
4. *A National Policy for Health Care: Principles and Positions*. Kansas City, Missouri: American Nurses' Association, 1977.
5. Krause, Elliott A. *Power & Illness*. New York: Elsevier North-Holland, Inc., 1977, 52–56.
6. *Ibid.*, 56.
7. Berg, *op. cit.*, 65.
8. Haley, Jay. *The Power Tactics of Jesus Christ and Other Essays*. New York: Grossman Publishers, 1969, 19–20.

9. Berle, *op. cit.,* 60.
10. Berg, *op. cit.,* 65.
11. Norris, Catherine M. *The Survival of Nursing 1975 and Beyond.* Paper presented to the California Nurses' Association, Region 10, Fort Ord, Calif., May 17, 1975.
12. *A National Policy, op. cit.*
13. Norris, *op. cit.*
14. Hamilton, William. Political cartoon. *San Francisco Examiner & Chronicle,* Sunday Punch, April 16, 1978.
15. Ginzberg, Eli. *The Limits of Health Reform.* New York: Basic Books, Inc., 1977, 6.
16. *Ibid.,* 22.
17. Dahl, Robert A. *Who Governs?* New Haven: Yale University Press, 1961, 257.
18. Ginzberg, *op. cit.,* 17.
19. *Ibid.,* 22.
20. Barritt, Evelyn R. *The Health Planning System—Its Impact on Nursing.* Paper presented at the National League for Nursing Convention, Anaheim, Calif., April 26, 1977.
21. Berle, *op. cit.,* 82.
22. Lerner, Max, in the introduction to Machiavelli, Niccolo. *The Prince and The Discourses.* New York: The Modern Library, 1950, xliii-xliv.
23. Berle, *op. cit.,* 20.
24. *Ibid.,* 122.

21 Patient Power and Powerlessness

Phyllis Beck Kritek

SEVERAL YEARS AGO I was employed as a scrub nurse in a small general hospital operating room. During that one year experience I often found myself wondering about the activity in which I was engaged. A recurring theme of my thoughts centered on the patient, a curiosity or uncertainty about how so intrusive an experience affected the person upon whom we operated. Many of the subjective experiences of surgical patients not only seemed somewhat mysterious to me, but also were not a clear part of "nursing knowledge" in a formal sense. These thoughts rushed back when I faced the fairly certain knowledge that I was about to experience that mystery. As a coping response, I decided to record carefully all the subjective experiences I was undergoing in the hope of identifying phenomena that would improve professional nursing's understanding of patients. This paper is an attempt to analyze the data collected, to make sense out of the diverse, sometimes contradictory, subjective experiences of one person as patient, and to place these data in some meaningful theoretical framework.

THE EVENT

One typical Friday night, our family, enjoying the closure of another hectic week, decided to go to a local family restaurant for a fish fry. I ate my meal with some abandon, forgetting that for several months I had some digestive problems with fried foods, cabbage and alcoholic beverages. Early Saturday morning I awoke with acute abdominal pain. By noon I was sitting in an emergency room doubled over, admitting to a family history of early gall bladder disease, confessing to months of half-denied symptoms and listening to tales of elevated serum amylase and WBC. I was admitted by one o'clock. After being tested and discussed for five days, my gall bladder was surgically removed. Five days later I was discharged. This paper is an analysis of my subjective experiences of that event.

THE METHODOLOGY

Somewhere between the emergency room and the admission X-ray, the decision to collect data on this experience took shape. I discussed my decision with my sister (also a nurse) who was waiting within the X-ray department. From that discussion, the focus of "patient powerlessness" emerged. Once admitted, I made the following additional decisions:

1. I would attempt to record subjective experiences of all phases of the hospitalization.
2. I would attempt to place in my field notes uncensored material, *i.e.*, I would write in journal fashion exactly what I experienced.

Reprinted with permission by *Supervisor Nurse: The Journal for Nursing Leadership and Management*, June 1981.

3. I would write field notes only when alone, attempting consciously to focus on and memorize events as they occurred and record them as soon as possible. I decided that since I was collecting data on my own experiences, with all their admitted subjective distortions, I would not identify myself as a researcher to the hospital personnel.

4. Although I would focus in particular on powerlessness as my subjective experience, to avoid censoring or losing important data, I also would record any event that seemed really important but which did not relate in terms of powerlessness. Such data could be dealt with later in the analysis state.

5. Because my level of feeling well, and therefore, my ability to take field notes might be uneven during the hospitalization, I would have to take notes as possible.

6. Although some analysis might occur during the experience, I would not initiate analysis early. I already sensed the stress I was experiencing and did not know how distorted such an analysis might become. In addition, I did not want premature analysis to lead to a censoring of important data.

These decisions set the stage for data collection. My sister brought the necessary materials and I wrote my initial field notes Saturday at 4:00 P.M. Some notes were recorded each day of the hospitalization except the day of surgery and the first postoperative day. The notes for the second and third postoperative days are somewhat sketchy; the fourth postoperative day writing was more extensive, including an effort to recall the previous four days. The most detailed notes are available for the day before surgery and the day before discharge. The former may have been a response to imminent surgery. The latter are very extensive because I spent most of this day recording anything I believed to be important, because the stimulus of my role as patient no longer would be available.

Some analysis occurred during this last day of hospitalization. After discharge, I avoided the notes for two weeks, largely because I was grappling with integrating the experience and its implications. When I finally read the notes I found myself somewhat embarrassed by some of them—and amazed at how many experiences I already had denied or distorted in my postoperative resolution.

Since that time until the writing of this report, I have repeatedly reread the notes, studied them and reconstructed and reconceptualized this experience in terms of the issue of patient powerlessness. I have shared the notes and analysis with many persons, both nurses and non-nurses, and a few other field researchers to assess my analysis for both distortions and clarity. This entire process has been influenced to a very high degree by the methodological protocols described by Schatzman and Strauss (1973), Webb *et al.* (1966), Lofland (1971), and Glaser and Strauss (1967).

LIMITATIONS OF THE STUDY

The issue of researching subjective experience runs the risk of a high degree of researcher bias. This risk seems more than balanced by the risk of continued nursing practice which negates or ignores patients' subjective experiences that threaten wellness. Increased awareness of these experiences could lead to substantive modifications in nursing care and to the identification of new avenues of nursing research.

In addition, some personal characteristics seemed important modifiers of researcher bias. The most influential is a tendency toward introspection and analysis of self as an object, enhanced by ten years of psychiatric nursing practice and educational experiences. Other factors within the research situation seem to function both as potential assets and potential limitations. They are recorded here to aid the reader in placing limits on the known researcher bias inherent in the study.

MY IDENTITY AS A NURSE

Although my identity as a nurse was advantageous in collecting data, understanding the experience of hospitalization and providing some natural links with personnel, it was also a deterrent to objectivity. It made my experiences somewhat atypical, both as they occurred and as I experienced them. I found myself in some instances sympathetic to hospital personnel because "I understood." Sometimes I resented having to be so sympathetic. Sometimes I was very critical *because* I understood.

My identity as a nurse was known to staff (I had been admitted both to ER and the unit by alumni of the school where I teach). The head nurse also noted that I was identified as a nurse educator on the chart. These facts doubtless colored my experiences, though it is difficult to ascertain clearly how and to what degree. It was my impression, and the impression of several visitors, that it seemed to increase avoidance behavior on the part of hospital personnel.

MY IDENTITY AS A PATIENT

In many respects, this factor seems most significant. First there is the inevitable bias, distortion flowing from being ill. However, since an attempt is made here to understand subjective experiences of a patient, these distortions become useful data about how patients distort. In addition, patient status can decrease access to information. Kardex, chart and nursing report information are to some degree, inaccessible. Interpersonal exchanges are given a one-person bias. Yet, again, these limitations clarify what patients do not know and how this affects them.

Finally, objective analysis of data depends on the postoperative integration of this experience. Adequate time for integration should have facilitated a relatively objective analysis of the experience.

MY ATTITUDE TOWARD POWER

Since, for many years, I have been concerned about maintaining power over my own personal existence and reluctant to relinquish control of my personal fate, this factor seems an important source of researcher bias. I knew that I would be very conscious of intrusions on or limitations of my personal control. On the other hand, there was the very real possibility that I would experience power issues where other patients would not. Acknowledging that quandary, I considered the fact that there are doubtless many levels of concern about power. My data would be useful to nurses caring for persons at my end of the spectrum. In addition, although many patients may not be conscious of or able to articulate power concerns, they still may experience and be influenced by such concerns.

CODING

In an effort to assure anonymity of the persons described in this report, all hospital personnel are identified by code only; the initials used are not their actual initials.

THEORETICAL FRAMEWORK

The theory of social power selected for this analysis is that of French and Raven [1]. Price notes that empirical efforts relative to the bases of power stem primarily from their work [2]. French and Raven were influenced by the work of Lewin for whom the concept of power was synonymous with influence [3]. Subsequent cooperative work with Cartwright, using Lewin's construct, also influenced French and Raven, who actually use Cartwright's definition of power as a starting point for their theory: "Power is a relation between two agents, O and P. It is concerned with the maximum influence which O can exert on P at a given time to change in a given direction" [4]. This definition of power is used to guide the data analysis.

The focus is placed on the social relationship or interaction involved in the exercise of power. As Warren states, "French and Raven defined the basis of power as the relationship between a person subject to power and an agent or person exercising that power" [5]. This description tends to create an image of a fairly strict dichotomy wherein the agent exercising power in the relationship remains constant, as does the agent subject to power. This is not, in fact, the case. In a later discussion of theory, Raven describes power as "potential influence" [6]. Either party in a social interaction has such potential, *i.e.,* "it is possible for O to have power to influence P and for P to have less power, equal power or greater power to influence O . . . Power is not inherently general and diffuse; locus and focus must be specified if predictions are to be made" [7].

French and Raven view the bases of power from P's perspective, *i.e.,* the bases of O's power as P perceives them. This particular vantage point is useful to the nature of this study. Although the data were collected by only the patient in the social power interchange, the data may describe the patient as either O or P in French and Raven's terms. Hence, where the patient functions as a person subject to power, the perceptions are direct; when the patient functions as an agent exercising the power, the perceptions of the health care system as P are inferred from the exchange.

Indeed, the data support this. With no previous knowledge of the above theoretical constructs, I recorded those factors which I viewed subjectively as either increasing or decreasing personal power in my new role as patient. In subsequent data analysis I discovered a trend. Those factors that I viewed as increasing my power focused primarily on means of controlling the health care system, *e.g.,* my knowledge base and organizational contacts. Those factors that I viewed as decreasing my power focused on the health care system, its demands and my feared inadequacy in meeting such demands, *e.g.,* fear of being a "bad" patient or of being independent and then abandoned. The picture shows a not-totally-powerless person versus the system. In retrospect, the interactions where the patient functions as a power-exercising agent appear minimally influential. Yet they provide some clue to the subjective interpretations of power that patients may generate for themselves.

The efforts of French and Raven were an attempt to refine further the social interaction conceptualization of power into a taxonomy of power that could provide a basis for further research. These five bases of O's power are [8]:

Reward power, based on P's perception that O has the ability to mediate rewards for him or her;

Coercive power, based on P's perception that O has the ability to mediate punishments for him or her;

Legitimate power, based on the perception by P that O has a legitimate right to prescribe behavior for him or her;

Table 21-1. Bases of Social Power Distribution (patient subject to power—health care system exercising power)

Power Base	No. of Incidents/Interactions	Percent of Total
Coercive	27	38
Legitimate	18	25
Referent	10	14
Expert	8	11
Reward	8	11
Total	71	99*

*Due to rounding error.

Referent power, based on P's identification with O;
Expert power, based on the perception that O has some special knowledge or expertness.

Based upon this category system, French and Raven have explicated further each type of power basis and explored empirically some of the relationships between the power bases. Their findings, where applicable, are related to the data analysis.

DATA ANALYSIS: THE PROCESS

Field notes recorded during the 11-day hospitalization were separated into discrete items on cards. Cards then were sorted according to French and Raven's taxonomy into incidents of interactions descriptive of one or another bases of power. This sorting was done for two types of O: the patient and the health care system. Each set was studied for common themes or patterns. The remainder of this paper discusses the results of that analysis. Because the majority of incidents or interactions were categorized as either coercive or legitimate power, these bases will be dealt with first. The remaining three bases will be discussed later. While not quantitatively sophisticated measures, Tables 21-1, 21-2, and 21-3 indicate the relative distribution of categorized interactions or incidents according to French and Raven's taxonomy.

Table 21-2. Bases of Social Power Distribution (health care system subject to power—patient exercising power)

Power Base	No. of Incidents/Interactions	Percent of Total
Coercive	13	33
Legitimate	10	26
Referent	6	15
Expert	6	15
Reward	4	10
Total	39	99*

*Due to rounding error.

Table 21-3. Bases of Social Power Distribution (total incidents)

Factor Subject to Power	No. of Incidents/Interactions	Percent of Total
Patient	71	65
Health care system	39	35
Total	110	100

COERCIVE POWER

"Coercive power is based on P's belief that O has the ability to mediate punishment for him" [9]. From the view of the health care system as O, the data indicate the largest number of incidents involve the system perceived as exercising considerable coercive power. A clear pattern emerges. Punishment was perceived by P, the patient, as unnecessary or unfair control—and the threat of its increase.

The most intense experiences of powerlessness as a patient centered around an inability to control the time of surgery. Admitted on Saturday, I had hoped for surgery by Wednesday at the latest. On Wednesday it was scheduled for Thursday. By Tuesday I felt consciously powerless. The field notes record repeated expressions of this. Tuesday's last entry reads "Very angry, very bitter, very trapped—hurt; up 'til 12:30." Interestingly, the notes also reflect a preoccupation with discharging myself. "In the case of threatened punishment, there will be a resultant force on P to leave the field entirely" [10].

I also perceived the health care system to be controlling my access to information. Although health care personnel were aware of my status as a nurse (which I erroneously had assumed would increase my access to information), I discovered that the physicians provided minimal responses to my questions and became somewhat irritated when I pushed for details. Nursing personnel, whom I also perceived as displeased with my questions, withheld information such as vital signs, even when it was solicited. I was afraid that they would withdraw from me further. My questions steadily diminished throughout the hospitalization. In the last few days I asked no questions and actively began to withhold information which I thought "they" might use to control me. Although I had abdominal muscle spasms and active evisceration fantasies, I feared that if I shared these facts they might make harmful judgments about me—and also withhold the information about the judgments.

Patient safety seems to be an obvious concern and yet, it may be perceived as a not so obvious expression of coercive power exercised by the health care systems in its relationships to patients. The patient P perceives the health care system O as possessing a significant degree of control over one's health status. At its extreme, this is perceived as control of one's life.

As the hospitalization wore on, the number of notes referring to this type of coercive power increased. On the third day of the hospitalization, I met the nurse assigned to my P.M. care through the following exchange.

NURSE: (cheery and smiling) "Hi, you're stuck with me tonight!"

ME: (taken aback, I emerged with my best sarcasm intact) "I like your direct appraisal of the situation."

The covert coerciveness of her message evoked my timed sarcasm, supporting French's contention that coercive power decreases attraction [11]. Two days later I recorded a second equally coercive exchange with Nurse L that took place the night before surgery.

NURSE: "So I don't forget, I wanted to remind you to be sure to cough and deep breathe after surgery. We've been kinda lax about that on this floor so we're really cracking down."

ME: "Oh, really" (noncommittal, using my best psychiatric nurse nonjudgmental tone of voice).

NURSE: "Yes, the last five choleys we've had on this floor had pneumonia so we're really working on getting our postops to cough and deep breathe."

ME: "Oh, really" (I'm keeping the same weird voice, but now I'm amazed).

NURSE: "Yeah, they never let us have surgicals but we insisted. Medical patients can get so boring."

ME: "Well, it's certainly a relief to know I'm not boring" (the sarcasm again).

NURSE: (Laughs) "Oh no, you're really pretty interesting. Well, I've gotta go."

I was offended and irritated by her comments. I perceived them as threatening to my health, musing peevishly that I was grateful that I wasn't scheduled for open heart surgery. Despite these intensely negative feelings toward Nurse L, I never communicated them to her. As Warren notes, "One of the key elements of coercive power is the indifference or opposition of those subjects to the wielder of coercive power. He is not likely to inspire attitudinal conformity so he must function in a high visibility condition for his authority to be effective" [12]. Interestingly, the notes also reflect that my major early postoperative preoccupation focused on coughing and deep-breathing. Indeed, my entire postoperative course of action was guided by doing precisely those things which assure one of a rapid recovery. I resented and feared these activities, yet performed them almost compulsively. This, too, supports researchers' claims about the effect of coercive power. "The extreme degree of conformity did not always correspond to acceptance of the supervision. In some cases hostility and personal rejection of the supervisor were accompanied by compliance. Where communication is restricted, overcompliance may be the only way of communicating disagreement with an order" [13].

The final major category of coercive power which I perceived the health care system to be exercising focused on sensory input and contacts. By the very fact of hospitalization, contacts were diminished and narrowed and sensory input decreased. As my world shrank, I felt increasingly unable to make judgments without distortion. I gradually felt forced to relinquish personal views, knowledge and expertise. Increasingly, I became *the patient*. Although originally I saw myself as fortunately deviant because I was a nurse-patient, by discharge this position had been eroded seriously. I increasingly conformed to the hospital's norms for patients. Raven discusses this deviate position and its erosion through social influence, where the deviate begins to "perceive selectively and distort items of content so that he perceives an ever increasing body of content supporting the group norm, and fewer items supporting his own initial position" [14]. Despite my firm intent to be an assertive patient, I had the following exchange with my day nurse, Nurse D, at discharge:

NURSE: "I wish all my patients were like you."

ME: "Really! Why do you say that?"

NURSE: (serious tone) "Oh, you were just so easy to take care of, and you got well so fast. So many of ours are so old and they never get better. You're really cheerful and fun too."

ME: (smiling sarcastically) "You like all that sarcasm, huh?"

NURSE: "Well, you took care of yourself. You weren't always asking for something. You know that lady down in (number of room given). She has me running the whole shift. You just can't keep her happy."

I envied the courage of the woman down the hall—such was the impact of the health care system's coercive power.

Reversing power roles, the notes indicate that the patient's exercise of coercive power fits quite logically into the picture just sketched. Although the largest number of patient power notes refer to coercive power, they show a remarkable sameness in behavioral pattern.

Repeatedly, my exercise of coercive power was precipitated by anger with the health care system. However, my anger was self-defeating and ultimately unsuccessful. On admission, I initially refused to let the nurse start an intravenous on me because it assaulted my "I'm not sick" denial system. Eventually she did start the intravenous. I tried to push several persons to set a time for surgery. Ultimately, they set it in their own way, at their own time. By the third day of my hospitalization, I defiantly ignored hospital rules and smoked in my room. For the remainder of the hospitalization I increasingly viewed this infraction as dangerous and behaved regressively about it and because I was worried about getting caught, hid my ashtray, I recorded "always close door, lots of guilt—back home, 12 years old. . . ." Each postoperative night I stayed up later and later and ignored offers for sedatives and kindly comments about the value of sleep. I acted defiant and regressive.

All of these entries speak to coercive power expressed through noncompliance. In retrospect, it seems a desperate, self-destructive attempt to maintain some sense of control, some capacity for decision-making. Given an adequate level of frustration and powerlessness, any exercise of control, even a self-defeating one, became attractive.

LEGITIMATE POWER

Incidents listed in the second major category of power were those connected with the exercise of legitimate power. "Legitimate power of O/P is here defined as that power which stems from internalized values in P which dictate that O has a legimate right to influence P and that P has an obligation to accept this influence" [15].

A certain amount of legitimate power was exercised by all members of the health team because I was a patient. As I gradually stopped denying that I was ill and took on the patient role (albeit reluctantly), more and more filed note entries refer to exchanges where I concede that one or another person is permitted to exercise control because, after all, I am a patient.

The first overt evidence of the gradual, pervasive impact of legitimate power was recorded on the third day of hospitalization when I received flowers from my work colleagues. I was upset and wrote "my self-concept is under assault." I was becoming a patient. The role of patient involved known, prescribed norms. In this way, as I increasingly acknowledged being a patient, I gradually conceded legitimate power to the health care system. In this sense, legitimate power was a relationship between roles. I eat distasteful food, live in a small room for several days, ingest or am injected with unknown chemicals, permit persons to cut open my abdomen, walk about with a cut-open abdomen and leave the hospital—all in response to others unexplained directives. Perhaps this is exemplified best by my self-initiated shift in postoperative pain medication. Sometime in the afternoon of my first day after surgery, I became aware that every time I received Demerol, nurses were offering me Percodan. I decided that that was something I was supposed to do soon after surgery, although I didn't really know their reasons. That night, I requested Percodan. I was commended, and never again saw Demerol.

This incident highlights and exemplifies Raven and French's distinction between legitimate and coercive power. "Legitimate and coercive power are similar in that each produces initial changes which are dependent upon O, the influencing agent. That is, even if P does not see the reason for the change, or accept the intrinsic value of the influence, he will nevertheless conform, in order to avoid punishment (coercive power) or because he accepts the right of O to influence him (legitimate power)" [16].

French and Raven refer to cultural values also serving as a basis for the exercise of legitimate power [17]. Several field notes are relevant to this contention. They relate to my culturally determined values about quality health care. One intern, three nurses and one aide effectively and consistently exercised legitimate power over me throughout my hospitalization because their behaviors were compatible with my values. The intern provided me with desperately wanted information about my likelihood for surgery. One nurse, a former student, showed a personal interest in and acceptance of my frustrated reaction to hospitalization, and provided me with an article about my rather uncommon diagnosis. The second nurse took a personal interest in my well-being in the recovery room because she was requested to do so by my sister who was also a nurse and had worked with her. The third nurse provided me with calm, competent, complete care the day of surgery. The aide gave me my only back rub during my hospitalization, and engaged me in a personal, interest-conveying conversation. My notes record extensive praise of and cooperation with these people. I was most unquestioningly compliant when interacting with these persons. I recall our interchanges vividly, but I had very brief encounters with each of them. Interestingly, Raven and French note that observability and visibility, while essential for coercive power, are not essential for the exercise of legitimate power [18].

The field notes show that when power agent roles were reversed, my exercise of legitimate power over the health care system was characterized by one overriding pattern. All examples are role related, *i.e.,* involve the legitimate exercise of power by a patient. Because I am a nurse, they were doubtless defined by experience of what the patient role entails. Thus, I exercised some control in a gradual modification of diet by griping about the liquid diet, an acceptable patient gripe. When the nursing personnel joked about my complaints, I would complain even more. Subsequently, my diet was modified. Far more irritating to me was the fact that three days of dirty linen piled up in my bathroom and no one removed it. This I did not gripe about. It was not role-appropriate in this hospital. French and Raven's observation is relevant here. "The attempted use of legitimate power which is outside of the range of legitimate power will decrease the legitimate power of the authority figure. Such use of power which is not legitimate will also decrease the attractiveness of O" [19].

Another of my attempts to exercise legitimate power speaks even more eloquently to this point. Nurse D, whom I affectionately referred to in my notes as "my invisible day nurse," came in with an OR permit the day before surgery. I began reading, viewing myself as exercising the legitimate power of the patient to protect her rights. She became overtly uncomfortable.

NURSE: (said rapidly, anxiously) "It's just a standard permit, there's nothing different in it."

ME: (Her comment angered me; I responded too sweetly, with a smile) "Never sign anything until you've read it . . . I'm sure you've heard that somewhere."

Nurse D seemed eager to "get out, to distance." She offered no information on surgery, so I began asking questions. I later recorded: "Tendency not to have clear answers—implied I don't need them or already have them; common line used: 'It's hard to tell.'" As she hurried out, she apologized saying that she had a great deal to do. "We've had so many people in today. Every time I look there's something else on the chart."

A second incident that evening again showed the effects of attempting to exercise legitimate power outside one's range of power. In this incident I was attempting to control the system's definition of my response to surgery. As I was about to retire, a religious sister who does "pastoral counseling" came to discuss my surgery with me. She was shy and tentative and I felt embarrassed for her. I tried overly much to be courteous.

SISTER W: "I guess you must be somewhat anxious about facing surgery."

 ME: "Not really; I think I'm a lot more concerned about my kids and their adjustment. The thing that's bothered me the most has been waiting here five days for the inevitable. I am really stir crazy."

SISTER W: "Well, sometimes when we're very anxious the only way to deal with our anxiety is to deny it. Do you think you might be doing that?"

 ME: "No, not really. I just don't like being here so long." (I'm feeling giggly—this is so bizarre!)

SISTER W: "How many children do you have?"

This exchange continued, essentially unchanged, with her persistent efforts to encourage me to admit my anxiety. My overwhelming response to surgery had been eagerness and relief, but it was not expected, so it was not legitimate.

These last two incidents demonstrate the effect of inadequate knowledge of the limits of the patient's legitimate exercise of power. Although I made a few comparable "errors" in judgment, the notes generally reflect that, as I began to identify with the patient role in this specific hospital, I became increasingly adept at exercising legitimate patient power. I often contrived these exchanges and settled for compromise in terms of my power needs, *e.g.,* enthusiastically and confidently requesting the written guidelines for post-discharge health behaviors while secretly harboring fear and ambivalence about discharge.

REFERENT POWER

Referent power has its basis in the identification of P with O. Although fewer notes refer to this power base, those that do have a common pattern—they all are contingent on my personal identity as a nurse. Thus, they probably are atypical. However, their characteristics seem noteworthy. As a nurse identifying with the health care system, I found myself, especially early and late in the hospitalization, tolerating inadequacies because I understood. I often resented this fact but persisted in understanding. My fourth day postoperative notes have two major focal points: the inadequacy of the health care system workers and my careful attempts not to tell them of their inadequacies. It appears that the reason these factors were so pronounced was due to my exercise of referent power over the system. The nursing personnel gave me an unusually high degree of control over my postoperative course of care—far more than I wanted. A persistent message was, "Well, you know that anyway," even when I said I didn't. Hence, my dressing went unchecked, my input and output unmonitored, my ambulation unsupervised, sometimes my medications uncharted. Although all of this angered me, I told no one. As Warren notes, "Visibility can be low because individuals subject to referent power share goals and need not be observed or supervised" [20].

The quandary secondary to a mutual exchange of referent power is reflected succinctly in one of my last field note entries before discharge. "As my power increases, I'm nicer, friendlier, convivial, humorous, one of the girls . . . *very empathic* . . . I keep saying these dumb things to the nursing staff about how well they're doing—commend them to excess all over the place—even makes me nauseous. Why do I feel a need to make them all so comfortable? I compose a letter of gratitude to the Director of Nursing Service in my head. I do it to protect them. I perceive them as needing it." According to Deutsch, "Referent power seems to be most diffuse and more likely than any of the other bases of power to enable the power wielder to affect a wide range of activities of the person being influenced" [21].

EXPERT POWER

Expert power is based on P's perception that O has superior knowledge and perception [22]. The range of expert power is somewhat limited since P evaluates O's expertness in relation to P's own knowledge as well as against an absolute standard [23]. My status as a nurse may explain why this category has few field note entries, a fact that may not be so readily reflected in the notes of a researcher without health care education or experience.

Health care personnel exercised expert power over me only when they demonstrated clearly that they possessed information which I did not have, or had skilled services to provide. In the latter instance, the informational control goes beyond the purely cognitive function French and Raven describe [24] to the actual skillful intervention based on the expert knowledge. Thus, the health care system exercised expert power over me not only in the fairly cognitive activity of diagnosing my illness, but in the far more powerful manipulation of my person through a surgical procedure and postoperative care. Some nurses exercised this power. More often than not, however, I interpreted the nurses as less expert than myself in terms of information. This seems particularly linked to the fact that I thought that none of the nurses ever collected enough data on me to make an accurate nursing diagnosis of my needs. Hence, I viewed their expertise as relatively useless to me.

On discharge, I was subject to self-doubt. I regretted that I really never had access to their expertise. I wrote: "Perhaps my eagerness to 'get out' was excessive, perhaps I couldn't handle it and I'd have a relapse." I also discovered that I still wanted the nurses somehow to intuit my needs and meet them. The essence of my discharge nursing was a congratulatory cheer on the fact that I was going home. I wrote: "Am ready to say goodbye to my jail—only partly. . . ." Although nurses exercised little expert power over me, I discovered I had very much wanted it.

My exercise of expert power over the health care system was linked again to my status as a nurse. The only entries relative to this are early in the hospitalization while I was still denying the possibility of surgery and "playing patient." I decided that playing patient was a lot like playing house—if you knew the rules. I decided I was an "in for diagnostic testing" patient. I washed up, brushed my teeth and hair, straightened the room a bit. I circled the rectangular unit several times. I greeted others cheerfully and politely. I watched my performance and commended myself on how well I played "in for diagnostic testing." I was able to exercise some temporary control over my fate largely because I knew the rules well enough to ritualize them and succeed. It was a temporary and ultimately ineffective, exercise of patient power.

REWARD POWER

Reward power refers to power whose basis is the ability to reward [25]. Warren notes that it requires a fairly high level of visibility [26]. French and Raven write that reward power is contingent on P's perception that O actually can and legitimately mediate the reward [27]. Given that very real constraint, little evidence of reward power is reflected in the field notes. The only clearly evident reward I perceived as available from the health care system was discharge, and I worked very actively to earn it. I was not aware of how intensely I sought this reward that I perceived as mediated by both nurses and physicians until the day before discharge when my internist stopped in to say goodbye. He commented that I had an excellent postop response and teased my husband about making sure I took it easy. He called me "Superwoman" throughout the discussion. The new label confused me. That afternoon several comparable messages were sent by nursing staff about my rapid recovery and what a wonderful patient I was. Only in retrospect did I recognize the extent of the reward power that the system exercised.

My attempts to exercise reward power as a patient generally were unsuccessful. I have several entries where I describe myself trying positively to reward health care givers whom I judged as effective. Thus, I commended the lab technician on a "good stick" when she was drawing blood. Her response was educative in nature—she gave me a mini-course in quality "sticks." Only in retrospect did I realize that patients cannot mediate positive rewards by congratulatory behavior. The only concrete reward I believe I successfully mediated was to leave. This discharge event appeared to please the staff, to make them feel successful. Once the order for discharge was written, staff members who previously had been relatively invisible suddenly began to stop by to congratulate me on my early discharge and to wish me luck. I was bemused, but this sudden enthusiasm for my departure and my apprehension was building: I had exercised reward power by getting well but had lost access to help. I also began to focus on my physical state. My evisceration fantasies persisted. My pain was minimal but I still had difficulty getting up and down in bed; I couldn't even imagine doing without bedrails. I still was having occasional muscle spasms which irritated me. As I calmly exercised reward power over the health care system, none of these problems was expressed—or met.

CONCLUSIONS

This study demonstrates that French and Raven's theory and taxonomy of social power may be a useful tool for analyzing patient-health care system power interactions and their characteristics. A second conclusion involves the distribution of power interactions. While quantitative strength of these data is limited by post-hoc categorization of complex interactions of a single case study, the high incidence of coercive power appears noteworthy as does the lower incidence of expert and reward power.

Some very specific patient control issues emerge from these data. Subjective experiences of patient powerlessness evolved around the health care system's control of time, scheduling, environmental stimuli, information and a patient's alterations of self-concept and roles. The patient most effectively exercised power when the patient role, as defined by a specific agency, was assumed and role expectations were met. Sensory deprivation appears to be a variable which strongly influences the exercise of patient power.

Relative to this, a patient who gradually is resuming power over self after its extensive diminishment may be quite ambivalent about such a resumption. Although regaining power may be actively sought, the sense of vulnerability created by a serious illness can influence a patient's perception of the attractiveness of that power.

A final obvious conclusion flows from the fact that nursing literature contains little empirical data about patients' subjective experiences of power and powerlessness. Given that this case study may be somewhat atypical, these data indicate that there is a rich array of empirical data available from patients and that these data could alter nurses' behaviors and attitudes.

IMPLICATIONS

The implications of this study are extensive and will not be exhausted. The most evident implications flow from the final conclusion. Nurse researchers could profit from exploring patient perceptions concerning power as a means of enhancing the profession's knowledge base and intervention repertoire. A useful theory and taxonomy of power already has been generated. What we need now are controlled, well-planned studies of patient powerlessness in terms of that theory and taxonomy. In addition, patient power and powerlessness could be studied as they relate to other variables as indicated in the study. These variables include the amount of patient-nurse contact, the level of patient sensory deprivation, patients' recovery rate, patients' perceptions of role changes, patients' length of hospitalization, nature of patients' illness and the extent of external patient resources. Certainly the patient not only can be, but "ought" to be a major data source in the nursing profession's efforts to add useful information to the growing body of knowledge that we call nursing science.

REFERENCES

1. French, John R.P., and B.H. Raven. "The Bases of Social Power." In Cartwright D. (Ed.). *Studies in Social Power*. University of Michigan Press, Ann Arbor, 1959, pp. 150-67.
2. Price, James L. *Handbook of Organizational Measurement*. D.C. Heath and Company, Lexington, Massachusetts, 1972.
3. Lewin, Kurt. "The Conceptual Representation and Measurement of Psychological Forces," *Contributions to Psychological Theory*, Vol. 1, No. 4, 1938, pp. 1-247.
4. Cartwright, Dorwin. "A Field Theoretical Conception of Power." In Cartwright D. (Ed.). *Studies in Social Power,* University of Michigan Press, Ann Arbor, 1959, p. 194.
5. Warren, Donald I. "The Effects of Power Bases and Peer Groups on Conformity in Formal Organizations," *Administrative Science Quarterly*, Vol. 14, No. 4, December, 1969, p. 545.
6. Raven, Bertram H. "Social Influence and Power." In Steiner I.D. and Fishbein M. (Eds.). *Current Studies in Social Psychology*. Holt, Rinehart and Winston, New York, p. 317.
7. Deutsch, Morton. "Field Theory in Social Psychology." In Lindzey, Gardner and Aronson, Elliot (Eds.). *The Handbook of Social Psychology: Vol. 1*. Addison-Wesley Publishing Company, Reading, Massachusetts, 1954, 2nd ed. 1968, p. 460.
8. French, John R.P., and Bertram H. Raven. "The Bases of Power." In Hollander, Edwin P. and Raymond G. Hunt (Eds.). *Current Perspectives in Social Psychology*. Oxford University Press, New York, 1963, 3rd ed. 1971, p. 525. (Excerpted from French and Raven, 1959).
9. Cartwright, Dorwin. "Influence, Leadership, Control." In March, James G. (Ed.). *Handbook of Organizations*. Rand McNally College Publishing Company, Chicago, 1965, p. 28.
10. French and Raven, 1965, *op. cit.*, p. 527.
11. French, John R.P. "Laboratory and Field Studies of Power." In Kohn, Robert L. and Elise Boulding. *Power and Conflict in Organizations*. Basic Books, Inc., New York, 1964, pp. 33-51.
12. Warren, 1969, *op. cit.*, p. 547.
13. Raven, Bertram H., and John R.P. French. "Group Support, Legitimate Power and Social Influence," *Journal of Personality*, Vol. 26, No. 1, March, 1958, p. 409.

14. Raven, Bertram H. "Social Influence on Opinions and the Communication of Related Content," *The Journal of Abnormal and Social Psychology,* 58 January 1959, p. 128.
15. French and Raven, 1963, *op. cit.,* p. 528.
16. *Ibid.*
17. *Ibid.*
18. Raven and French, 1958a, *op. cit.,* p. 84.
19. French and Raven, 1963, *op. cit.,* p. 529.
20. Warren, 1969, *op. cit.,* p. 548.
21. Deutsch, 1968, *op. cit.,* p. 400.
22. French, John R.P. "A Formal Theory of Social Power," *Psychological Review,* vol. 63, No. 3, 1956, p. 184.
23. French and Raven, 1963, *op. cit.,* p. 531.
24. *Ibid.,* p. 532.
25. *Ibid.,* p. 525.
26. Warren, 1969, *op. cit.,* p. 548.
27. French and Raven, 1963, *op. cit.*

Section 5
Politics

22 Power in Structured Misogyny

IMPLICATIONS FOR THE POLITICS OF CARE

Jo Ann Ashley

So while I do not pray for anybody or any party to
Commit outrages,
Still do I pray, and that earnestly and constantly,
For some terrific shock
To startle the women of this nation into self respect
Which will compel them to see the abject degradation of
Their present position;
Which will make them proclaim their allegiance to women
First;
Which will enable them to see that man can no more feel,
Speak, or act for woman than could the old slave holder
For his slave.
The fact is, women are in chains,
And their servitude is all the more debasing because they
Do not realize it.
O, to compel them to see and feel.
And to give them the courage and conscience to speak and
Act for their own freedom,
Though they face the scorn and contempt of all the world
For doing it.

SUSAN B. ANTHONY, 1870

INTRODUCTION

The purpose of this article is to show how misogyny, or the hatred of women, has been historically structured throughout human experience and to interpret how this structured misogyny affects our current politics of care. In confronting destructive elements in patriarchy, nurses must intellectually and emotionally come to grips with the extent to which patriarchal ideas, institutions and practice weaken and destroy nursing's power, practice and ability to exercise effective politics in care. Coming to grips with the damaging effects of patriarchy is necessary before nurses can begin to visualize new ways of thinking, acting and being at home and at work.

Within patriarchy the power of structured misogyny keeps women in their role of glorified servants to men—keeps them oppressed in subjugated domestic roles living out

Reprinted from *Advances in Nursing Science* by Jo Ann Ashley by permission of Aspen Systems Corporation, © April 1980.

the cult of true womanhood. Great women scholars and writers have for centuries recognized and analyzed this basic fact and its effect on the course of human history. The present generation of women scholars has built on this heritage and is now showing more clearly than ever how misogyny has been structured into patriarchal relations, philosophies, theories, myths, language and totality of human experience. They have shown how misogyny has contributed to the destructive course of history and why we now seem to be at the end of a patriarchally founded civilization.

Since the vast majority of nurses are women, our first concern must be that of analyzing the various forms of violence leading to the constant destruction of the mental and physical health of women. Remaining deaf, dumb and blind to the suffering and destruction of our own kind is agreeing to the political dominance of those who wish to continue destroying the strengths of women.

EARTHLY AND HUMAN DEVASTATION

We are living in a time period when the exhaustion of the earth's resources, when disregard for human and nonhuman life are rapidly leading to forms of earthly and human devastation, such as dehumanization by computerization and nuclear destruction, which are hard to imagine by the American mind. We live in a society that no longer values the capacity to care for human life. Our society values technology, machines and its structures of steel and concrete more than it values life itself [1].

Humans are not made of steel. They are not made of cement or of concrete. They live. They breathe. They feel. Humans are not made of wood or of iron. They bleed when cut. They cry when badly hurt. They fear when fright takes hold of their hearts. The structure of the human body and mind is such that it requires nourishment to survive. Both body and mind require an atmosphere and environment conducive to the maintenance of life. We live in a society that negates this. Our society overlooks the nature of human beings and the nature of the earth on which we live [1; 2, p. xi].

Slowly but surely, writers and scholars are beginning to take note of the limits (i.e., the seeming inability of people in general to reverse the exploitation) surrounding the exploitation of the earth's resources and of human life. As one cultural historian puts it, "we have already entered the era of limits, and with industrial expansion at its limit, people are beginning to look to other things for the meaning of life. It is time to move on to other visions of the meaning of human culture . . ." [1]. This male historian notes that the 21st century "will see all the worst nightmares of the ecologists come true in epidemics of environmentally caused diseases which will recall the Black Death of medieval times" [1].

Feminist scholars are currently pinpointing the origins of the runaway course of earthly and human destruction observed in society [1; 2, p. xi; 3, pp. 103–4; 4, pp. 12–13]. Rosemary Ruether explains that "only today have large numbers of people begun to suspect that patriarchy, which has shaped human history until now, is unviable for future development and indeed is fast proving unable to maintain the survival of humankind on the planet" [2, p. xi]. In other words, patriarchal ideas have given shape and form to social institutions, life styles and governments that are now proving inadequate to preserve human life and the earth itself.

DEATH IN LIFE

Although in most of our present life experiences it appears that the sources of patriarchal institutions remain powerful and strong, a close historical analysis reveals that our present civilization is crumbling. Most of recorded history reveals that men are, and always have been, dominant in this world [2, p. xi; 3, pp. 103–4; 5]. As a result, our life styles and our social institutions are built on sand. The patriarchal foundations, which are grounded in marriage and the nuclear family, are not firm. Indeed the foundations are shaking. They are feeble, frail and falling. It is past the time for patriarchy to cease being dominant. Valuing patriarchy has meant death in life—malaise, apathy, depression and general destruction of the human spirit—for many, and in the future it promises to mean death in life for many more. It is questionable whether the well-intentioned people of this earth can reverse the human political and environmental destruction that patriarchy has left behind [3, pp. 103–4].

The death in life resulting from patriarchy has tremendous implications for the politics of care. Nursing will have to prepare itself to care for the victims of epidemics of environmentally caused diseases and the Black Death of the future [1]. The patriarchy has done little and is doing little to stop the evils causing these diseases and this death [2, p. xi; 3, pp. 103–4; 6, p. 221].

As the recent Three Mile Island incident clearly demonstrates, our civilization faces widespread and possibly lethal outcomes from the uses of nuclear energy, and seems unable to come to grips with how to reverse or stop the events leading to destruction. As radical feminist Mary Daly clearly points out, the patriarchal leaders are unable or unwilling to stop their own destructive games [3, pp. 103–4]. Daly stresses the fact that our society is necrophilic, in love with death and unconcerned about life. Patriarchal scientists and leaders "through the 'peaceful use of nuclear energy' and other forms of pure pollution . . . have paved the way for planetary plagues causing disgusting and virulent sores—radiation sickness and various forms of cancer" [3, pp. 103–4]. From a political and caring standpoint, nurses would be wise to actively and publicly oppose the forces giving rise to the ultimate destruction of human health on this earth.

ROOTS OF STRUCTURED MISOGYNY IN RELIGION AND PHILOSOPHY

Misogyny and hatred of the expansion of women's potential beyond the male-defined limits of serving males find their greatest support in religious ideas, traditions and institutions. As Ruether explains: "The religion of patriarchal culture validates the auxiliary status of women in various ways. . . . In the creation story, generic humanity is envisioned as male, the essential and original autonomous human person. Woman was created second as a derivative being [4, pp. 12–13]. Myths surrounding the cult of true womanhood permeate patriarchal history. Because of myths accompanying pervasive misogyny, nurses are still the servants of physicians and secretaries the servants of business executives.

WOMAN AS EVIL

In patriarchal religion, men alone were created in the image of God. Misogynous myths portray women as evil instead of being created in God's image. The biblical "misogynist tradition goes beyond the definitions of women in terms of property, dependency and service. It defines women as the source of evil and, in somes sense, inherently evil. This of course is suggested in the stories that make Eve not only secondary in creation but the source of sin in the world, either through the fall from Paradise or by the seduction of the angels through which the demonic beings were born" [4, p. 14].

The association of women with evil is a predominant thought in all written history and mythology [2, p. xi; 4, pp. 12–13]. According to Simone de Beauvoir, "That is why religions and codes of law treat women with such hostility as they do. . . . Eve, given to Adam to be his companion, worked the ruin of mankind; when they wish to wreak vengeance upon man, the pagan gods invent woman; and it is the first-born of these female creatures, Pandora, who lets loose all the ills of suffering humanity. The Other—she is passivity confronting activity, diversity that destroys unity, matter as opposed to form, disorder against order. Woman is thus dedicated to Evil" [5].

WOMAN AS INFERIOR

Eleanor Commo McLaughlin, a church historian, emphasizes the "evidence is overwhelming that the medieval Christian theological tradition and the symbols that it generated . . . did provide important stimuli and a convenient ideology for the dehumanization of the female sex [7, p. 78]. Although their work has been buried and silenced until the present women's movement, early feminists were acutely aware of the damaging effects of religious beliefs on the health and welfare of women. In 1837 Sarah M. Grimke declared that "Woman, instead of being elevated by her union with man, which might be expected from an alliance with a superior being, is in reality lowered. She generally loses her individuality, her independent character, her moral being [7, p. 99].

Further reacting to the biblical notion that the male was created as a being superior to the female, Grimke expressed her views on the matter: "The idea that man, as man is superior to woman involves an absurdity so gross, that I really wonder how any man of reflection can receive it as of divine origin; and I can only account for it, by that passion for supremacy, which characterizes man as a corrupt and fallen creature [7, p. 69].

However absurd the idea, prominent philosophers have wholeheartedly subscribed to the notion of male superiority. St. Thomas Aquinas, as a voice of the masculine age, argued that "woman is defective and misbegotten, for the active force in the male seed tends to the production of a perfect . . . masculine sex; while the production of woman comes from a defect in the active force or from some material indisposition . . ." [7, p. 69].

WOMAN AS SERVANT

In *The Church and the Second Sex,* Daly has commented that St. Thomas shared the commonly held view that women are not quite human. According to Daly, Thomas viewed women as having an intellectual inferiority that necessitated their also having social inferiority. Since women were inferior, their subjection to men was a "natural" state. As Daly explains, Thomas's view was that women should have no autonomy. The most a woman could hope for "even in the best of worlds, would be a kind of eternal childhood, in which she would be subject to man 'for her own benefit' " [8, p. 93].

Another philosopher, Rousseau, a male supremacist of the worst kind, argued that "since women are made to please men and be useful to them, the entire education of the female should be directed toward that end" [7, p. 106]. Rousseau taught that women "must be subject, all their lives, to the most severe restraint." He believed women should never be permitted "for a moment to perceive themselves entirely freed from restraint" [7, p. 113]. In elaborating on the need to restrain women, he noted: "There results from this habitual restraint a tractableness which the women have occasion for during their whole lives, as they constantly remain either under subjection to the men, or to the opinions of mankind; and are never permitted to set themselves above those opinions" [7, p. 114].

Rousseau further argued that women should quietly, with a mild disposition, suffer injustice, insults and believe in false religions in order to remain rightfully subjected, pleasing and useful to men. He thought the "criminality" of women's errors would be overlooked by God, since women were too defective to make judgments for themselves [7, p. 117].

Aristotle, who argued that man is a political being and that order in a society depended on the determination of what was just, also argued that man alone was fit to command and woman was made to obey. He concluded that women could not be good in the same sense that a man could be good [7, pp. 41–45].

There is no end to the misogynous beliefs expressed in religious and philosophical writings. Historical writings of males repeatedly set forth arguments that women are defective, inferior and have no sense of justice. One final example from a philosopher provides reason enough for women to examine the nature of the politics of care to determine why patriarchal dominance has depleted the human capacity to care. In declaring that the "fundamental fault of the female character is that it has no sense of justice," Schopenhauer noted that "The weakness of their reasoning faculty also explains why it is that women show more sympathy for the unfortunate than men do, and so treat them with more kindness and interest; and why it is that . . . they are inferior to men in point of justice, and less honourable and conscientious" [7, p. 214].

Here, Schopenhauer is really finding fault with women's capacity to care and is attributing this capacity to their ineffective reasoning ability or their intellectual inferiority. Religious teachers and philosophers have overwhelmingly argued that it was women's nature to be kind, gentle, loving and nurturing, but many at the same time argued that this behavior was an outgrowth of their defective nature.

The early feminist philosopher, Mary Wollstonecraft, expressed an acute sense of injustice when she proclaimed in reaction to misogynous views about women: "How grossly do they insult us who thus advise us only to render ourselves gentle, domestic brutes!" [9, p. 50]. In acknowledging that women had been socially and politically conditioned into a state of inferiority, she identified the influence of men as the major cause of women's inability to grow beyond this state. In her words: "I shall only insist that men have increased that inferiority til women are almost sunk below the standard of rational creatures" [9, p. 70]. Wollstonecraft was indignant about the fallacious and hate-filled ideas that enslaved the minds and bodies of the female sex.

POWER OF STRUCTURED MISOGYNY

Misogynous beliefs did not originate with women. They originated with men and have served the purpose of causing both women and men to hold deep-seated misogynous notions about women [2, p. xi; 3, pp. 103–4; 6, p. 221]. The power in these structured beliefs has led to longstanding hatred and denigration of women and to the societal worship of the male phallus. Just as patriarchal religions center around the worship of a male god, our societal institutions exist to honor and worship male performance. Male dominance and the worship of males go hand in hand [2, p. xi; 3, pp. 103–4; 4, pp. 12–13]. Daly has accurately labeled our society phallocratic, noting that "patriarchy is itself the prevailing religion of the entire planet" [3, p. 39].

STRUCTURED MISOGYNY IN THEORY

In analyzing existing psychological theory, there is clear evidence that patriarchal systems of belief measure all human existence from the standpoint of the existence or lack of existence of male genitals. Within these systems of belief, women are, of course, found lacking and appear as mutilated defectives horrifying to the human mind and eye [2, p. xi; 3, pp. 103–4; 8]. This picture of woman stands out blatantly in psychological theories in common use by nurses.

Ruether gives Freud the distinction of being "the founder of the sexist perversion of psychoanalytic interpretation [2, p. 138]. Although in my opinion this is quite true where psychoanalytic interpretation is concerned, in his theory Freud was merely repeating the basic misogynous beliefs espoused by male religious leaders and philosophers. His limited vision, influenced solely by a society that embraced only misogynous beliefs, could not conceive of woman as being anything other than what men had always thought her to be.

Freud accepted without questioning the ancient religious and philosophic view that women are biologically defective. For Freud, this limits and conditions the entire course of women's psychological development, and keeps women from reaching higher realms of intelligence and moral discipline. Freud's theory explicitly states that male genital characteristics are the normative foundation of full humanity, against which norm women are found to be defined as deprived or "castrated." Freud even goes to what I consider the ridiculous length, seldom questioned by nurses, to state that very young girls realize their "castrated" state and feel inferior because of it [2, p. xi; 4, pp. 12–13].

Freud's misogynistic beliefs entirely pervade his theory, presenting a view of woman's lifelong development as a no-win, completely inferior prospect. According to Freud, once the young girl realizes her "castrated" condition, she turns away from the mother to the more powerful father in hope of receiving a penis, which the father has and the mother lacks. The young girl's psychic development thereafter is a frustrated quest to receive from males, most often the father, husband, or a son, the potency that she has been deprived of by nature [2, p. xi; 4, pp. 12–13].

FREUD'S "NORMAL" WOMAN

According to Freud, the lifelong quest to make up for their inherent deficiency leads women to three possible types of development. The first two types Freud views as pathological. The third, which *is* pathological, Freud views as "normal." First, women can withdraw into neurosis or resentment, burying feelings of deprivation in a refusal to relate to others to any great extent.

Second, women can refuse to accept the fact of their "castrated" nature and organize their personality around their clitoris, or rudimentary penis, which gave them pleasure and was the basis of their oedipal desires as an infant. This second option Freud called the masculinity complex, which gives rise to a woman's attempt to emulate men and to pretend that they have exactly the same nature as men. Freud viewed the aggressive, professional or intellectual woman as this type of infantile, clitoral woman, her behavior arising from her refusal to accept her "castrated" nature. Freud viewed women who entered psychoanalysis as doing so because of their penis envy, seeking to obtain from the psychoanalyst-father what their own fathers had failed to give them.

The third option Freud sees as possible for women's lifelong development reflects the most subtle/blatant and damaging form of misogyny. The woman accepts the fact of her "castrated," inferior and defective nature, and essentially worships her father, husband, son and other men because they have male genitals. For Freud, this type of personality development is "normal," and follows a course of gradual acceptance by the woman of her biological fate. The woman then resigns herself to her secondary and dependent destiny, wasting her personal life in pursuit of having a man of one sort or another. Freud's description of this course of development, while ridiculous in the extreme, and indeed perverse as Ruether calls it, reflects ancient patriarchal myths about feminine sexuality.

According to Freud, the "normal" woman must shift the source of her desires from the active libido in the clitoris to the vagina, where she awaits penetration by the male as the source of her feminine fulfillment. This shift requires giving up her drive to grow and develop her potential and demands her acceptance that her true biological destiny requires that she remain a passive, dependent orifice that waits for masculine activity and penetration. It is in making this regressive, growth-denying shift that the woman finally achieves compensation for her deprivation—a baby [2, p. xi]. As Ruether points out in analyzing Freud's position, "Of course, not just any baby will do. What women desire primarily is a boy-baby—the penis-baby through which they possess, vicariously in their son, what they have been deprived of in themselves. To produce a girl-baby is to create just another mutilation" [2, p. 140].

Freud's views about penis-babies are similar to those of St. Thomas Aquinas who believed that the male seed tended to reproduce itself only, that is, only male children were normal reproductive products. If a child was born female, it was because something drastic had gone wrong [2, p. xi]. When analyzed, Freud's theory is a form of structured misogyny having tremendous power over the shaping of modern social thought and action. Such theories should be viewed as having raped the minds and spirits of nurses and of women, generally serving no good purpose for women, only the purpose of forcing women to worship males and their phallocentric ideations, institutions and practices, however demeaning these are to women.

PERPETUATING MISOGYNOUS BELIEFS IN NURSING

Curricula in schools of nursing all over this country perpetuate misogynous views of women by teaching the theories similar to those analyzed in this article and then expect nurses to consider themselves educated, self-confident and qualified enough to help women achieve healthy minds and bodies. As I have observed, most nurses who have master's or doctoral degrees in the field of mental health and psychiatric nursing were taught to accept, absorb and believe that Freudian and neo-Freudian theories made sense. To illustrate the damage to nurses, most undergraduate programs in nursing encourage students to read the works of Maslow because he has written a good deal about so-called "health" and self-actualization. Following is a quotation that speaks volumes about Maslow's real beliefs on the health of women. In writing about healthy individuals, Maslow says it is essential for a woman:

to be able to adore a man, to look up to him as once she looked up to her father, to be able to lean on him, to be able to trust him, to feel him to be reliable, to feel him to be strong enough so that she can feel precious, delicate, dainty, and so that she can trustfully snuggle down on his lap and let him take care of her and the babies, and the world, and everything else outside the home. This is especially so when she's pregnant, or when she's raising small infants and children. Then she most needs a man around to take care of her, to protect her, and to mediate between her and the world. . . . If she cannot perceive in him the ultimate, eternal, B-masculine qualities, she must be profoundly and deeply unhappy as any woman without a man must be. [10, pp. 107–8]

Maslow's indirectly expressed hatred and ambivalence toward women is more clearly evident when he writes about the nature of man's "love" for woman:

Now the truth is that any woman, especially to the perceptive eye, to the sensitive man, to the more aesthetic man, to the more intelligent man, to the more healthy man, can be seen in a B-way, with B-cognition, however much a prostitute or a psychopath or a gold digger or a hateful murderess or a witch she may be. The truth is that at some moments she will suddenly flip into her goddess-like aspect, most especially when she's fulfilling those biological functions that men see as basically female; nursing, feeding, giving birth, taking care of children, cleaning the baby, being beautiful, sexually exciting, etc. [10, p. 110]

As the reader should note, Maslow says nothing derogatory about men. He uses no words that might cause the imagination to conceive of a man as ever having a fault. According to Maslow's view, men are obviously nearly perfect all the time. He strongly emphasizes that men must overlook the basic nature of evil in women in order to "love" them. This comes from a theorist who argues that human nature is basically and intrinsically good. Maslow's belief about women as being all evil (or good and saintlike in rare moments) aptly describes the contradictory images of the nurse. Nurses are commonly portrayed as witches, bitches and whores or saintly angels of mercy.

Without careful efforts to point out the misogynous content inherent in their words, I believe educators in nursing must refuse to teach ideas, such as Maslow's and Freud's, that are grossly denigrating to women. If nurses are to effectively analyze the politics of care, if they are to change education and practice in a favorable direction, all practitioners in nursing must become increasingly aware of the subtle ways hatred of women is communicated in patriarchal institutions and settings. Certainly, huge amounts of nurses' time and energy need to be devoted to research designed to analyze and correct misogynous ideas inherent in theories and bodies of knowledge widely used by professionals and consumers of health care. Until nurses have begun this research task, we will not have taken the first step toward an adequate resolution of the problems surrounding the politics of care in this country.

LIVING POWER OF WORDS, IDEAS AND MYTHS

Religion, philosophy and theory create myths and ideas that shape human experience. The political and social roles of language and ideas have not received much attention in nursing literature. However, language and ideas are alive, having constant effects and shaping the lives of individuals, nations and the human race. Lewis Thomas reminds us that "the gift of language is the single human trait that marks us all genetically, setting us apart from all the rest of life." He further notes: "Language, once it comes alive, behaves like an active, motile organism." Like life itself, "parts of it are always being changed, by a ceaseless activity" [11].

The energy to maintain psychological and social life comes from words and ideas that give meaning and nourishment to life. To understand the politics of any society, the living words and the language of the people are of primary importance. Without language and words that renew the energies of life, we literally die spiritually with much disease caused by the blockage of free-flowing psychic and physical energy necessary for maintaining a healthy organism [11; 12, p. 155].

The myth of male superiority, of phallic superiority, is alive and survives in religion and in major theories or systems of belief purporting to be scientific in origin [2, p. xi; 3, pp. 103–4].

Religion is, of course, supposed to be based on meaningful myths, but the substance of scientific theory is assumed to go beyond mythical supposition and embody truths when possible. Myths often hide truths, and as James Hillman points out, "The myth that is alive is not noticed as mythical until seen through" [12, p. 155]. In a careful analysis of language and ideas, nurses can begin to see through the myth of phallic superiority, finally beginning to understand most, if not all, of the energy-draining issues sapping the spirits of nurses. Confronting the political nature of the myth of phallic superiority will shed much light on the detrimental ways in which this myth enables men to continue exercising male power over women. Presently, and historically, the psychic and physical health of women has been undermined. The survival of women's psychic and physical health is now at stake more than ever, making it a necessity to create new words and ideas that will reenergize women.

We need to know, and to have written in our nursing literature, the effects words and ideas have on our thoughts and behaviors. Then, as women, we can start thinking differently and acting differently. As observed everywhere, in the written word, in films and drama, in verbal conversations, in the real, practical world where nurses live and work, nurses are put down and degraded. This degradation arises from nurses' attachment to and involvement with the cult of "true womanhood"—defined in our misogynous society as serving, pleasing and seeking approval of males. Nurses are, on the surface, praised, rewarded and given token but subversive gains because of their "womanly" service. Yet that very service and cult works to keep nurses subjugated, powerless and politically impotent. This cult and all the definitions we know of womanhood have all grown out of phallic worship.

Men recognize that if they do not use their power (in misogyny) to keep women politically impotent, the balance of power would change and they would lose their privileged position in society. Therefore, men fear change in women, and this fear runs as deep as the misogynous beliefs perpetuated about women in our society [2, p. xi; 3, pp. 103–4; 4, pp. 12–13; 5, 13]. Feminist scholars make a good case supporting the view that men do not want women to become healthy holistically, no longer victims of misogyny, a view having a great deal to do with the politics of care and the issue of whether men have the capacity to care for women. Rich makes it clear that men fear healthy change in women because they think that "in becoming whole human beings, women will cease to mother men, to provide the breast, the lullaby, the continuous attention associated by the infant with the mother. Much male fear . . . is infantilism—the longing to remain the mother's son, to possess a woman who exists purely for him" [6, p. 221].

Words and ideologies are followed by action, by policy and by the formation of laws and social institutions. The old saying that actions speak louder than words is not really true. Actions are always preceded by words. Actions take shape after words have been thought, spoken and written. This is why education is valued. It shapes minds, spirits and actions. Hillman makes the interesting observation that "words, too, burn and become flesh as we speak" [12, p. 9]. If this is true, nurses would do well to spend a good deal of time trying to imagine what the battered, scarred and bruised souls and minds of women, our own and that of our neighbor, must look like.

Hillman further elaborates on the power and politics of words:

We need to recall that we do not just make words up or learn them in school, or ever have them fully under control. Words . . . are powers which have invisible power over us. They are personal presences which have whole mythologies: genders, genealogies . . . histories, and vogues, and their own guarding, blaspheming, creating, and annihilating effects. For words are persons. This aspect of the word transcends their nominalistic definitions and contexts and evokes in our souls a universal resonance. Without the inherence of soul in words, speech would not move us, words would not provide forms for carrying our lives and giving sense to our deaths. [12, p. 9]

MISOGYNY EXPRESSED IN OPPOSITION TO WOMEN'S EDUCATION AND DEVELOPMENT

The power and political use of words cannot be overemphasized. Men have always been aware of this power. It is a power they have never wanted women to gain [13]. Thus their strong historical opposition to women obtaining an education that would enlighten their minds and enable them to create their own thoughts and words, thoughts and words not originating with men.

Virginia Woolf tells of a woman who applied for admission to the Royal College of Surgeons in Edinburgh in 1869. At the time, medical students gathered in a group, howling with laughter, singing merry songs of ridicule. Of course, the male authorities did not permit women to enter their college [13].

Where attitudes toward women are concerned, the times have not changed much since 1869. In today's society, women who choose to enter male-dominated sciences are cruelly insulted, and males overtly attempt to destroy their psychological health. Evelyn Fox Keller reports on her experiences while trying to obtain a degree in physics at Harvard. She was in essence told that she was not "good enough" to be in the field. She was watched constantly, psychologically and socially isolated, subjected to rude male laughter, to "unmitigated provocation, insult and denial" [14, p. 78–91].

In my analysis, Keller remained sane only because she was a strong woman. Both the educated and uneducated men at Harvard displayed their incapacity to care for this woman and her potential. Instead they did all they could possibly do to drive her insane. The men overtly denied her perceptions, her values and her ambitions, forcing her into a state of complete demoralization. From her experiences with male hatred and hostility, Keller concluded that if she had been more politically and socially astute she would not have persisted in searching for affirmation from males who had no capacity to give her any [14, pp. 78–91].

DOCUMENTATION OF MISOGYNY

As women in the male sciences begin to relate and document their experiences, the horrors women confront in the male sciences reveal themselves to have no end. One such experience is related by Naomi Weisstein, in telling of her experiences in experimental psychology. She reports that this male-dominated profession considered her research activity an "outrageous violation of the social order" and "against the laws of nature" only because she was a woman. On the day of her arrival at graduate school, one of the "star" male professors, while puffing on his pipe, told her that women do not belong in graduate school [14, pp. 242–50]. Following the role model of the professor, the male graduate students "as if by prearranged signal, then leaned back in their chairs, puffed on their newly bought pipes, nodded, and assented: "Yeah." "Yeah," said the male graduate students. "No man is going to want you. No man wants a woman who is more intelligent than he is. . . . You are out of your *natural* role: You are no longer feminine [14, p. 243].

Weisstein concluded that "the most painful of the appalling working conditions for women in science is the peculiar kind of social-sexual assault women sustain. . . . When feminists say that women are treated as sex objects, we are compressing into a single, perhaps rhetorical phrase, an enormous area of discomfort, pain, harassment, and humiliation" [14, pp. 248–49].

As Weisstein's experience illustrates, the misogyny of the language in psychological theories does not remain in theoretical form; it is alive and overtly manifested in the behavior of male psychologists [2, p. xi; 3, pp. 103–4; 4, pp. 12–13]. As Weisstein further relates:

I have been at too many professional meetings where the "joke" slide was a woman's body, dressed or undressed. A woman in a bikini is a favorite with past ... presidents of psychological associations. Hake showed such a slide in his presidential address to the Midwestern Psychological Association, and Harlow, past president of the American Psychological Association, has a whole set of such slides, which he shows at the various colloquia to which he is invited. This business of making jokes at women's bodies constitutes a primary social-sexual assault. The ensuing raucous laughter expresses the shared understanding of what is assumed to be women's primary function—to which we can always be reduced. Showing pictures of nude and sexy women insults us: it puts us in our place. You may think you are a scientist, it is saying, but what you really are is an object for our pleasure and amusement. Don't forget it. [14, p. 249]

THE POLITICS OF CARE AND FEMINIST CONSCIOUSNESS

Coming to intellectual and emotional grips with the politics of care means coming to grips with the damage done to women by the political use of misogynous ideas commonly expressed in male myths, scientific theories and male behavior. In a book entitled *For Her Own Good: 150 Years of the Experts' Advice to Women*, Barbara Ehrenreich and Deirdre English carefully examine the nature of advice given to women by professional experts. These authors document their conclusions that the advice of professional experts has been most damaging to women. They provide clear evidence that "the male professional hoarded up his knowledge as a kind of property, to be dispensed to wealthy patrons or sold on the market as a commodity. His goal was not to spread the skills of healing, but to concentrate them within the elite interest group" he represented [15].

Ehrenreich and English place special emphasis on the fact that medicine defined women as "sick" because they had a uterus and ovaries and then set out to reinforce that "sickness" by exploiting women with the medical treatments they dispensed that actually induced illness and kept them physically and psychologically less powerful. At the present time, this making of sick women is a social problem of massive proportions [3, pp. 103–4; 15]. With feminists questioning the saneness and rationality of this approach to women's health, members of the traditional health professions are losing their credibility as health professionals and as a result will ultimately lose all of their powers over the minds and bodies of women as they lose the power granted by their profession.

MEN CARING FOR WOMEN

In analyzing the historical evidence, it is clear that the traditional "health" professions have not demonstrated that they are interested in health [3, pp. 103–4; 15]. Since these professions have been dominated by males, we must raise the serious question of whether men have the capacity to care for women at all. There is an abundant amount of evidence indicating that this capacity is limited, if it does exist. We must therefore question man's ability to change the position of women in this system.

In maintaining a close and longstanding relationship to medicine, psychiatry, gynecology, psychology and many other male-dominated groups in the health field, which are based on the noncapacity to care for women, nursing has done great damage to itself, destroying its potential for power, prostituting the practice of nursing and killing the moral consciousness of nurses. In clinging to these male-dominated groups in various interdisciplinary relationships, nurses have swallowed whole and live out the mythical beliefs and realities inherent in the cult of true womanhood as defined by men. Women in the nursing profession have not begun to examine the destructive nature of these relationships.

Rich clearly explains why women can no longer ignore the power in and the detrimental effects of patriarchal thinking:

Patriarchal man is in dangerous confusion about his "private" interest. For centuries, patriarchy has maintained itself by asking what was good for males, has assumed male norms and values as universal ones, has allowed the differences of "otherness," the division of male and female consciousness, to become a terrifying dissociation of sensibility. The idea of woman exists at a strangely primitive level in the male psyche. She remains, for all his psychological self-consciousness, the object-figure on which can be projected all that man does not understand, all that he needs, all that he dreads, in his own experience. (Erich Neumann . . . went so far as to say that man's consequent fear and hatred of woman has been so deep that were it not for his sexual need of women they could have been extirpated as a group.) Denying his own feminine aspects, always associating his manhood with his ability to possess and dominate women, man the patriarch has slowly, imperceptibly, over time, achieved a degree of self-estrangement, self-hatred, and self-mutilation which is coming to have almost irreversible effects on human relationships and on the natural world. [6, pp. 110–11]

Man's projection of self-hatred and self-mutilation onto woman actually results in the real mutilation and destruction of women. Indeed, power structures and relationships built on male misogyny are highly destructive for both women and men. Identification with these structures and relationships has resulted in the fragmentation of women's power, interests, work, health, and capacity to care for self and for other women. Despite fragmentation, women (especially those who identify with the cult of "true womanhood" as defined by men) still strive for the graspable *illusion* of power, rather than the difficult to obtain "real thing," by attaching to men as the sustainers, supporters or assistants of men in accomplishing men's work.

NURSES AS "TOKEN TORTURERS"

In such a role in the male-dominated "health" professions, nurses have the very serious problem of being publicly identified as the "token torturers" of other women. Daly elaborates on this problem:

The medical employment of women as token torturers is evident in the use of nurses, physiotherapists, and token women doctors. In the field of body-gynecology, the nurse, trained to be totally obedient to the Olympian Doctor, functions as the proximate and visible agent of painful and destructive treatment. Nurses shave women about to give birth and given enemas to women in labor. It is they who give injections and it is they who withhold pain medication begged for by the patient. Programmed not to answer women's questions, they sometimes magnify suffering by unreasonable silence and degrading nonanswers . . .

most unpleasant procedures which nurses perform . . . are done while the woman is awake and aware of being hurt, whereas the deepest wounding—cutting in surgery—which is performed by doctors, is done under anaesthesia. Thus . . . within the hospital situation most procedures experienced as painful are by women, whereas the doctors' actions—prescribing drugs which often have harmful effects, issuing orders from on high—are often not directly perceived. The nurse, then, functions as token torturer in the primary sense of the term token, that is, an outward indication or expression. She is both weapon and shield for the divine doctor. [3, pp. 276–77]

Thoughtful, insightful and perceptive feminists are finally seeing through the myths that surround abusive medical practices directed toward women patients. As Daly notes, the rituals of medicine are more often than not sadistic and "the processions of necrophilic medicine are endless" [3, p. 274].

Fragmentation and the illusion of power on the part of many nurses who have accepted the patriarchal structure of their profession have created a wide gulf that generally separates them from the experiences of women. In other words, nurses who have struggled to become "professionals" have by that patriarchal definition of "professional" been forced to leave behind their true identity as women. Many nurses are deaf, dumb and blind to the needs of women; nurses are often cruel and abusive to women and to other nurses. In pursuit of male approval, this group of nurses will lie to, cheat, steal from and kill the spirits of women in order to support and serve the purposes of male professionals. The fact that many nurses do this out of ignorance does not excuse the guilt of participating in destructive behavior originating with males.

THE PERSONAL IS POLITICAL

The liberation and freeing of women from the grip of structured misogyny is an idea whose time has come. This liberation and freeing has psychological and physical dimensions. The psychological includes personal and spiritual components of being; the physical encompasses political and social factors forming limiting boundaries around the public and private activities of women. All of these problematic facets serve to restrict and inhibit the being of women [3, pp. 103–4].

Since the destruction of the mental and physical health of women is constant in our society, it is time for all nurses, from licensed practical nurses to nurses with doctorates, to seize the opportunity for beginning their journey into an exploration of the politics of care. Where nurses are concerned, issues surrounding nursing and health care generally cannot be separated from feminist issues. For the individual, the need for health and nursing care and efforts to obtain these boil down to a personal concern. Women have coined the phrase that the personal is political [16–18]. This phrase and its meaning have tremendous implications for the social stance most likely to be successful in analyzing the politics of care.

Identifying the personal as political is a means of providing women with an avenue for examining the personal aspects of women's lives in political terms. The necessity of taking this approach seems obvious, since women's experience has been centrally concerned with the personal, private dimensions of human life. Within patriarchal society, women have been largely excluded from public life, left primarily to care for the personal concerns of men and children within the context of the family. As illustrated in this article, when women have engaged in the activities of public life, they have been grossly ignored, negated and de-valued. Operating within the realm of the personal, it is only logical that women's devalued personal world be subjected to political analysis, opening a door to an extensive examination of how that which is personal provides the foundations of political and social superstructures controlling the lives of women, a control that remains mostly uninfluenced by women.

THE MYTH OF PROFESSIONALIZATION

In a mad rush of confusion, confronting contradictions and illusions, we nurses have mistakenly pursued the myth of professionalization, hoping that the public achievement of this state would provide us with the prestige, recognition and acceptance traditionally accorded male professionals. In our haste to imitate male professionals, we have overlooked the political implications of our personal pursuits. Writing some time ago, Woolf raised the question of why women would want to enter male professions or become like male professionals. She noted that the professions made the men who practiced them "possessive, jealous of any infringement of their rights, and highly combative if anyone dares dispute them" [13]. Moreover, Woolf was not unaware of the egotism and greed that characterize educated men who spend their time in "committee rooms, soliciting favours, assuming a mask of reverence to cloak ridicule" [16].

Nurses would do well to follow Woolf's example of seriously considering the effect the professions have on those who practice them. Women are just now beginning to look at the effects the professions have had on society, and the conclusions are not very praiseworthy. Certainly from a political standpoint, we nurses, in our efforts to model our profession after male-defined concepts have overlooked the extent to which this model has repeatedly negated the value of nursing and its scientific/artistic development. As nurses, we have grossly overlooked the fact that in a patriarchal society the means of nurturing the personal development of women's potential is not a priority. Patriarchal religion, philosophy and theory have created the reality of women's personal world and personal views of themselves, yielding women almost totally powerless in both personal and political experience.

For the care and development of women's potential to become a reality, all women must learn to care first for women. In doing this we will not model ourselves or our profession after male ideations or standards. I have illustrated the fact that males and male professionals have only a limited capacity to care for women, if they have this capacity at all. This male limitation must be understood before we can begin to get a clear picture of the meaning of the politics of care.

NURSING—THE TURNING POINT

For many years we have heard that nursing is at the crossroads. Nursing never seems to get over being at a crossroads. Indeed, nursing has been at a crossroads many times, but instead of taking a new road, leaders in the profession always choose to continue bearing the burden of continuing to live out the subservient role under the patriarchal system, rather than taking a new road that can lead beyond patriarchy. Nursing is no longer at a crossroads. It is at a turning point. It needs to turn away from being the "token torturer" of itself and other women. It needs to turn toward the health awaiting women in a woman-defined, woman-created world that lies beyond patriarchal ideas and institutions [2, p. xi; 6, p. 221].

Finally, after more than a century of existence, the nursing profession needs to become a self-directing, honorable profession, unashamed of its efforts and its aims, rightly divining the word of truth where it can be found. In order to become self-directing, honorable and unashamed of searching for its own truth, nursing must shed its petty and childish fears of feminism and begin to embrace the powerful knowledge and insights to be gained from feminist literature. I believe nursing cannot become self-directing or effective in the politics of care without embracing feminism and all it stands for.

VALIDATING NURSING EXPERIENCE

If nursing is to become self-directing and effective in the politics of care, nurses cannot continue to identify with male-dominated professions for the reasons I have already outlined, ignoring the problems of real, live nurses and the problems of women in general. Rich speaks to this issue:

For if, in trying to join the common world of men, the professions molded by a primarily masculine consciousness, we split ourselves off from the common life of women and deny our female heritage and identity in our work, we lose touch with our real powers and with the essential condition for all fully realized work: community.

Feminism begins but cannot end with the discovery by an individual of her self-consciousness as a woman. It is not, finally, even the recognition of her reasons for anger, or the decision to change her life, go back to school, leave a marriage. . . . Feminism means finally that we renounce our obedience to the fathers and recognize that the world they have described is not the whole world. Masculine ideologies are the creation of masculine subjectivity; they are neither objective, nor value-free, nor inclusively "human." Feminism implies that we recognize fully the inadequacy for us, the distortion, of male-created ideologies, and that we proceed to think, and act, out of that recognition. [6, p. 207]

When analyzed, medical ideology and all the ideologies of the traditional health professions are masculine ideologies. As such, they negate the very existence of nursing as a separate and valid profession with much of value to offer society, a service that goes beyond mere treatment of disease to the provision of needed care for the health of people.

In accepting the token generosity of fatherly figures in the medical profession and in other fields of male scholarship, nurses negate the validity of their own experiences, thereby losing the power they might have by identifying with the needs and concerns of all women. In the future, nursing practice should focus all of its attention on validating the experiences of women. Women comprise 70% to 80% of all consumers of health care services, and women make up at least 75% of the work force in all health care settings [19]. Since women risk their health by going to male professionals, nurses have the large task of warning women that this risk is real and dangerous. The professional obligation of the nurse as an advocate of the woman client is that of explaining the risks involved and helping her to safeguard her health by finding competent and reliable practitioners who will meet her needs for humane care. From a sound political and ethical standpoint, nurses cannot avoid undermining the unwarranted confidence that women tend to place in unscrupulous professionals.

NURSES CARING FOR NURSES

In examining the politics of care, nurses should also examine their own profession. The nursing profession is divided into various levels of women workers. To date, organized nursing has done little toward studying the specific problems of these various groups of women workers. Instead, nurses support the patriarchal phenomena of divide and conquer, which continues to succeed in splitting and fragmenting the efforts of all nurses. Nurses remain psychologically and socially isolated from one another. Their loyalties remain false and misplaced.

The hostility nurses feel toward other nurses is overtly expressed. Nurses have never examined the male origins of this hostility, which arises from all the misogynous beliefs held about women. Men have despised the work of women, devaluing it and giving it no real place in history. Taking place largely as a form of servitude, women's work and its value have gone unnoticed. Modeling themselves after males, women also devalue the work of other women, particularly women who are viewed as "the other" because of different levels of educational preparation.

It is truly a shameful thing that professionally prepared nurses cannot care for and value the lives and experiences of nurses' aides, practical nurses, associate degree and diploma graduates. It is shameful that no connection or sense of community exists between these groups of women. If nurses would begin to care for other nurses, the profession would have more than enough power necessary for controlling its practice and its destiny. The effective use of a caring kind of politics will not become a reality until nurses begin to make meaningful connections with the lives of other nurses and women, establishing a community of shared caring. This is the type of politics that is feared by the patriarchy and that can be personally and publicly effective in overcoming the damages wrought by the same patriarchy.

The power, the politics and the practice of feminism are devoted to the preservation of human life and to its nourishment. Feminism is devoted to the preservation of the earth's resources as a necessity for the preservation of human life and health. These goals should be the goals of any politics of care. And these should be the goals of nursing practice both now and in the future. Exploring, examining, embracing and employing the ideas, beliefs, values and actions of feminism can provide nurses with a new and vital source of energy—energy that is absolutely necessary for healthy performance in women's lives. Women nurses are *women* first. If we consistently remember this, accepting our heritage and strengths as women, our politics of care can begin.

REFERENCES

1. Thompson, W. I. *Darkness and Scattered Light* (Garden City, N.Y.: Anchor Press 1978) p. 44.
2. Ruether, R. R. *New Woman New Earth: Sexist Ideologies and Human Liberation* (New York: The Seabury Press 1975).
3. Daly, M. *Gyn/Ecology: The Metaethics of Radical Feminism* (Boston: Beacon Press 1978).
4. Bianchi, E. C., and Ruether, R. R. *From Machismo to Mutuality: Woman-Man Liberation* (New York: Paulist Press 1976).
5. de Beauvoir, S. *The Second Sex,* trans. and ed. H. M. Parshley (New York: Alfred A. Knopf 1976).
6. Rich, A. *On Lies, Secrets, and Silence* (New York: W. W. Norton & Co. 1979).
7. Osborne, M. L., ed. *Woman in Western Thought* (New York: Random House 1979).
8. Daly, M. *The Church and the Second Sex* (New York: Harper & Row, Publishers 1968) p. 93.
9. Wollstonecraft, M. *A Vindication of the Rights of Woman* (New York: W. W. Norton & Co. 1971).

10. Maslow, A. H. *Religion, Values, and Peak Experiences* (New York: Penguin Books 1964) pp. 107–108.
11. Lewis, T. *The Lives of a Cell* (New York: Bantam Books 1975) pp. 105–106.
12. Hillman, J. *Re-Visioning Psychology* (New York: Harper & Row, Publishers 1975).
13. Woolf, V. *Three Guineas* (New York: Harcourt, Brace and World 1938) p. 66.
14. Weisstein, N. Y. " 'How Can a Little Girl Like You Teach a Great Big Class of Men?' the Chairman said, and Other Adventures of a Woman in Science," in Ruddick, S. and Daniels, P., eds. *Working it Out: 23 Women Writers, Artists, Scientists, and Scholars Talk About Their Lives and Work* (New York: Pantheon Books 1977).
15. Ehrenreich, B., and English, D. *For Her Own Good: 150 Years of the Experts' Advice to Women* (Garden City, N.Y.: Anchor Press 1978) p. 30.
16. Koedt, A., Levine, E. and Rapone, A., eds. *Radical Feminism* (New York: Quadrangle 1973).
17. Morgan, R. *Going Too Far* (New York: Vintage Books 1978).
18. Firestone, S. *The Dialectic of Sex: The Case for Feminist Revolution* (New York: Bantam Books 1970).
19. Hackett, O. P. "Women and the Health System: A Case Study in Feminist Praxis." *Radical Religion* 3:2 (1977) pp. 36–43.

BIBLIOGRAPHY

Berkin, C. R., and Norton, M. B. *Women of America: A History* (Boston: Houghton Mifflin Co. 1979).

Brownmiller, S. *Against Our Will: Men, Women and Rape* (New York: Simon & Schuster 1975).

Clark, E., and Richardson, H., eds. *Women and Religion* (New York: Harper & Row, Publishers 1977).

Corea, G. *The Hidden Malpractice* (New York: Jove Publications 1977).

Daly, M. *Beyond God the Father* (Boston: Beacon Press 1973).

David, D. S., and Brannon, R., eds. *The Forty-Nine Percent Majority: The Male Sex Role* (Menlo Park, Calif.: Addison-Wesley Publishing Co. 1976).

DeCrow, K. *Sexist Justice* (New York: Vintage Books 1975).

Dinnerstein, D. *The Mermaid and the Minotaur* (New York: Harper & Row, Publishers 1977).

Dworkin, A. *Woman Hating* (New York: E. P. Dutton & Co. 1974).

Frankfort, E. *Vaginal Politics* (New York: Bantam Books 1972).

Goldenberg, N. *Changing of the Gods* (Boston: Beacon Press 1979).

Greer, G. *The Female Eunuch* (New York: Bantam Books 1971).

Griffin, S. *Rape: The Power of Consciousness* (New York: Harper & Row, Publishers 1979).

Griffin, S. *Woman and Nature* (New York: Harper & Row, Publishers 1978).

Lederer, W. *The Fear of Women* (New York: Harcourt Brace Jovanovich 1968).

Mackinnon, C. A. *Sexual Harassment of Working Women* (New Haven, Conn.: Yale University Press 1979).

Nies, J. *Seven Women: Portraits from the American Radical Tradition* (New York: Penguin Books 1978).

Oakley, M. B. *Elizabeth Cady Stanton* (New York: The Feminist Press 1972).

Pomeroy, S. B. *Goddesses, Whores, Wives and Slaves* (New York: Schocken Books 1975).

Ruether, R. *Liberation Theology* (New York: Paulist Press 1972).

Sangiuliano, I. *In Her Time* (New York: William Morrow & Co. 1978).

Sochen, J. *Movers and Shakers: American Women Thinkers and Activists, 1900–1970* (New York: Quadrangle/The New York Times Book Co. 1973).

Tolson, A. *The Limits of Masculinity* (New York: Harper & Row, Publishers 1977).

23 A Discourse on the Politics of Nursing

Beatrice J. Kalisch and Philip A. Kalisch

IN OBSERVING THAT "the mass of men lead lives of quiet desperation," Thoreau used the traditional masculine gender, but astute observers today will have to admit that "quiet desperation" aptly describes the political life and status of the nurse.

Nurses belong to one of the largest (850,000 active RNs) and most neglected groups in our voting population. Politically, most nurses are unorganized; they are neither joiners nor participants. The nurse does not usually have the time, the energy, the available resources, the self-direction, the confidence, the assertiveness, or the will to move into active roles in our government. No nurse has ever been elected to Congress and, so far as the writers know, none have attempted such a challenge. Only a handful have served in state legislatures and in local government. Yet nursing is inevitably becoming more and more shaped by political decisions.

Nursing and politics have ordinarily been studied as separate subjects; when political decisions affect nursing programs, such separation is no longer possible. Of course most nurses abhor the idea that politics could ever be involved in any of their policies, deliberations, or activities. Nursing must indeed always be above the various confines of favoritism, corruption, or specialized interest. It must be in the "patient's interest." But such conceptions are merely the products of the language of symbolism used. Decisions are not made in a patient-interest vacuum. The symbols serve to ornament the prose rather than to inform one about objective reality.

WHAT IS POLITICS?

The heart of politics concerns power and the allocation of scarce resources. To be sure, many nurses will react to "politics" as though it were a dirty word. Such a feeling is not without justification. Politics is a hard and cruel business, especially so when related to health care and matters of life and death. It is cruel because it involves conflict, and in any competitive struggle for scarce resources not everyone can emerge victorious.

Since nursing is constantly subjected to the constraints of scarce resources, politics inevitably enters into all phases of the nurse's life, realized or not, with its implication of a severe form of favoritism or corruption. For example, when a nurse hears that politics was involved in an arbitrary decision to freeze nurses' wages, she might automatically conclude that some other group or category received a favor or benefit to which it was not entitled. Now if the

Reprinted by permission from "A Discourse on the Politics of Nursing" by Beatrice J. Kalisch and Philip A. Kalisch, *Journal of Nursing Administration,* Volume 6, Number 2, 1976.

benefit or favor was outside the limits of the law, corruption was obviously involved; if legal requirements were met, then the appropriate label would simply be "power politics."

Politics concerns the promotion of one's interest group and the *use* of whatever resources are available to protect and advance that interest. Such activity may or may not involve corruption, favoritism, and collusion. Nursing is a political matter, and those who take the responsibility to understand all that this implies are better off than those who undertake their work without knowledge of nursing's political dimensions. The way that nurses have been manipulated, historically, both from within and outside the profession, often reminds one of a hot knife cutting through butter.

Traditional worship of authority, still sometimes inculcated through the educational process, the socialization of the young nurse in the mores of the institution, the reliance on those above to make the right decision, the fear of questioning and generating open controversy—all combine historically and currently for political naiveté in nurses as a class. In addition, nurses are often young women, many of whom eventually leave the profession altogether, or severely limit their interest and participation after they become married and begin to rear families. From the professional interest group point of view, this turnover in membership is a debilitating factor in terms of maintaining a cohesive, active membership base as a political resource with which to advance the meritorious and to discourage eroding factors.

The benign neglect of political factors in the education of nurses fosters the omission of a critical element in understanding, planning and executing nursing services. A simple course in American government as part of a general education requirement is no substitute; nursing is unique insofar as applying the principles of politics is concerned, and a course in "politics of nursing" is desperately needed. For whether they like it or not, student nurses will be increasingly involved in a political environment as they embark upon their professional careers. The ones who succeed will be the ones who learn to understand it, adjust to it, and turn it to the advantage of their profession. This is not to imply that schools of nursing should consign their curricula to such a study, but political factors in nursing should not entirely be ignored.

Politics also includes all efforts to influence public policy, which is to say the decisions and actions of public officers and employees. Legislative, executive, and judicial bodies are not unified forces. "The Congress" simply does not exist in reality. Congress is composed of numerous subgroups, particularly committees, which exert power in the policy-determining process.

THE CONSEQUENCES OF POLITICAL NEGLECT

The communication most state legislators or congressmen have with their districts inevitably puts them in touch with organized groups and with individuals who are relatively well-informed. The representative knows his constituents mostly from dealing with people *who do* write letters, *who will* attend meetings, *who have* an interest in his legislative stance. Thus his sample of contacts with a constituency of several thousands or several hundred thousand people is heavily biased; even the contacts he apparently makes at random are likely to be with people who grossly overrepresent the degree of political information and interest in the constituency as a whole. Are nurses, despite their large numbers and potential political clout, likely to be considered as long as they continue to remain relatively silent?

As an example of politics in action, the outright disdain that the nation's most powerful politician has for nursing was amply documented in the President's veto of the Nurse

Training Bill on January 2, 1975, and again on July 25, 1975. He arbitrarily determined that the "measure would authorize excessive appropriations levels—more than $650 million over the three fiscal years covered by the bill. Such high federal spending for nursing education would be intolerable at a time when even high priority activities are being pressed to justify their existence."

Such reasoning is hard to believe when Americans are spending over $115 billion annually for all health services and nursing education is valiantly attempting to pull itself up and into the mainstream of meeting its demands. Also without apparent foundation was the additional statement that:

This act inappropriately proposes large amounts of student and construction support for schools of nursing. Without any additional federal stimulation, we expect that the number of active duty registered nurses will increase by over 50 percent during this decade.

Such an increase suggests that our incentives for expansion have been successful, and that continuation of the current federal program is likely to be of less benefit to the nation than using these scarce resources in other ways. One result of this expansion has been scattered but persistent reports of registered nurse unemployment, particularly among graduates of associate degree training programs.

That unemployment in the auto industry was excessive no one would deny, but all across the nation help wanted ads for nurses remained consistently high according to a March 1975 survey by the American Hospital Association.

Although the second Presidential veto was quickly overridden by Congress, it was obvious that the vetoes of the Nurse Training Acts of 1974 and 1975 were political decisions and nurses were again being acted upon rather than acting upon. They were expendable and a whole host of much less justifiable politically "sacred cows" were not. As long as politics is treated by nurses as a forbidden field, misinformed outsiders professionally skilled in its mysteries can impose their will on nursing. Thus defeat of proposals that seem reasonable to nurses may continue to appear like an infuriating, indefensible betrayal of "patient interest" rather than as an adjustment or trade-off among a variety of competing claims.

INSTITUTIONAL POLITICS

Institutional politics, based on many of the same principles, plays a large role in the nurse's daily life and also deserves close attention. Hospitals and schools of nursing are political structures. They provide the framework for health care professionals to develop careers and therefore provide platforms for the expression of individual interests and motives. The advancement of a nurse's career, particularly at the higher administrative levels, depends upon the accumulation of power as the vehicle for transforming individual interest into activities which influence other people. "Selling out nursing" from a professional standpoint in order to attain and maintain professional advancement is frequently regarded as necessary for an ambitious nurse to move up the political pyramid of the hospital or university, given the locker-room mentality of the political elite in health care.

A LESSON FROM MACHIAVELLI

We can learn something along these lines by harkening back more than 460 years to 1513, when Niccolo Machiavelli, an Italian patriot deeply involved in the diverse political maneuvers of sixteenth century Italy, addressed pertinent advice to Lorenzo de' Medici which was later published as *The Prince* five years after his death. In this short book Machiavelli undertook to treat politics scientifically, judging men by an estimate of how in fact they do behave as political animals rather than by ideal standards concerned with how they out to act. The hardheadedly consistent refusal of the author to submit political behavior to moral tests has earned the name "Machiavellian" for amoral instances of power relations among nation states and other organized groups.

Machiavelli understood how success is always a minimal condition of political greatness. In *The Prince* he presents a manual of advice on the winning and retention of power. He never pretended that his book was a guide for the virtuous. On the other hand, he did not set out to prescribe the way to wickedness. He meant his account to be a practical guide to political power. Machiavelli realized that men seldom get to choose the circumstances most favorable to their political hopes. They must settle for what is possible rather than for the ideal.

In reading the following extracts from *The Prince,* substitute "physician," "hospital administrator," "nursing service director," or "dean" for "Prince" and apply these Machiavellian maxims to authoritarian situations in health care delivery and nursing education and service:

A Prince should be concerned for the people he governs only to the extent that such concern strengthens his hold. . . .

A Princes good Counsell ought to proceed from his owne wisedome.

A Prince above all things ought to wish and desire to bee esteemed Devout, although he be not so indeed.

A Prince ought to sustaine and confirme that which is false . . . , if so be it turne to the favour thereof.

A Prince need not care to be accounted Cruell, if so be that hee can make himselfe to be obeyed thereby.

A Prince ought not to trust in the amitie [good] of men.

It is better for a Prince to be feared than loved.

Cruelty which tendeth and is done to a good end, is not be to be reprehended.

A Prince ought to exercise Crueltie all at once: and to doe pleasures by little and little.

A vertuous Tyrant, to maintaine his tyrannie, ought to maintaine partialities and factions amongst his subjects.

A Prince ought alwaies to nourish some enemie against himself, to this end, that when he hath oppressed him, he may be accounted the more mightie and terrible.

A Prince ought to know how to wind and turne mens minds, that he may deceive and circumvent them.

A Prince ought to have his mind disposed to turne after every wind and variation of Fortune. [A man for all seasons].

A Prince in the time of peace, maintaining discords and partialities amongst his subjects, may the more easily use them at his pleasure.

The meanes to keepe subjects in peace and union, and to hould them from rebellion, is to keepe them always poore.

A Prince ought to commit to another those affaires which are subject to hatred and envie, and reserve to himselfe such as depend upon his grace and favour.

Fear of introducing a more democratic climate in nursing education and service is evidenced by such typical occurrences as:

Selection of deans of schools of nursing and directors of nursing service by committees dominated (overtly or covertly) by physicians, hospital administrators, and others rather than by a democratic consensus among the nurses.

Failure to consider the vital issues of administration, such as the budget, in open meetings and instead concentrating on relatively meaningless trivia.

Unquestioned acceptance of all directives from above and the expectation of the absolute acceptance of directives given to those below (the military model of command).

Excessive obedience and worship of authority by staff nurses and faculty members and the lack of open constructive criticism of administrative policies even though the interest of patients is involved.

THE DESIRABILITY OF DEMOCRACY

Nursing and patient care will enormously benefit by greater use of democratic principles such as: delegating specific authority to specific nurses for specific tasks by democratic procedures; requiring all those to whom authority has been delegated to be responsible to those who selected them; distributing authority among as many nurses as is reasonably possible; rotating tasks among individuals; communicating the vital information as frequently as possible; and providing equal access and open allocation of scarce resources. When such principles are applied, they insure that the political structures that are developed will be controlled by and responsible to *all* the nurses. The Machiavellian nurse administrator will be forestalled as those occupying positions of authority will be more "open," flexible, and subject to votes of confidence. They will not be able to accrue power and become authoritarian, because ultimate decisions will be made by the group at large.

Unquestioned support of the status quo implies that nurses accept such incongruous facts as the continuation of the physician as the last of the big time private entrepreneurs in addition to his practicing medicine. As long as the great gulf remains between the power of physicians and nurses, as long as physicians exercise power politics and nurses abhor politics, the opportunity for nurses to participate responsibly on the American medical care scene will be muted. What is more, the junctures between nursing and national, state, and local politics will be governed overwhelmingly by forces external to the profession.

The price of silence is deadly high. Health care in the United States is currently in a drastic state of flux. Nurses are under attack from both above and below. The emerging allied health professions encroach upon responsibilities that were once exclusively those of the nurse. At the same time schools of nursing and related governmental offices are pyramided with such bureaucratic structures as a "college of health professions" or a "department of health manpower," diluted of much of their power, and placed under the direct jurisdiction of a non-nurse. In addition, the coordination between the nurse practitioner and the physician's assistant or associate remains unresolved. What is more, the exact form and nature of impending national health insurance legislation needs a larger nursing input.

THE CHALLENGE AT HAND

Greater political consciousness will occur as there is an increase in the number of single nurses, unlike their predecessors in the 1940s and 1950s who married young, became mothers early, and had no opportunity to see themselves in any way but in relation to parents, husband, or children and not as professionals. Political consciousness raising for nurses has had some small beginnings such as the birth of Nurses' Coalition for Action in Politics (N-CAP). Indeed it may be further fed by the social ripples of the activities of such women's liberation or rights groups as the National Organization for Women (NOW) and the Women's Equity Action League (WEAL). Waiting for such external forces, however, is not the solution. Nurses' Coalition for Action in Politics and ANA's lobbying activities are proper openings for developing greater intelligence and action concerning effective political pressure points on behalf of nursing.

Inevitably, tens of thousands, perhaps hundreds of thousands, of nurses will still retain a detachment, apathy, or outright hostility to anything associated with politics. Many of these nurses are so caught in their present mindset as nurses, women, and mothers, as to be prevented from gaining a true political consciousness or having the time or energy to do anything even if their consciousness were raised. What is more, development of such an outlook runs counter to numerous strong interest groups.

Politically speaking, the model nurse is not the quiet, submissive, hardworking individual who makes the best of every situation, but the cold, calculating professional who uses all available resources to advance the health care world around her. The model nurse seeks power: the capacity to help determine her own and others' action for improving patient care in all its dimensions. Perhaps the most important political change, which an alteration in the nurse's role portends, is the possibility of an improvement in the lopsided balance between values of power and cooperation among the nurse and physician groups. When physicians and other political elites are resocialized to some of the nurse's values, greater cooperation in decision making will subject outmoded constraints of the nurse to the glaring light of objectivity and promote open analysis of roles and responsibilities as the basis of costs and benefits to the public.

The failure of nurses to become a viable political force as a group is only a reflection of broader trends. Any area in which women have dominated has generally been considered nonpolitical. Since politics by definition is concerned with the interplay of power relationships, and involvement with power is somehow a masculine attribute, most nurses will tread on foreign ground. But if the political manipulation of nurses becomes apparent to the rank and file, the results are likely to have an effect that is opposite to that intended. Previously nonpolitical subjects will almost always become political when reality comes to be perceptibly discordant with social myths and when an interchange of information creates organizational action. In recent years, action on the part of women has brought into the political arena such topics as birth control, abortion, and child rearing and freed them from the traditional role prescription and psychological terms in which they were formerly enmeshed.

Politics is an art and not a science. The "rules and regulations" are guidelines only, and within the guidelines there is wide latitude for flexibility and maneuver. The art of advancing nursing depends upon people, timing, and events; personalities, luck, and know-how are as important as the rules and regulations. Opportunism, compromise, trade-offs, and timing are not necessary evils, but the basic and legitimate principles of operation. The employment of practical politics by nurses cannot accomplish for nursing that which is not within the material or intellectual capacities of nurses. It is at once the weakness and strength of politics in a democracy that the fate of its members lies largely in their own hands. Where power rests ultimately upon the political participation of all nurses, it is their wisdom, collectively formed and expressed, that will determine its degree of success.

SUGGESTED READINGS

The challenge at hand is the education and mastery of the art of politics as it relates to both internal and external factors in nursing. The following readings are suggested as a means of introducing the nurse in search of such knowledge to this foreign field.

Adorno, T., *et al. The Authoritarian Personality.* New York: Harper and Row, 1950.

Aggar, R. E., *et al. The Rulers and the Ruled: Political Power and Importance in American Communities.* New York: John Wiley, 1964.

Amundson, K. *The Silenced Majority.* Englewood Cliffs, N.J.: Prentice-Hall, 1971.

Banfield, E. C. *Political Influence.* Glencoe, Ill.: Free Press, 1961.

Banfield, E. C., and Wilson, J. Q. *City Politics.* Cambridge, Mass.: MIT and Harvard University Press, 1963.

Barnard, J. *Women and the Public Interest: An Essay on Policy and Protest.* Chicago: Aldine, 1971.

Barone, M. *et al. The Almanac of American Politics, 1974.* Boston: Gambit Incorporated, 1973.

Barrer, M. E., Ed. *Women's Organization & Leaders: 1973 Directory.* Washington: Today Publications & News Service, Incorporated, 1973.

Bell, D. V. *Power Influence and Authority.* New York: Oxford University Press, 1975.

Bell, R., *et al. Political Power: A Reader in Theory and Research.* New York: Free Press, 1969.

Bird, C. *Born Female: The High Cost of Keeping Women Down.* New York: McKay, 1968.

Boyarski, B., and Boyarski, N. *Backroom Politics.* New York: Hawthorne, 1974.

Cantril, H. *Human Nature and Political Systems.* New Brunswick, N.J.: Rutgers University Press, 1961.

Carden, M. L. *The New Feminist Movement.* New York: Russell Sage Foundation, 1974.

Charlesworth, J. C., Ed. *Contemporary Political Analysis.* New York: Free Press, 1967.

Chu, F. D., and Trotter, S. *The Madness Establishment: Ralph Nader's Study Group Report on the National Institute of Mental Health.* New York: Grossman, 1974.

Congressional Quarterly Incorporated. *Washington Information Directory 1975–76.* New York: Quadrangle/The New York Times Book Co., 1975.

Dahl, R. A. *Modern Political Analysis.* Englewood Cliffs, N.J.: Prentice-Hall, 1963.

Dahl, R. A. *Who Governs?* New Haven: Yale University Press, 1961.

Davies, J. C. *Human Nature in Politics: The Dynamics of Political Behavior.* New York: John Wiley, 1963.

Deloughery, G. L., and Gebbie, K. M. *Political Dynamics: Impact on Nurses and Nursing.* St. Louis: C. V. Mosby Company, 1975.

Deutsch, K. W. *The Nerves of Government.* New Haven: Yale University Press, 1963.

Easton, D. *A Framework for Political Analysis.* Englewood Cliffs, N.J.: Prentice-Hall, 1965.

Eulau, H. *The Behavioral Persuasion in Politics.* New York: Random House, 1963.

Fenno, R. F. *The Power of the Purse: Appropriations Politics in Congress.* Boston: Little, Brown and Company, 1966.

Flexner, E. *Century of Struggle: The Woman's Rights Movement in the United States.* Cambridge: Belknap Press of Harvard University Press, 1959.

Frankfurt, E. *Vaginal Politics.* New York: Quadrangle, 1972.

Freeman, J. *The Politics of Women's Liberation: A Case Study of an Emerging Social Movement and its Relation to the Policy Process.* New York: David McKay, 1975.

Friedrich, C. J. *Man and His Government: An Empirical Theory of Politics.* New York: McGraw-Hill, 1963.

Froman, L. A., Jr. *The Congressional Process: Strategies, Rules and Procedures.* Boston: Little, Brown and Company, 1967.

Gager, N., Ed. *Women's Rights Almanac, 1974.* Bethesda, Md.: Elizabeth Cady Stanton Publishing Company, 1974.

Gornick, V., and Moran, B. K., Eds. *Women in Sexist Society: Studies in Power and Powerlessness.* New York: Basic Books, 1971.

Gruberg, M. *Women in American Politics.* Oshkosh, Wisc.: Academic Press, 1968.

Hacker, A. *The Study of Politics: The Western Tradition and American Origins.* New York: McGraw-Hill, 1963.

Hall, D. R. *Cooperative Lobbying—The Power of Pressure*. Tucson: University of Arizona Press, 1969.

Haveman, R. H., and Margolis, J., Eds. *Public Expenditures and Policy Analysis*. Chicago: Markham, 1970.

Hess, R. D., and Torney, J. *The Development of Political Attitudes in Children*. Chicago: Aldine, 1967.

Howe, F. (Editor). *Women and the Power to Change*. New York: McGraw-Hill Company, 1975.

Hunter, F. *Community Power Structure; A Study of Decision Makers*. Chapel Hill: University of North Carolina Press, 1953.

Jacob, H., and Vines, K., Eds. *Politics in the American States, A Comparative Analysis*. Boston: Little, Brown and Company, 1965.

Jaquette, J. S., Ed. *Women in Politics*. New York: John Wiley, 1974.

Jennings, M. K., and Niemi, R. G. The division of political labor between mothers and fathers, *American Political Science Review*, Vol. 65, March, 1971, 69–82.

Kalisch, B. J., and Kalisch, P. A. "Congress Copes with the Nurse Shortage: Dynamics of Congressional Nurse Education Policy Formulation," in the Proceedings of the *American Nurses' Association, Ninth Nursing Research Conference*. Kansas City: American Nurses' Association, 1974, 317–377.

Key, V. O. *American State Politics: An Introduction*. New York: Alfred Knopf, 1966.

Kirkpatrick, J. J. *Political Woman*. New York: Basic Books, 1974.

Lamson, P. *Few Are Chosen: American Women in Political Life Today*. Boston: Houghton Mifflin, 1968.

Lane, R. E. *Political Life: Why People Get Involved in Politics*. Glencoe, Ill.: Free Press, 1959.

Lasswell, H. D., Ed. *A Study of Power*. Glencoe, Ill.: Free Press, 1950.

Lasswell, H. D. *Power and Personality*. New York: Norton, 1948.

Lipset, S. M. *Political Man*. New York: Doubleday, 1959.

Lowenstein, K. *Power and the Governmental Process*. 2d ed. Chicago: University of Chicago Press, 1965.

Magnuson, Sen. W. G. *How Much for Health?* New York: Luce, 1974.

Meehan, E. J. *The Theory and Method of Political Analysis*. Homewood, Ill.: Dorsey, 1965.

Merriam, C. E. *Political Power*. New York: Collier, 1964.

Millet, K. *Sexual Politics*. New York: Doubleday, 1970.

Morrow, W. L. *Congressional Committees*. New York: Scribner, 1969.

Murphy, I. L. *Public Policy on the Status of Women: Agenda and Strategy for the 70's*. Boston: D. C. Heath Publishers, 1974.

Nigro, F. A. *Modern Public Administration*. 2d ed. New York: Harper and Row, 1970.

Olson, M. *The Logic of Collective Action; Public Goods and the Theory of Groups*. Cambridge: Harvard University Press, 1965.

Presthus, R. *Men at the Top: A Study in Community Power*. New York: Oxford University Press, 1964.

Ralph Nader Congress Project. *Citizens Look at Congress*. New York: Grossman, 1972.

Riker, W. H. *The Theory of Political Coalitions*. New Haven: Yale University Press, 1962.

Ripley, R. B. *Congress*. New York: Norton, 1975.

Saloma, J. S., III. *Congress and the New Politics*. Boston: Little, Brown and Company, 1969.

Sharkansky, I. *Policy Analysis in Political Science*. Chicago: Markham, 1969.

Sharkansky, I. *Spending in the American States*. Chicago: Rand McNally, 1968.

Shively, W. P. *The Craft of Political Research: A Primer*. Englewood Cliffs, N.J.: Prentice-Hall, 1974.

Simon, H. A. *Models of Man; Social and Rational*. New York: John Wiley, 1957.

Spiro, H. J. *Politics as the Master Science: From Plato to Mao*. New York: Harper, 1970.

Tanenbaum, S. Montesque, and Mme. de Stael. The Woman as a factor in political analysis, *Political Theory*, Vol. 1 February, 1973, 92–103.

Tolchin, S., and Tolchin, M. *Clout: Womanpower and Politics.* New York: Coward, 1974.

Torrence, S. W. *Grassroots Government: The County in American Politics.* New York: Luce, 1974.

Trohan, W. *Political Animals.* New York: Doubleday, 1974.

Truman, D. B. *The Governmental Process.* New York: Alfred Knopf, 1951.

U.S. Congress, *Congressional Record.*

U.S. Congress, Hearings.

Example:

U.S. Congress. House. Committee on Interstate and Foreign Commerce. *Health Manpower Programs.* Hearings, 94th Cong., 1st sess., on bills to amend the Public Health Service Act to revise and extend the programs of assistance for training in the health and allied health professions, for nurse training, to revise the National Health Service Corps program and for other purposes. Washington: Government Printing Office, 1975.

U.S. Congress, Reports.

Example:

U.S. Congress. House. Committee on Interstate and Foreign Commerce. *Nurse Training Act of 1975*; report to accompany H.R. 4115. Washington: Government Printing Office, 1975 (94th Cong., 1st sess. House Report No. 94-143).

U.S. General Services Administration, *The Federal Register.*

Ware, C. *Woman Power: The Movement for Women's Liberation.* New York: Tower, 1970.

Washington Report on Medicine and Health.

Ziegler, H. *Interest Groups in American Society.* Englewood Cliffs, N.J.: Prentice-Hall, 1964.

24 Motivating Nurses to Be Politically Aware

Marilyn Bagwell

MANY FACETS of the multi-billion-dollar health care industry are regulated by the U.S. Congress and State legislatures. Since nurses comprise the largest single professional group in the health care industry, they are a logical group to influence the legislatures' decisions on the health policies which affect the profession of nursing and, ultimately, the consumer. Nurses, having direct responsibility for much of the patient care, see the health care system as few others are able to see it. In the process, they have accumulated valuable data about consumers and health care services. To communicate this data to the various legislators, nurses must become involved in the legislative process concerning health care policies.

Involvement in this legislative process requires that a nurse first be motivated to become politically aware. Motivation, according to Jung [1], includes terms "that refer to such diverse states as desires, wishes, plans, goals, intents, impulses, and purposes." Confer [2] defines motivation as "being equated with the reasons for behavior, the explanatory principle above all others." Thus, a general discussion of motivation refers to the causes or reasons that underlie a given behavior.

In nursing, Maslow's hierarchy of needs is the most widely accepted holistic approach to explain human motivation. According to Lysaught [3], most nurses probably find it difficult to meet their lower-level needs for security and, beyond those, to satisfy their psychosocial needs for greater contribution, acceptance, recognition, and fulfillment. In addition, Lysaught states that nursing has two major facts which inhibit nursing motivation: Most nurses are women, and nursing has been an altruistic profession. However, nurses must make an effort to overcome obstacles in becoming politically motivated. Today's society is beginning to require that nursing priorities include preventive care as well as patient care. Both priorities are affected by the political arena as state and national governments debate the health delivery system.

Consequently, the need for nurses to become politically aware is critical. Mullane [4], in discussing the need for nurses to contribute their knowledge to government policies concerning health care facilities for all, stresses the importance of nurses recognizing and utilizing their valuable political skills as well as their clinical skills. Deloughery and Gebbie [5] state that "all nurses are a part of political dynamics every day and that many of them are becoming aware that they understand but little of the political process in which they are involved or the ways in which they react to it."

In actuality, this understanding is not difficult to achieve. It can begin on an individual level or a group level. One method for the nurse to use in becoming more politically aware

Reprinted with permission of Charles B. Slack, Inc., from *Nursing Leadership,* Volume 3, Number 4, December 1980.

on a national or state level is for her to identify what legislative district she resides in and who are the representatives and senators of her district. Once she has identified these legislators, she should try to meet them if possible. One way of meeting the legislators is to call their offices to make an appointment. Most legislators will be quite willing to inform her about health care legislation in process. Another method is to invite the legislators in for "coffee and donuts" with a group of nurses and health care professionals. Identifying her legislators and initiating contact with them lowers the barrier which frequently exists between a legislator and his constituents, thereby enabling the nurse to be less hesitant in contacting the legislator about bills in which she and other health care professionals are interested.

A nurse can use several resources to identify her national and state districts. In most states, as in Arizona, the Secretary of State's office has maps that outline the national districts. For the state districts, the Mountain Bell Telephone Company and other telephone companies provide a directory of the legislature which includes: names, addresses, telephone numbers, committee memberships, chairmanships, and a map of the legislative districts. Several states have a newspaper, such as Arizona's *Legislative Review*, which is usually available in the local library or by subscription and provides information on current legislators. Another resource is the League of Women Voters, which has a chapter in every state and which is always willing to help citizens identify their districts and to give out information about current legislative issues.

After identifying the district she represents, the nurse might begin asking her co-workers what legislative districts they live in and helping those who are not able to identify their districts to do so. She could then compile a listing of the districts, which would be invaluable when the group might decide to contact their individual legislators about a specific bill. Once individual nurses and then groups of nurses have knowledge of their legislative districts, they may become more interested in what their legislators are doing and what bills are being presented in the legislature.

Nurses who live in a state capital can attend sessions and get copies of bills; however, the majority of nurses will need to use other resources to keep abreast of legislation. The local newspaper generally lists the current legislation, as do the specialty newspapers like the *Arizona Legislative Review*. Another resource is the listing of all the current bills being introduced to the legislature for that particular week. This listing is called the *Legislature Digest* in Arizona but is utilized by most state legislatures. The nurse can get on this mailing list by requesting it from her legislator and when she scans this list, will become more aware of the many decisions about health care and nursing that are made in the legislative branch of government.

Once nurses are aware of their legislative district, the names of their representatives, and the current bills, they are ready to follow a bill through the legislative process. It would be helpful at this time if the nurse could have an inservice or workshop available on legislative process conducted by either a legislator or a nurse who is well informed about the process. Such information would give the nurse or nursing groups an opportunity to become more familiar and comfortable with the process.

Whether a bill is local or national, its process usually follows a pattern once it has been introduced into the House or Senate. The bill is introduced by a legislative member, a group of members, or a standing committee. It is assigned a number, read (First Reading), referred to appropriate standing committees, and then printed and distributed. The standing committees consider the bill, which may include hearings, expert testimony, reports, and recommendations from citizens. After the bill leaves the standing committees, it goes to the committee on rules, which determines if the bill is constitutional and in proper form. The bill is then read (Second Reading) before the committee of the whole: all members of either the House or Senate. This group debates, amends and makes recommendations. Following the final reading (Third Reading), a roll call vote is taken. Every member present must vote. If after the final reading the bill passes one house, it goes to the other house, and the process is repeated, except in Nebraska which is a unicameral, or one-house, legislature.

The fate of a bill depends upon the support it has in the committees to which the bill is assigned. The chairman of a standing committee controls whether or not the bill assigned will be heard and discussed by the committee. The bill will not leave a committee unless a majority of the committee favors the bill. However, a bill which doesn't pass committee might be attached by amendment to another bill coming up before the committee of the whole.

If the bill passes out of the second house with no changes, it will pass to the governor or President for his signature or veto. If the bill isn't identical to that passed by the first house, it goes back to the original house to be accepted in its new form or to be rejected and sent to Conference Committee, which comprises members from both houses and works for a compromise. If the committee succeeds, the bill is sent back to each house and upon acceptance by both houses goes to the governor or President.

The governor or President will either approve or veto a bill. The legislature may override the veto by a two-thirds vote of both houses if they are in session. When the bill becomes law, it will become part of the state or national statutes.

Now the nurse who has begun to sharpen her political knowledge, skills, and awareness by the above methods and who already has a large amount of data concerning consumers and health care services can select a bill that has implication for health care and nursing. She can determine which committees will consider the bill and how much support the bill has in the legislature. She will be able to assess the support by either calling her legislators and asking them for a vote count or by contacting the nurse lobbyist in her state. Upon request, the Secretary of State of individual states will furnish the names of registered lobbyists, which will include the nurse lobbyist.

The nurse is now prepared to write a letter, telephone, or wire her legislator and other key legislators about her position on the bill; however, it is important to remember when writing or calling to be well informed on the issue.

When writing a letter try to keep it to one page, accurately describe the position being supported, and offer any assistance to the legislator for additional facts that may be needed to make a decision on this particular piece of legislation. The letter doesn't have to be typed; correct details about the pending legislation will be sufficiently influential. Most legislators will respond to the letter by providing feedback on their position. Writing, telephoning, or wiring legislative representatives is another step in becoming politically astute.

Information about a particular bill or the position politicians are taking on health issues is knowledge which nurses need to share with other nurses and health care professionals. A legislative bulletin board is a method which can be utilized in any health care agency, hospital, or school setting. It is a resource for posting important materials and for visually stimulating others to the importance of legislation on health care issues.

A Health Issues Today Committee (HIT) is also a method of sharing information on pending state and national legislation. The purpose of the HIT committee is to inform other nurses and health care professionals about health-related issues at the local, state, and federal levels. The membership of the committee should represent a cross section of the nurses and health care professionals who work in the agency, hospital, or school setting.

When the bill a nurse or nursing group has been supporting becomes law, be sure to write or call the legislator or legislators who were responsible for the passage and give them approval. This type of feedback encourages the legislators and confirms the genuine interest in that particular piece of legislation. It may also induce them to consider seriously the nurse's or group's objections or support for other bills.

In motivating nurses to become politically aware, the methods of identifying and getting acquainted with their legislators, knowing the legislative process, and writing or calling their legislators will be a major step. The individual nurse can spearhead the Health Issues Today Committee and a legislative bulletin board in her agency, activities which will ultimately involve other nurses and health care professionals in the process of getting legislation passed that benefits the profession and the consumer.

The nurses or nursing groups taking the initial steps toward involvement with the political process are going to be the ones who influence future health care legislation. Remember, the stakes of nursing are imbedded in the health policy legislation that will be passed in the national and state legislatures.

REFERENCES

1. Jung J: *Human Motivation—A Cognitive Approach.* New York, Macmillan Publishing Co, Inc.
2. Confer CN: *Motivation and Emotion.* Glenview, Illinois, Scott Foresman & Co, 1972.
3. Lysaught JP: *Action in Nursing Progress in Professional Purpose.* New York, McGraw-Hill Book Co, 1974.
4. Mullane MK: Nursing care and the political arena. *Nurs Outlook* 23(11), November 1975.
5. Deloughery G, Gebbie K: *Political Dynamics—Impact on Nurses and Nursing.* St. Louis, CV Mosby Co, 1975.

Section 6
Collective Action

25 Collective Action

THE BASIS FOR PROFESSIONALISM

Ada Jacox

THE NOTION that organizing for the purpose of collective bargaining is somehow not professional has been persistent in nursing. Such a statement reflects a basic misunderstanding of the concept of profession and its relationship to collective action.

The question "Do labor organization activities decrease professionalism?" is comparable to the question, "Does having an administrative hierarchy in a department of professionals decrease the quality of professional service given?" The anwer to both questions is "Sometimes" or "It depends on who is doing the bargaining or the administration." Both collective bargaining and administration are means to an end. In collective bargaining or collective action by professionals, the ends are improvement in the quality of professional service delivered and in the economic and general welfare of the professionals. Administration of a department of professionals is the efficient and effective use of resources to facilitate delivery of a high quality of professional service. Both processes, when used by professionals, share the goal of promoting delivery of a high quality of professional service. They are two mechanisms or means for achieving that common goal.

In both collective bargaining and administration, the means can be misunderstood or misused so as to negate the purposes for which they are meant. It is true that the leadership in some unions becomes caught up in the politics of the conflict and in their own self interest to the detriment of the welfare and concerns of those represented. It is also true that some administrators abuse their power and do not act in the best interest of the organization or of the employees. The fact that some persons or groups, including nurses and nurse administrators, abuse mechanisms for achieving certain ends does not make the mechanisms themselves wrong. It is the use that people make of them that is right or wrong. In exploring this issue more fully, I will address the following points:

The nature of a profession and its relationship to collective bargaining
Modifications in use of the collective bargaining process with professionals
The desirability of a professional association or a non-nurses' labor union as the bargaining agent for nurses
The importance of a unified nursing community.

PROFESSIONALS AND COLLECTIVE BARGAINING

The two major characteristics of a profession are a long period of specialized education and a service orientation. A third characteristic based on these two is autonomy, which means

Reprinted with permission by *Supervisor Nurse: The Journal for Nursing Leadership and Management,* September 1980.

that members of the profession are self-regulating and have control of their functions in the work situation. The concept of autonomy is in direct opposition to the concept of obedience, on which nursing traditionally has placed a high value. Nurses have been expected to follow unquestioningly the orders of doctors and their "superiors" in nursing. In nursing service departments authority was and still is, for the most part, vested in administrative position rather than in the professional's expert knowledge.

Occupations can be arranged along a continuum of professionalism according to the degree to which they are characterized by the above attributes. It is difficult to say where any given occupation lies along this continuum, but a number of sociologists have directed their attentions specifically to the degree of autonomy experienced by an occupation and how this influences its status as a profession. Etzioni, for example, suggests that one way in which semi-professions are distinguished from full professions is that they have less autonomy from supervision than do the full fledged professions [1]. Others have observed that teaching, social work and nursing are all semi-professions organized along bureaucratic lines with regulation and supervision coming from administrators rather than along professional lines with regulation and supervision coming from knowledgeable peers [2]. They claim that this happens because semi-professionals lack the degree of specialized knowledge around which professionals build collegial authority patterns. These authors suggest that the fact that most semi-professionals are women seems to increase the tendency for these occupations to be organized along bureaucratic lines. "The public is less willing to grant professional autonomy to women than to men, and . . . women are less likely than men to develop attitudes favorable to professionalism, because most of them are oriented more toward family roles than toward work roles."

I'm spending considerable time discussing the concept of autonomy in a professional because it is at the basis of the argument regarding whether or not professionals should organize for collective bargaining purposes. Nurses traditionally have not experienced much autonomy. As noted above, they have been expected to follow the orders or directions of physicians and nurse administrators, rather than to exercise their own professional judgment. Such an attitude is reinforced in the writings of some nurse administrators who suggest that it is the nurse administrator who is responsible for the quality of nursing practice given. The idea that a single administrator can or should be solely responsible for the quality of service given by a group of professionals is misguided and anti-professional. The nurse administrator, the medical administrator, the hospital administrator, other administrators, and the governing board all share some responsibility for the quality of health care provided to patients. However, it is the collective responsibility of the professionals who provide a service to determine the standards of practice—the quality of service delivered. This is acknowledged in the case of physicians who, as a medical staff, determine the standards for medical care to be given in an agency. It is no less true of professional nurses, who collectively are responsible to assure that a high quality of nursing care is delivered. It is the professionals themselves who give the care and who must have the major role in determining the standards of practice and seeing that they are implemented. The authority of the group of professionals based on their specialized knowledge, cannot be delegated or relegated to an administrator. The fact is that many nursing departments have not acknowledged that nurses are professionals and that the authority for practice rests with the professionals collectively. It is only recently that nurses have begun to adopt such ideas as audit committees, peer review of practice, and committees composed of representatives of practicing nurses to set standards for practice. The prerogatives and responsibilities of professionals have not been accepted by nurses generally. Instead, practice standards have been determined by administrators and administrators sometimes have had sole responsibility for evaluating the practice of the individual nurse. Serious acceptance of autonomy—that is, both the authority and responsibility for their own practice—by professional nurses is long overdue. One way that nurses are beginning to gain this autonomy is by organizing for collective bargaining purposes.

Professionals traditionally have used their collective strength to achieve certain kinds of professional goals. One form of collective action is joining a professional association, which lobbies lawmakers and governmental agencies for the development of laws and regulatory procedures that have a direct impact on the delivery of the professional service, collectively determining through professional associations what the standards of education and practice of the profession will be, and organizing collective bargaining units to improve salaries and the conditions of professional practice. While the latter kind of collective action is relatively new for the professions, its newness does not make it any the less desirable as a mechanism for professionals to use in achieving their goals. Although collective bargaining is associated in the minds of some with the skilled and semi-skilled trades, for the last several decades it has been used increasingly by salaried professionals. These professionals include teachers, physicians, engineers, nurses, airline pilots and university faculties.

MODIFICATION IN USE OF COLLECTIVE BARGAINING WITH PROFESSIONALS

The legal definition of collective bargaining is "the performance of the mutual obligation of the employer and the representatives of the employees to meet at reasonable times and confer in good faith with respect to wages, hours, and other terms and conditions of employment, or the negotiation of any agreement, or any question arising thereunder" [3]. The last clause provides the opportunity for professionals to negotiate about conditions that directly affect the quality of their practice. This kind of focus in bargaining activities is one of the ways in which collective bargaining by professionals differs from collective bargaining by traditional labor unions, which generally negotiate about salaries and fringe benefits. The process used is the same, whether the bargaining is done by professionals or traditional labor unions. It is the issues over which bargaining takes place that are different. For professional nurses, negotiations related to practice issues have included the establishment of practice committees on which practicing nurses serve, provision for adequate staff development including orientation and preparation for working in specialty units, the addition of equipment deemed necessary for patient safety on units, adoption of specific standards of practice such as requiring that adequate means for communicating about patients and their care plans be established, provision for practicing nurses to be evaluated by their peers, and similar mechanisms intended to improve the quality of nursing care delivered. When collective bargaining is used by professional nurses in this way, it is one of the clearest possible expressions of professionalism. Nurses behaving in this way are seriously seeking to achieve professional autonomy—control over their own practice in the work setting.

WHO SHOULD REPRESENT NURSES IN COLLECTIVE BARGAINING?

For the past 34 years, the American Nurses' Association (ANA), the professional association for nurses, has had a program of economic and general welfare for nurses. Support for the program has varied by state, by time periods and by general social conditions. The House of

Delegates, which is composed totally of professional nurses elected by their peers to represent them, has consistently and repeatedly given strong endorsement to the program. The House of Delegates also has considered and set policy for the numerous other concerns of a multipurpose professional association. These issues have included those clearly related to nursing practice, such as adopting a code of ethics, and setting standards for education, nursing practice and the administration of nursing services. They also have included taking firm stands on issues affecting the health and well being of the population and on issues affecting the welfare of those employed in health care settings. The scope of concerns to which a professional association necessarily must give attention is broad, because the concerns of professionals are many and varied. Unfortunately, this has meant that all issues do not always receive the full and undivided attention of the association, which must shift its priorities as the needs of professional nurses and society in general change.

During the past 12 years, I have been a vocal advocate of a strong program of collective bargaining by ANA. It has been distressing to note the apathy and even antagonism of many nurses who have not understood that collective bargaining can be a strong and appropriate mechanism for nurses to use to improve nursing practice and their own economic and general welfare. Time after time, attempts by state nurses' associations to organize nurses for collective bargaining have not been successful because nurses themselves voted not to organize. They believed, mistakenly in my opinion, that such activity was not "professional." Some state associations have been reluctant to develop strong economic and general welfare programs, because they also hold the same mistaken notion that it is somehow unprofessional.

Now, fortunately, that notion is being dispelled. There is increasing recognition by nurses of the various positive, constructive and *professional* uses of collective bargaining. What is *unfortunate* is that some nurses are seeking to be organized by unions that are composed of and run by non-nurses. During the past few years, it seems that all sorts of groups from retail clerks to teachers to butchers suddenly have developed an interest in organizing nurses. The fact that their unions are composed of a wide variety of workers with diverse backgrounds and interests is ignored by them and by the nurses willing to join them. The American Federation of Teachers (AFT), for example, has a membership of approximately 500,000 persons, which includes deputy sheriffs, custodians and janitors, photographers, bus drivers, ambulance attendants, antialcoholic and drug-abuse workers, radiation safety specialists, data and computer technicians, transportation workers, attorneys, and schoolteachers. This union, originally established to represent teachers, has been remarkably *unsuccessful* in attracting teachers to its ranks. By contrast, the National Education Association, which is AFT's major competitor in representing teachers, represents 1.8 million. It is unfortunate that some nurses seeking to be represented are not looking beyond the immediate promises of what these unions will do for nurses to their record of performance with their own groups.

At the heart of the controversy over who is best able to represent professional nurses in collective bargaining is the relationship of collective bargaining to the other activities of a professional association. *Because issues of economic and general welfare of professional nurses and issues related to professional practice are so inextricably related, both in collective bargaining and in the total functions of a profession, it is inappropriate for any organization composed of and controlled by non-nurses to represent professional nurses in collective bargaining.* The American Nurses' Association is comprised only of professional nurses, and policy decisions are made by professional nurses elected by other professional nurses. This is not so with any of the unions seeking to represent nurses, and it is not likely that nurses will have much influence in these diverse, polyglot organizations. If it is difficult to deal with the multi-purposes and diverse interest within a professional association comprised entirely of nurses, think how much more difficult it will be to achieve nurses' professional goals within a still more varied group of people and concerns.

The answer for nurses who are now finally ready to use collective bargaining to improve their practice and their salaries, is not to ask a labor union of non-nurses to do this for them. That smacks too much of expecting physicians, hospital administrators, or other groups to act in the best interest of nurses. We have been disappointed too often when we've held such expectations.

THE IMPORTANCE OF A UNIFIED NURSING COMMUNITY

The answer is to join the professional association, elect representatives supportive of collective bargaining and *insist* that the association increase enormously its collective bargaining activities. Constituents of the ANA now represent over 100,000 nurses in collective bargaining. That number should increase tenfold. If the ANA were to represent the 1,000,000 nurses in collective bargaining and in all other areas related to the practice of professional nursing, think of what an effective force nurses could be in improving health care in this country—as well as in improving nurses' economic status.

If professional nurses in all settings and positions could acknowledge that our common interest in improving patient care is considerably more important than those intraprofessional issues that often divide us, we could have the positive impact on patient care that we wish. Organizing for the purpose of collective bargaining does not decrease professionalism. To the contrary, it is one of the strongest mechanisms by which nurses can achieve professionalism. However, it must be done by an organization of professional nurses, controlled by professional nurses and acting in the best interest of nurses and nursing practice. It is time for professional nurses to claim professional autonomy in an appropriate and responsible way, by joining their professional association, controlling its directions and priorities and *insisting* on being well represented in collective bargaining.

REFERENCES

1. Etzioni, Amitai. (Editor) *The Semi-Professions and Their Organization.* New York: The Free Press, 1969.
2. Simpson, Richard L., and Ida Harper Simpson, "Women and Bureaucracy in the Semi-Professions," in *The Semi-Professions and Their Organization,* Amitai Etzioni, editor. New York: The Free Press, 1969.
3. Labor Management Relations Act, 1947, sec 8(d).

26 The Professional Association and Collective Bargaining

Margaret Colangelo

FOR TOO LONG, action through collective bargaining by workers in white collar jobs and other occupations variously termed semi- and quasi-professional has been held in disrepute. While the use of collective bargaining to promote their own ends and welfare has been assumed to be not only the exclusive right but also the distinctive mark of blue collar workers, any collective action by segments of the work force other than the blue collar workers is represented as "beneath their dignity." When applied to the trades, unionism is an acceptable movement, philosophy, and method, but the same methods adopted by the class of workers enjoying a social position between the true professional and the blue collar worker immediately makes them suspect. Both their public and self-image become marred, they are accused of being less than professional (a status denied them anyway), and any attempt to demand the same privileges accorded to others throughout the economy is somehow supposed to be demeaning.

Collective action under the guise of cohesion and unity often is viewed with respect and awe when undertaken by members of the professions as an indication of their stature and high degree of their commitment. However, the white collar and semi-professional workers are expected to prove their "professional" commitment in individual and collective acts of self-sacrifice. On the other hand, blue collar workers are accorded the privilege of collective action through unionism (albeit reluctantly) as a just reward for and protection of their labor. They have achieved a degree of recognition and respect through the very success of such efforts. As a consequence this very large and important segment of the working public is caught in the squeeze between the professionals who, by unilateral and largely unquestioned action, control their own destiny, and the blue collar workers who call their tune through united action backed up by threats which, when carried out, can drastically affect the nation's economy.

The squeeze upon the salaried segment of the working force has become tighter and tighter until it appears that this middle group will demand more elbow room in one direction or the other or both—in whatever manner they can get it. It is an issue critical to all areas of our economy and social structure whether these groups should, can, or will: (1) adopt the philosophy and methodology of the labor union as presently organized, (2) attempt to achieve professional and autonomous control of their occupations, or (3) arrive at a form of collective action somewhere in between.

Reprinted with permission by *Supervisor Nurse: The Journal for Nursing Leadership and Management,* September 1980.

NURSES AS QUASI-PROFESSIONALS

In no other single class of workers is this force more evident and more understandable than in the field of nursing. This paper will examine the status of nursing and the context in which the main body of its practice occurs. It will describe the forces which hinder and favor organization for collective action and it will suggest some guidelines for the future. The author's principal thesis is that the right of the American public to an acceptable standard of health care—of which nursing is an essential part—cannot be achieved apart from the right of nurses to engage in collective action to determine their own conditions of employment and to set standards for practice. I have concluded that the American Nurses' Association must play the major role in bringing about these changes.

Instead of chastising themselves for lack of unity and aggression, nurses must begin to understand that they are a product of their history. In this light, it is possible to marvel at the steps the nursing profession has taken already to become self-directive and free itself of some of the chains that have held it captive for so long. Today's nurses can make even greater strides in adapting to current demands and in taking the initiative in determining and interpreting what nursing has to offer to the whole health care field if they are given the freedom to do so.

One cannot attempt to analyze the forces moving nurses toward any form of collective action without first considering the factors which have brought about the present situation. One must concur with Etzioni that nurses must realize that "what they consider 'their' problem is shared by other semi-professionals and is, in part, socially induced" [1].

It is not within the purpose of this paper to discuss the struggle of nursing to achieve professional status, so it is important to acknowledge the validity of the viewpoint of sociologists in making a distinction between profession and semi- or quasi-profession. Within the context of such definitions [2], the author recognizes that nursing is placed among the semiprofessions, along with social work and teaching. Thus, when the term or concept of "profession" as pertaining to nursing is used in this paper, it is intended to convey the semiprofessional status described in sociological literature [3].

THE NURSE AND THE HOSPITAL

A number of distinct and overlapping forces account for the total situation in which nursing is practiced today, and these also help to explain the fact that nursing has made no greater strides than it has in achieving more control over its own practice. The religious and military aura surrounding the origins of both primitive and modern nursing quite naturally led to great value being placed on the personal virtues of obedience, dedication, conformity, and even chastity. Such values were reinforced when a lack of respectability came to be associated with early movements in secular nursing. These influences were coupled with the natural or inherent attraction of women to nursing's nurturing function and a social climate in which any form of livelihood for women enjoyed limited respectability. These factors resulted in nursing's being seen as a subordinate, submissive role and destined it to become a predominantly female occupation. Out of this background the nurse-hospital administrator and nurse-doctor relationships arose and they continue to this day to mirror typical male-female roles in our society [4].

Lacking its own body of other than intuitive knowledge, nursing developed under the aegis of the medical profession. While the nursing profession gained some control of the educational content as schools of nursing developed in the nineteenth century, the educational system itself remained under hospital and medical management. A natural exploitation of students occurred since emphasis was placed on the needs of the hospital system for service rather than the needs of the student for education and experience. This in time led to a low rate of employment of graduates by hospitals; therefore many of the early graduates practiced private duty nursing. Unfortunately, the profession did not seize this opportunity to proclaim its autonomy.

After World War I, additional employment opportunities in fields outside the hospital helped to absorb the oversupply of nurses which continued until the advent of World War II. What happened during this period to alleviate the critical shortage of skilled nurses has had a profound and lasting effect on nursing. The precedent then established of employing less qualified nurses to provide direct patient care rather than increasing the rewards of the professional nurse for continuing her unique nursing function was an early capitulation of professional authority derived from knowledge to a "managerial" authority derived from position in the hospital bureaucracy. Hospital management continued to place emphasis, especially through promotion, on coordination-type duties and thus enhanced the pattern of advancement for those who excelled in managerial functions, rather than in professional nursing functions.

Exemption from labor relations laws further provided hospital management with its legal justification for not improving the economic conditions of nurses, thus perpetuating the pattern of employing less skilled persons for direct patient care and promoting the professional nurse away from direct care. Through a completely unchallenged last minute amendment to the Taft-Hartley Act in 1947, nonprofit hospitals remained exempt from mandatory recognition of employee groups. Employees were thus prohibited from requesting representation elections, from filing unfair labor practice charges with the National Labor Relations Board, and from having recourse to any federal agency until they had first gained voluntary recognition by the employer. This, of course, required that they have overwhelming support of their cause. Since then, in regard to labor relations in hospitals, conventional wisdom, "that structure of ideas based on acceptability," has prevailed, even though it is obsolete [5].

The resistance of hospital administrators to giving voluntary recognition to hospital employees and negotiating in collective bargaining has been justified in many ways. The claim is made that they should be immune from the threat of strike so as not to risk interruption of their mission. Their nonprofit status makes funds for bargaining unavailable. The notion that nonprofit status provides them with an *a priori* right to refuse to negotiate on a voluntary basis is offered as justification for the legal exemption and *vice versa* [6].

However, the reasons they give for refusing voluntary recognition and negotiations are untenable. Hospital employees are entitled to the same rights as members of other sectors of the economy and they cannot be expected to subsidize increasing health care costs. The continued resistance to voluntary and legally mandated recognition really is an attempt to deny the existence and prevent the emergence of conflict over control of the function of the employed professional. Does the authority of a position come from the management hierarchy or should this authority be derived from professional knowledge and competence? The director of nursing service is the epitome of both types of authority and, for this reason, is in an especially vulnerable position. Recognizing this, the hospital administrator has attempted (and largely succeeded) in preventing collective action on the part of nurses through control of this position and threats to the individual in it [7].

Nurses increasingly recognize that a perpetuation of the system under which the vast majority of them practice is no longer tenable or consistent with acceptable nursing practice standards. The increasing amount of collective action that has occurred in the past decade, particularly since 1966, is indicative of this growing concern.

In the milieu described in the beginning of this paper, which has been implicitly sanctioned by law, it is not surprising that nurses who have engaged in or thought of engaging in collective action have been beset with feelings of mixed loyalty and even of guilt. The odds against which these scattered groups of nurses have had to work include legislative exemptions; loyalties to themselves, peers, and supervisors, especially to nursing service directors; the paternalistic attitude of hospital administrators and the attitudes of nurses which derive from traditions of self-sacrifice and service.

Paternalism certainly characterizes the relationship between the nurse and the employer, although nurses may be reluctant to admit the fact. To the objective observer, however, it is obvious that many nurses are satisfied to accept uncritically the subordinate, dependent position in an authoritarian relationship [8]. Through a paternalistic attitude hospital administrators often project an image of benevolence, purporting to have gone to great lengths to satisfy professional demands. They become the "injured party" when faced with expressed nursing concerns. While hospital administrators cannot order members of a professional group to behave in ways that are contrary to their professional ethics, they can and often do intimidate the entire nursing staff through their power to discharge the director of nursing and any dissident nurses. They have succeeded all too well in this intimidation of predominantly female workers. "Employeeism," that set of beliefs leading employees to rely on employer benevolence to protect their interests, together with the image of the nurse projected by "Nightingalism" may be the strongest deterrents to the spread of professional collectivism and the success of the ANA Economic Security Program [9].

After 25 years the American Hospital Association acts as though collective bargaining to help combat the appalling employment problems besetting the nursing profession is a whole new idea [10]. Through the hospital association they capitalize on the dilemma of the director of nurses and use their influence to alienate nurses from the ANA. As a result many nurses have withdrawn from the professional organization. Nurses providing direct patient care and in charge of the management of patient care units are conditioned to believe that they must have the sanction of the director of nursing to engage in organized activity [11].

Since it threatens the unilateral control of administration, collective bargaining is labeled unprofesional and undignified, another technique for controlling the behavior of those who prize the term "professional" and any behavior that supposedly validates it. However, there is no evidence that collective bargaining adversely affects the performance of the professional function or the dignity with which it is carried out. Collective bargaining, as such, is irrelevant to whether or not an occupational group maintains professional standards [12].

FACTORS ENCOURAGING COLLECTIVE BARGAINING

Factors which encourage collective action by nurses are, of course, the opposite of those enumerated as obstacles. As long as legislative attempts to amend the Taft-Hartley Law to eliminate the exclusion of nonprofit hospitals failed, it was necessary to work through state legislatures and the courts. Success in some states with passage of laws mandating recognition of employee organizations and favorable court rulings upholding collective actions encouraged the early efforts of nurses in uniting for action. For example, in 1967 the Connecticut Board of Labor ruled that "the Connecticut Nurses' Association is a proper bargaining agent" when challenged on conflict-of-interest grounds. The Michigan Nurses'

Association was cleared of unfair labor practice charges filed in 1970 on similar grounds involving the role of supervisory nurses in a bargaining unit [13]. Further indication of official concern for the status and working conditions of nurses is the instrument on Personnel Practices on Conditions of Work and Life of Nursing Personnel drawn up jointly by the International Labor Organization and the World Health Organization and recommended for adoption worldwide "to fight major obstacles to effective health care—extreme shortage, maldistribution and poor utilization of nurses" [14].

Finally, after many attempts and against formidable opposition, the last legal barrier to the right of a large majority of nurses has been removed by the 1974 amendment to the Taft-Hartley Act. This amendment guarantees to employees of nonprofit hospitals the same rights of recognition and collective actions as have been considered a legal right of other workers, guaranteed by law for 25 years. "The continued exemption of large numbers of health care employees from jurisdiction of labor relations laws perpetuated a gross inequity. In the absence of voluntary recognition and agreement, the employees faced the choice of relinquishing their right to engage in self-organization and collective bargaining, or resorting to the strike and picket line" [15]. Collective bargaining thus has become not only possible, but probable. Past experience has demonstrated that the results include better salaries and benefits and more control over practice. However, where successful such gains have been accomplished by the very methods that nurses were attempting to avoid in order to gain the same ends, i.e., strikes, picket lines, and mass resignations. The impetus the amendment will give to employee organizations within the hospital must not be underestimated. Unions have been responsible for great advancement in the working conditions and rewards of millions of workers. That they can and will do the same for hospital employees, including nurses, is not difficult to predict.

NURSES SEEK REPRESENTATION

Should nurses seek representation through collective action, including collective bargaining? Are they doing so? It is no longer a matter of whether or not nurses should seek representation; the question is, by whom? The social and legislative climate is such that if nurses do not organize on their own initiative to engage in collective action, someone else will do it for them, and the question of their status will be resolved by default. The choice is whether nurses should organize along the pattern of the craft unions or of the industrial unions. The time is at hand for nurses to take the action they see necessary to accomplish their goals, and this includes a clear understanding of what the choices involve.

If nurses choose union representation they should do so with the full realization that they are organizing along the lines of industrial unions. Their special and unique needs and functions will be subject to consideration and negotiation within the framework of the total hospital employee unit representing diverse functions and working conditions. Not only will such organization interfere with advancement toward any autonomy, it will overshadow their current semiprofessional status and identity.

On the other hand, organizing along the lines of medieval guilds and present craft unions would mean representation by the professional association, the American Nurses' Association and its constituents. To question the appropriateness of such a role by a professional organization no longer is relevant. The charge that a professional organization becomes "nothing but a union" and thereby exposes itself to charges of nonprofessionalism is a smoke screen used to draw attention away from the issue of control of practice [16]. What is important is the determination of whether or not nurses want and will accept primary authority over what constitutes (1) competent nursing practice and (2) the conditions under which members of the profession will practice.

THE AMERICAN NURSES' ASSOCIATION

Perhaps the most encouraging and also the most controversial factor presently favoring collective action is involvement of the professional nursing organization with its many strengths. The American Nurses' Association must gear itself for a major all-out effort; and, in fact, it has taken recent action to that end. Now that the legal climate is more favorable, there are indications of increased union efforts to organize in all hospitals. Previously, where unions have entered hospitals, they have had only limited success in organizing registered nurses. Industrial unions work within the bureaucratic management system; in fact, they are part of it. As such, they cannot achieve for nurses the improvements in the control of their own practice and working conditions such as those accomplished by the professional organization in Cook County [17], New York City, and elsewhere [18]. In collective bargaining, the professional organization can focus on the authority system residing within the profession and its knowledge base. Recognizing this, nurses in San Francisco in 1967 [19], in Cedars of Lebanon in 1969 [20], and currently in the other hospitals have rejected unionization because they want and need the direct involvement available under the professional organization. The present status of ANA involvement in economic security includes:

firm commitment to collective bargaining as the best method for dealing with job and professional problems
good public support for collective bargaining
realization of the feeling among employed RNs who show deep dissatisfaction over job and economic conditions and increased belief that they can do something about them
steps by state associations to develop expert negotiators
good marriage between the economic status of the worker and purely professional problems of education and standards of professional practice. [21]

While the American Nurses' Association membership includes only about 28 percent of all registered nurses, it is nevertheless the single dominant organization representing nurses in their job-related and professional problems. No other professional organization should offer significant opposition to this representation [22]. If nurses believe they should be represented by an organization paralleling a craft union whose sole interest is exclusive representation of one craft or trade, they must be aware of and accept the fact that their professional organization is indeed that "union." Many nurses shy away from this term, but it is time they understand the consequences of the alternatives: (1) no action at all, (2) collective action under the control of labor organizations, or (3) professional collective action.

The role of the professional nursing organization in employer-employee relationships and negotiations dates back to 1944 when the ANA ruled that state nurses' associations might engage in collective bargaining [23]. However, the Economic Security and General Welfare program was adopted in 1946 with the provision of a "no strike or use of similar coercive devise clause." Thus nurses entered the collective bargaining, but without the ability to bring hospital management to the bargaining table [24]. In the first 20 years of the

ANA's Economic and General Welfare program (1946–1966) only modest gains were made in the economic conditions of nursing. An average annual salary of $5,200 prevailed, compared to $2,100 in 1946. In 1948 the ANA called upon state associations to refrain from engaging in joint economic security programs with hospital management to avoid charges of company unionism. The association saw no conflict between the ethical codes of the nursing profession and collective bargaining as an ethical imperative to help nursing achieve a truly professional status. In 1950, the "no strike clause" was reaffirmed.

In spite of this position, there was only sporadic activity or achievement until 1966. In that year both in New York City and in San Francisco, concerted action by nurses brought rather dramatic gains [25]. About the same time, the House of Delegates of the ANA adopted unanimously a nationwide salary goal for 1966 of $6,500. Great strides were made toward achieving this goal in various sections of the country. However, in other instances recognition was achieved slowly and only by threatening to use, or using, force. Thus, in 1966, the state associations of California and Pennsylvania, followed by the national association in 1968, revoked the no strike pledge. While progress has been slow, it is a wonder that so few could accomplish so much against such odds.

Immediately prior to and following the national salary goal set for 1966, activity was spurred throughout the nation. In New York City 1,500 RNs (one-half of the total) submitted resignations in protest of unsatisfactory employer proposals. Five days prior to the effective date of the resignations, minimum salaries were increased from $5,150 to $6,400. In San Francisco, there was a move to join the AFL-CIO, but the California Nurses' Association (CNA) won out [26]. Informal picket lines were formed. The decision to turn in mass resignations forced the CNA to revoke its no strike policy. Contracts were finally awarded which provided for increasing salaries from $5,280 to $7,200. Similar events occurred across the country following unanimous adoption of the national salary goal. During the remainder of the year, in 143 situations 19,000 nurses joined together to negotiate for better salaries and working conditions [27].

In 1968 the ANA rescinded its no strike clause and pledged support to efforts of state nurses' associations, which would undertake concerted economic pressures lawful and consistent with the nurses' professional responsibility. Meanwhile a study of organizing efforts a year earlier showed that the number of hospitals with contracts had doubled since 1961 [28]. Meanwhile in Ohio in 1966 and in California in 1969 when nurses went out on strike, sympathetic unions offered their support to the striking nurses [29]. At the same time, hospitals organized to combat unionism and collective bargaining in any form. Hospitals in Southern California joined to fix wages and no hospital union has yet been powerful enough to combat the Southern Hospital Council of the CHA. While the Cedars of Lebanon nurses succeeded in getting partial recognition of their Professional Performance Committee (the equivalent to a local unit), the CNA was not recognized as a bargaining agent for salaries and fringe benefits.

In 1973 ANA once again testified that the Taft-Hartley exemption had resulted in a substandard wage structure throughout the hospital industry [30]. In 1974 at a Council of Representatives of State Constituents, ANA launched a drive to organize the nation's 600,000 nurses for collective action for quality care. It determined that it would commit substantial resources to the 52 constituent nurses' associations to bring about collective bargaining in each health care facility. Its continued lobby to end nonprofit hospital exemption from collective bargaining and to clarify the term "supervisor" as applied to nurses finally was successful [31].

DISCUSSION

On the basis of this previous review and analysis, I conclude that the only ethical, professional, and pragmatic alternative available to nurses is to unite in expending every effort to make the national, state, and local nursing organizations the collective bargaining agent for all nurses. It is their moral imperative, consistent with their professional concern for quality nursing care, the Patient's Bill of Rights [32], and the Code for Nurses [33]. To carry out this imperative, nurses must combat the divisive techniques that have separated them. It should not matter that there are splinter nursing organizations organized to meet the unique needs of specialized categories of nurses. It is fortunate that these exist, so that the ANA can concentrate its resources on a single purpose.

No other organization replaces or duplicates what the ANA does and should continue to do for nurses. It is the voice of the profession on both national and state levels. It is within the power of the professional organization to make this economic and general welfare program its primary commitment. It must expand staff for collective bargaining and educate nurses in the negotiating relationships between management and labor. It must take the lead in making public the details of hospital financing. Some unions have even suggested that hospitals be classified as public utilities and become subject to regulations of the Public Utility Commission.

At the least the nonprofit status of the hospitals no longer should continue to be used as a ploy to justify the employees' subsidizing of capital improvements through substandard wages. Nurses should see to it that nursing care and services are visible in patients' bills, as are x-ray, laboratory, central supply, or pharmacy charges, rather than being lumped under a daily board and room charge which serves as an umbrella for such sundry costs as housekeeping, dietary, and professional nursing services.

THE SUPERVISOR AND DNS

Through its organization the nursing profession must come to grips with the dilemma of the nursing service director and associated supervisory personnel. In addition to collective bargaining for the nurse providing direct patient care or managing a nursing unit or team, there must be attention and support given to those nurses classified as supervisory and administrative personnel. Steps must be taken to implement the positions described in "The Role of the Director of an Organized Nursing Service in Collective Bargaining" [35]. Hospital management has been successful in imposing its social philosophy on its managerial staff, including the director of nursing and, in turn, on the total nursing staff. Nurses must realize that collective bargaining is essentially a decision-making process that is available to them as it is to other workers.

The nursing profession must forget, at least for now, concern over whether it has achieved true professional status and address itself to the urgent issues which face it, especially control over its own practice. Only then can nursing be prepared to determine its destiny rather than simply to await it. The fact that nursing is one of those occupations striving for professional status, but which in reality has an employee relationship within a bureaucratic system that confers upon it only semiprofessional status, shows the futility of pursuing or arguing the point. As Goode states, "Within the set of dependent relations or tensions among autonomy, service and knowledge there are three extreme outcomes which aspiring professions try to guard against, but over which they have little control: (a) The occupation may achieve some cohesion but expend this greater strength in merely improving incomes, with little concern about the ideal of service; (b) the occupation may, as its knowledge base grows, simply split into numerous sub-associations so that little cohesion develops; and (c) because the occupation can be superseded by a bureaucracy and the substance of its work requires little autonomy, it is simply absorbed into high level bureaucratic positions" [36].

No nurse would welcome any of these outcomes and, perhaps it is not too late to exert some control and bring about some balance between the bureaucratic and professional management systems within which nursing operates. There seems to be no real danger from the first, but there is definite threat from the second and third. United action through the professional organization may be the only hope of avoiding all three. Certainly, going the way of industrial unionism will only hasten these outcomes, either directly or by default.

REFERENCES

1. Etzioni, Amitai, ed. *The Semi-Professions and Their Organization,* The Free Press, New York, 1969.
2. *Ibid.*
3. Katz, Fred, "Nurses," *The Semi-Professions and Their Organization,* pp. 82–140.
4. Bullough, Bonnie, "The New Militancy in Nursing," *Nursing Forum,* Vol. 10, No. 3, 1971, p. 273.
5. McCormick, William, "Labor Relations in Hospital," *American Journal of Nursing,* Vol. 70, No. 12, December, 1970, pp. 2606 ff.
6. *Ibid.,* p. 2607.
7. ANA Position, "The Role of The Director of Organized Nursing Service in Collective Bargaining," *American Journal of Nursing,* Vol. 70, No. 3, March, 1970, pp. 551–556.
8. Sheppard, Harold K. and Audrey P. Sheppard, "Paternalism in Employer-Employee Relationships," *American Journal of Nursing,* Vol. 51, No. 1, January, 1951.
9. Grand, Norma K., "Nightingalism, Employeeism, and Professional Collectivism," *American Journal of Nursing,* Vol. 10, No. 3, March, 1971, p. 289.
10. Conta, A. Lionne, "Bargaining by Professionals," *American Journal of Nursing,* Vol. 72, No. 2, February, 1972, p. 209.
11. *Op. cit.,* ANA position, p. 552.
12. Kleingartner, Archie. *Professionalism and Salaried Worker Organization: Industrial Relations Institute,* University of Wisconsin, Madison, 1967.
13. News, "Connecticut Nurses End Year Long Negotiations," "Michigan Association Cleared of Unfair Labor Practice Charge," *American Journal of Nursing,* Vol. 72, No. 11, November, 1972, p. 1964.
14. News, "Taft-Hartley Hospital Exemption May End," *American Journal of Nursing,* Vol. 72, No. 10, October, 1972, p. 1772.
15. News, "ILO/WHO Draws Up Instrument on Personnel Practices for Adoption for Nurses Worldwide," *American Journal of Nursing,* Vol. 74, No. 2, February, 1974, p. 189.
16. Kleingartner, Archie, "Nurses, Collective Bargaining and Labor Legislation," *Labor Law Journal,* Vol. 18, April, 1967, p. 240.
17. News, "Strike Over Practice Issue Wins Gains, Nurses Win Battle to Keep RN Performance Committee," *American Journal of Nursing,* Vol. 73, No. 5, May, 1973, p. 784.
18. News, "New York City Nurses Switch Non-Nursing Functions to Implement New Law and New Position Discrepancies," *American Journal of Nursing,* Vol. 72, No. 12, December, 1972, p. 2135.
19. Miltman, Ben and Beatrice Bumgarner, "What Happened in San Francisco?" *American Journal of Nursing,* Vol. 67, No. 1, January, 1967, pp. 80–84.
20. Lewis, Edith P., "Cedars of Lebanon Story," *American Journal of Nursing,* Vol. 69, No. 11, November, 1969, pp. 2385–2390.

21. *Op. cit.,* Kleingartner, p. 224.
22. Jacox, Ada, "Collective Action and Control of Practice by Professionals," *Nursing Forum,* Vol. 10, No. 3, 1971, p. 239.
23. Belote, Martha, "Nurses are Making It Happen," *American Journal of Nursing,* Vol. 67, No. 2, February, 1967, pp. 285–289.
24. *Op. cit.,* Bullough, p. 273.
25. *Op. cit.,* Bullough, p. 275.
26. *Op. cit.,* Belote, p. 273.
27. *Op. cit.,* Bullough, p. 273.
28. *Op. cit.,* Bullough, p. 273.
29. *Op. cit.,* Lewis, p. 2385.
30. News, "ANA Testifies in Taft-Hartley Exemption," *American Journal of Nursing,* Vol. 73, No. 10, October, 1973, p. 1667.
31. News, "ANA Launches Drive to Organize Nurses for Collective Action in Quality Care," *American Journal of Nursing,* Vol. 73, No. 1, January, 1974, p. 7.
32. Statement on a Patient's Bill of Rights, affirmed by the AHA Board of Trustees, November, 1972.
33. Code for Nurses with Interpretive Statements, ANA Committee on Ethical, Legal and Professional Standards.
34. Klassen, Kathryn, "The Nurse's Right for Self-Determination in Professional Practice," *Nursing Forum,* Vol. 10, No. 3, 1970, p. 322.
35. *Op. cit.,* ANA position, pp. 551–556.
36. Goode, William J., "The Theoretical Limits of Professionalization," *The Semi-Professions and Their Organization,* p. 300.

27 The Grievance Process

Elaine E. Beletz and Mary T. Meng

THE SUCCESSFUL NEGOTIATION of the labor-management contract is not the end of the negotiating process. The contract simply states broad guidelines which both parties have agreed to live with. It cannot include every situation which will arise. For this reason, the grievance procedure is vital.

It is the heart of any contract. Without it, the contract may become a useless piece of paper. The grievance procedure is necessary for the administration and intepretation of the contract—it makes the contract a dynamic and viable document.

Although contract language has been agreed upon by both parties, each side will interpret every contract sentence in terms of protection of its own rights and interests. If, as a result, a dispute arises, it can be resolved through the grievance procedure.

There are obvious benefits in the grievance process for the employee. It gives him a voice in resolving problems and a vehicle for adjusting disputes arising out of the interpretation and application of the collective bargaining agreement. It might provide a way to continue the negotiating process without having to renegotiate an entirely new contract. For management, the grievance procedure is an avenue for communication and may provide the impetus for instituting change and discovering needs for policy reform.

There will never be an entirely content and satisfied employee staff. This would be utopia. Having a few grievances is considered to be quite healthy [1].

A grievance may be caused by an alleged violation of a contract provision, a change in a past practice, or an employer decision which is considered arbitrary, capricious, unreasonable, unfair, or discriminatory. Gripes, personality differences, or generalized, nonspecific, malcontent complaints do not constitute grievances.

Precedents and past practices are frequently not enumerated in contracts. A precedent is a decision that serves as an example, reason, or justification for future responses to similar grievances. It establishes a rule of behavior. A past practice is a mutually accepted behavior or response that has continued to recur over a significant period of time, is considered the appropriate practice within the institution. A grievance might result if, for example, the institution always let employees go home one hour early on Fridays and suddenly stops the practice.

Generally speaking, most grievances are initially handled informally by the employee, and/or his representative, and the employee's immediate supervisor. If the grievance is not settled, the employee and/or his representative advances the grievance to people in successively higher levels of management as specified in the contract. The day-to-day administrators of the contract, therefore, are the employee's representative, who may be the head of

Copyright © 1977, American Journal of Nursing Company. Reproduced, with permission, from *American Journal of Nursing,* February, Volume 77, Number 2.

the local unit or other designated individual as a grievance chairman or delegate, and the first-line supervisor [2].

The delegate, also called shop steward or shop committeeman, is the vital connecting link between the certified representative for collective bargaining, for example, the state nurses' association, or the union and the employer. He or she is elected by the employees to be their spokesman in the day-to-day contract administration. As the employees' advocate, his main function is to protect the rights of the members of the bargaining unit through conduct of the grievance process.

Within the nursing hierarchy, a supervisor may be the head nurse, supervisor, nursing care coordinator, assistant director, or director, depending on the position of the aggrieved employee and the authority delegated to resolve grievances to each of the positions mentioned. Federal labor law generally defines a supervisor as one who has the authority to effectively resolve grievances as well as having other powers commensurate with the position.

The primary role of the supervisor in relation to the contract is to keep formal grievances to a minimum, while establishing a cooperative relationship with the bargaining unit and its representatives. When members of the bargaining unit are professionals, the first-line supervisor may have greater identification with the employee than with administration. Such an individual will feel personal conflict when faced with a grievance. Often, supervisors feel that their abilities are judged by the number of grievances received and these are viewed as employee expressions of discontent. This may then add to their personal conflicts in resolving grievances [3].

A frequent concern of such supervisors is that they will not receive administrative backing or that their decisions will be reversed. Many, in defense, may not resolve a grievance, but allow it to go to the next step.

In relation to management backing, Von Bleiken emphasizes:

It must be understood by an individual on the line of mid-management level that top management may be faced with situations where, although the supervisor's action is technically correct, extenuating and far-reaching circumstances may dictate that it is greater wisdom for management to reverse the supervisor's decision. . . . However, management has an obligation to the respective supervisor, either to inform him to that effect prior to publishing the decision, and giving him the reasons why, or to allow the supervisor to reverse his own decision. [4]

It is our practice to discuss decisions made by supervisors with them and, if a reversal is necessary, we explain why and allow them to reverse the decision themselves. We believe that this maintains the authority of the supervisor.

The grievance procedure itself is negotiated and clearly described in the contract. Ideally, it provides for a series of progressive steps and time limits for submission and resolution of unresolved grievances to higher and more authoritative management levels. The grievance procedure also will define what a grievance is and the manner of its presentation. This is to guard against emotional excesses on the part of either party [5].

In our institution, we go through the following process:

INFORMAL DISCUSSION

This is just a talking stage during which employee informally presents his complaint to the supervisor, usually as soon as possible after the violation has occurred. The collective bargaining agent has the right to be present.

STEP 1

If the grievance is not adjusted by informal discussion, written notice of the grievance is given within 5 to 10 workdays to the supervisor. A written response from this level of authority should be received within 3 to 5 workdays. Many institutions have forms upon which formal grievances are submitted. The employee, delegate, and supervisor are present for any discussions at this time.

STEP 2

If the response to Step 1 is not satisfactory, a written appeal may be submitted within 10 workdays to the director of nursing or her designee. Parties to discussions at this stage are the employee, SNA representative, grievance chairman and/or delegate, and the director of nursing or designee. Again, written response will be provided in 5 workdays subsequent to these meetings. In the bargaining units with which we are acquainted, the positions of delegate and grievance chairman are separated. Generally, the grievance chairman is an officer in the bargaining unit, and though she is apprised of the grievance at the early stages, she may become more actively involved at the later stages. Whether the person is a delegate or grievance chairman will depend on how the bargaining unit is structured.

STEP 3

The employee, SNA representative, grievance chairman, and/or delegate, director of nursing, and director of personnel meet for discussions. The 10- and 5-day time limits for appeal and answer are again observed.

STEP 4

This final step is arbitration. It is invoked when no solution suggested is acceptable at all. Present at these meetings are an arbitrator who is a neutral third party selected by both parties involved, the SNA representatives, employee and hospital representatives, and any others who may be called as witnesses. The submission of a grievance to this step may be required in 15 days of Step 3.

In some contracts that we are familiar with, there is a step between 3 and 4 which provides that the grievance be taken to someone in hospital management before going to arbitration; however, this is not usual.

Often a statement included in each of the steps states that if the time limits are not observed by one party, the grievance may be considered resolved and further action barred. The contract also usually specifies how an arbitrator is selected. One should remember that, in some cases, the employer also has the right to state a grievance and use the procedure to resolve it.

The handling of a grievance places the delegate and the supervisor into adversary positions. Each is expected to vigorously defend the interests he or she represents [6]. The supervisor represents the goals and objectives of management. The delegate represents the interests of the employees and, if the group belongs to a professional association, may be representing the goals and objectives of the profession. Even though the goals and objectives of management and employees may be the same, the translation of those goals into day-to-day activities may cause conflict.

The conceptual frames of reference for management and the bargaining group are somewhat different. Managements usually assume a profit-maximizing posture. However, in such nonprofit service institutions as hospitals, the management's frame of reference may be efficiency. Within the framework of efficiency, managements will seek to maximize the work force and provide a proper mix in allocating resources between labor and fixed capital [7]. Management behavior also is geared toward maintaining the right to exercise administrative initiative. This right is frequently stated in management's rights clauses of contracts [8].

Historically, collective bargaining groups have had to fight to maintain employee security and membership within the certified unit [9]. Therefore, bargaining unit integrity is a major concern of the employee group. As an advocate for the employee, the bargaining unit exercises the right to protest and appeal as well as to improve working conditions. A bargaining unit of professionals also may seek to advance the goals and objectives of the profession.

Whether one serves as supervisor or delegate, certain rules apply:

Any grievance should be approached as soluble.
Every grievance should be considered with the knowledge that it may go to arbitration.
A dispute is to be resolved, not a difference in personalities.
Knowledge of the contract is a must, and familiarity with past practice, arbitration awards, and decisions rendered in similar grievances is important.

Data collection of the facts must answer the questions of who, what, when, where, why, and how. The answers to these questions can generally provide a factual and objective description of just what the issue is.

Who relates to the grievant. *What* defines the grievance. *When* is the time it occurred, and *where* the place of occurrence. *Why* designates the reason for the grievance, which is usually stated in terms of clause and section of the contract, or the policy or rule violated, or why a decision is considered unfair. *How* prescribes what will rectify the situation—this is the response that is requested from the employer. It is not so much a matter of who is right and who is wrong, but *what* is right. The goal is to reach an equitable solution. Grievances should be negotiated on their own merits. They are all important to the individual employees involved.

During such negotiations, acting timid and defensive is not successful; nor is being offensive. Both parties should hear each other out, stick to the main points of the grievance, and not become sidetracked by superfluous, irrelevant statements, situations, facts, or emotions. Successful labor relations are based on negotiations in good faith, honesty, and respect.

There are times when a satisfactory solution cannot be reached by the parties. When such a situation occurs, the final step in the grievance process, arbitration, is invoked. The most common type of arbitration is voluntary arbitration—whereby the two parties submit a dispute to a neutral third party who will render a judgment which both parties have agreed would be final and binding. In this type of arbitration, the awards are confined to interpretation and application of the language already agreed to in the contract.

The powers of an arbitrator are set forth in a contract clause which often states that the arbitrator can neither add to nor delete any clause in the agreement. Some contracts limit the arbitrator's powers to specific issues and clauses in the contract [10]. Some contracts specifically call for a definite method of selecting an arbitrator. If no method is defined, the American Arbitration Association (AAA), if contacted, will provide a list of arbitrators, selected on the basis of the nature of the dispute [11]. (Suggestions for arbitrators may also be obtained from the Federal Mediation and Conciliation Service or from the individual state mediation and conciliation boards [12].)

Each of the disputing parties deletes any names it objects to from the list, and rank orders the others in terms of preference. One criterion used in making the selection is how the arbitrator has rendered decisions in the past. Obviously, each side is inclined to choose someone who is supportive of, and familiar with, their position. This should not be construed that arbitrators show bias. The most important asset of an arbitrator is his impartiality. Hopefully, the parties will be able to make a mutually acceptable choice. If not, the AAA will make an administrative appointment [11].

Arbitration proceedings are analogous to informal courts, where arguments are presented, briefs and evidence are submitted, witnesses can be sworn, and cross-examination occurs. As the representative of the grievant, the bargaining unit speaks first, except in the case of discharge of an employee, where the burden of proof is on the employer. There is no jury present and arbitrators are not bound by precedents in similar cases. The cost of the arbitrator is shared equally by both parties, and generally the cost is high. Some contracts might even provide for payment by the losing party [13].

The major function of the arbitrator is the interpretation of a clause in the collective bargaining agreement. During negotiations, items are agreed to with specific intent, though the intent may not be readily obvious in the language of the contract. Delegates and supervisors must be aware of the intent of their respective parties in adjusting grievances. Arbitrators give careful consideration to the intent of the contracting parties, as well as analyzing the specific contract language.

The arbitrator also will have to decide whether the particular dispute is arbitrable under the terms of the contract. If an arbitrator exceeds his jurisdiction, the rendered award can be reversed by a court of law.

Occasionally, a bargaining unit and management will disagree as to whether a dispute is arbitrable. This, in fact, may be what is determined in an arbitration procedure.

Frequently, the management rights clause is invoked as a restriction to arbitration. However, a dispute may be rendered arbitrable under the implied covenant of good faith in bargaining [14].

The grievance and arbitration process is political in nature. In institutions where collective bargaining is new to the employees and management, or a new bargaining group has formed, the number of grievances may be greater than in situations where labor and management have had years to learn to work with one another. This may be an attempt to right all alleged wrongs at once. The adjustment of grievances takes time, which means one is not about the specific job he was hired to do. Both parties generally prefer harmony, which is enhanced with successful employee-management relationships.

Occasionally, a flood of grievances will be used as a "slow-down" weapon, or the actual grievances may not be stated, causing similar grievances to be filed [15]. This may be used as a means of bargaining for more advantageous conditions than the contract provides. At times, a grievance is taken to arbitration (when both parties can fairly well anticipate the award) because it is politically advantageous to do so, either for the bargaining unit or for management.

The militaristic and religious models that have molded nursing have consistently stressed obedience. Obedience is not to question why, nor is it to complain. Obedience is complying with directives issued by one in a higher position.

Because of this, many grievances are never revealed. One may be afraid of reprisals, antagonizing one's supervisor, or being labeled troublemaker. The grievance machinery should provide an atmosphere in which one need not fear reprisals. Too often, nurses do not exhibit the candor and perseverance needed to carry grievances through to a resolution with which they can live. In such a case, objective representation by delegates who are not emotionally involved in the situation can provide the supportive backup needed.

Nurses who are supervisors may have that sudden feeling in the pit of the stomach and that sudden urge to run when involved in a grievance. This will be especially true if the grievance is caused by a directive she has issued, or if she is new at grievance adjustment. Or it may be prompted by anger at having her authority questioned or dismay because she thought she followed "all the right rules."

The supervisor needs the same degree of tenacity, perseverance, objectivity, and flexibility, that the grievant needs. If she is unsure, she may wish to have a peer member in attendance during grievance sessions. However, it is best not to make this a practice; it may undermine or negate her authority in the employee's eyes.

The last advice one can give supervisors is to use good judgment in assessing problems and refer those beyond your scope of responsibility to persons with authority to resolve them. Handle those problems which fall in your domain with equanimity and a sense of humor.

Ultimately, the grievance and arbitration process should be viewed as a means of democratic expression and involvement within a health care institution.

REFERENCES

1. Clelland, Rod. Grievance procedures: outlet for employee insight for management. *Hospitals* 41:58-60, Aug. 1, 1967.
2. Metzger, Norman, and Pointer, D. D. *Labor Management Relations in the Health Services Industry.* New York, Science and Health Publishers, 1972, p. 202.
3. Clelland, *op. cit.,* p. 58.
4. Heyel, Carl. *Handbook of Modern Office Management and Administrative Services.* New York, McGraw-Hill Book Co., 1972, pp. 8-47.
5. *Ibid.,* p. 8-38.
6. Baer, W. E. *Grievance Handling: 101 Guides for Supervisors.* New York, American Management Association, 1970, p. 48.
7. McConnell, C. R. *Economics, Principles, Problems and Policies.* 3d ed. New York, McGraw-Hill Book Co., 1966, p. 480.
8. Stessin, Lawrence. *Employee Discipline.* Washington, D.C., Bureau of National Affairs, Inc., 1960, p. 22.
9. Cohen, Sanford. *Labor in the United States,* 4th ed. Columbus, Ohio, Charles E. Merrill Publishing Co., 1975, p. 88.
10. Metzger and Pointer, *op. cit.,* p. 212.
11. Stone, Morris. Using arbitration to settle disputes. *Hosp. Prog.* 50:55, Apr. 1969.
12. Trotta, M. S. *Arbitration of Labor-Management Disputes.* New York, American Management Association, 1974, p. 55.
13. *Ibid.,* p. 75.
14. *Ibid.,* p. 87.
15. Cohen, *op. cit.,* p. 71.

28 Mediation—What It Is, What It Does

Bonnie Graczyk Castrey and Robert T. Castrey

THE COLLECTIVE BARGAINING process provides a structure within which employees and management can negotiate agreements on employment issues, such as wages, hours, and working conditions. In nursing and in other professions, such as teaching, control over professional practice is most often a subject of negotiation as well.

Although the provisions of collective bargaining oblige both parties to bargain in good faith, the law does not compel the parties to reach agreement. Participants may sometimes reach a deadlock with regard to certain topics or issues, at which point agreement seems unlikely. Should this occur, there are four alternatives for resolving the differences: mediation, fact-finding, arbitration, and strike.

Because health care providers perform functions that are vital to the health and welfare of the community, a strike among such employees creates a crucial situation, and should be carefully avoided. It is important for nursing administrators involved in collective bargaining situations to know what measures can be taken to avoid a strike.

This article discusses one such measure, mediation. The discussion focuses particularly on the services provided by the Federal Mediation and Conciliation Service (FMCS), an independent government agency which assists in preventing and settling labor disputes.

MEDIATION, FACT-FINDING, ARBITRATION

Mediation is a process whereby a neutral third party assists labor and management in seeking alternative solutions to their problems. The third party acts as a catalyst, bringing the two sides together to reach their own agreement.

Mediation is distinguished from fact-finding and arbitration in that the mediator makes no decisions as to the substantive terms of resolution. Mediation is actually an extension of collective bargaining and facilitates the bargaining process between the parties.

In fact-finding, a neutral third party investigates the issues in dispute, makes findings of fact, and issues nonmandatory recommendations on the terms of settlement in a written report to the parties.

Arbitration takes two forms and is the most formal kind of third party intervention. When unresolved collective bargaining issues are submitted to an arbitrator for determination, the process is defined as *interest* arbitration. The arbitration of a dispute over the application or interpretation of an existing agreement is defined as *rights* arbitration. In both cases, the issues are heard by an arbitrator who then presents a decision that is binding on the parties.

Reprinted by permission from "Mediation—What It Is, What It Does" by Bonnie Graczyk Castrey and Robert T. Castrey, *Journal of Nursing Administration*, Volume 10, Number 11, 1980.

NOTIFICATION REQUIREMENTS

When Public Law 93–360 (The Health Care Act of 1974) amended the National Labor Relations Act by removing the exclusion of nonprofit hospitals and adding other health care institutions, it brought the industry under the same federal labor laws as other businesses throughout the United States, with some exceptions. The second part of the Act placed certain limitations and restrictions on the collective bargaining process beyond those that govern negotiations in the private sector industries. Essentially, the restrictions consist of longer notification periods both prior to negotiating changes in existing agreements and in the event of a dispute that brings threat of a strike. Congress imposed these additional requirements to assure all possible efforts to resolve labor disputes with minimal disruption in health care delivery.

Specifically, 90 days prior to the expiration date of an existing agreement, one or both parties to the agreement must serve written notice to the other party stating that they intend to modify or terminate the existing agreement. Additionally, the parties are required to notify the Federal Mediation and Conciliation Service at least 60 days prior to the expiration date of the contract if the parties have not concluded an agreement by that time. In the private sector, parties must deliver a 60-day notice of intent followed by a 30-day notice to FMCS.

In the case of certification or recognition of a newly formed bargaining unit, 30 days' notice must be given to the Federal Mediation and Conciliation Service. Additionally, in both the 60-day and 30-day notice situations a further 10-day notice of intent to strike is required. In the private sector, notice is not required in the case of certification or recognition of a newly formed bargaining unit and the 10-day notice of strike is not required in either situation.

FEDERAL MEDIATION AND CONCILIATION SERVICE

The FMCS was formed to provide a structure and process through which bargaining parties can obtain the assistance of a neutral third party when negotiations break down. The Taft-Hartley Act, which amended the NLRA in 1947, created the FMCS as an independent agency in the Executive Branch.

The work of the Service is carried out by a staff of over 300 commissioners in approximately 80 major cities in the United States. These mediators are experienced negotiators with special skills in conflict management. One criterion for appointment is seven years of direct experience at the bargaining table. The commissioners are appointed by Wayne L. Horvitz, Director of FMCS, who is appointed by the President.

INITIAL INVESTIGATION

FMCS involvement in the negotiating process begins with receipt of a notice from one or both parties in compliance with the notification requirements described earlier.

When the Regional Office of the FMCS receives the appropriate notice, an assignment is made to a mediator stationed in the geographical area where the health care institution is located. The mediator then contacts both of the principal spokespersons, either by telephone or in person, to assess the impact of a work stoppage on the delivery of health care to the community and to learn the current status of bargaining.

To determine the potential effect of a strike on the community, the mediator will ask questions regarding the number of beds in the facility, the number currently in use, the total number of employees, whether the institution is independent or part of a multihospital system, the kind of care provided (acute, longterm, outpatient), special services (for example, ICU, CCU, dialysis), and other facilities in the area that provide similar services and their distance from the institution. He or she will also want to know whether other employees in the institution are organized, which unions represent them, when their contracts expire, and the number of employees in each bargaining unit.

To determine the status of bargaining, the mediator will ask other pertinent questions, such as, Have the parties met? Have you exchanged proposals? What are the outstanding issues? What is your prognosis? What is your meeting schedule? Describe your relationship with the other party. How many grievances were filed and how many went to arbitration? In an initial contract bargaining situation additional questions may be asked about the election campaign.

The mediator will also answer your questions about the function of mediation in the bargaining process and arrange procedures for maintaining contact with you as the negotiations proceed.

BOARD OF INQUIRY

In addition to requiring increased notice time, Congress authorized the director of FMCS to appoint an impartial Board of Inquiry (BOI) to engage in fact-finding in those cases where a strike would substantially interrupt the delivery of health care in the locality concerned.

After the mediator has gathered all the pertinent information from both parties, he or she will submit an evaluation to the director of FMCS who will determine whether to appoint a BOI. There is no comparable statutory fact-finding procedure at this level for dispute resolution in other private sector industries covered by the National Labor Relations Act.

The director of FMCS has the unilateral right to appoint a BOI within the 30 days following receipt of a 60-day contract renewal notice and within 10 days where the bargaining is for an initial agreement following certification.

If the director decides to appoint a BOI, the parties are notified by telegram of the Board's identity and date of appointment. The Board may consist of one or more persons but most often only one. These persons are usually selected from the roster of arbitrators maintained by FMCS.

The BOI has 15 days after appointment in which to conduct hearings and issue a written report of the facts and its recommendations for resolving the issues in dispute. The objective of this procedure is to assist the parties in reaching a prompt, peaceful, and just settlement. The parties may accept or reject the recommendations in toto or in part, or use them as a basis for settling the issues.

The fees and expenses of the BOI are paid by the FMCS. Each party pays the costs and expenses for its witnesses, documents, and other information it may submit.

Whether or not a BOI is appointed, the mediator will maintain frequent contact with both parties to stay in touch with the progress being made at the bargaining table. In fact, mediation may have begun prior to the BOI appointment and if so, the mediator will probably be in attendance at the hearings. Many times mediation moves ahead while the BOI report is being prepared. In other cases the mediator may not enter the negotiations until later, perhaps when the 10-day strike notice is filed (this notice will be discussed later in the article). The determination of when to actively intervene is made on a case-by-case basis either by request of one or both parties or by the mediator based on his or her assessment of bargaining status.

THE MEDIATION PROCESS

When the mediator joins the parties at the bargaining table, the following is an example of what you might expect to happen.

The mediator will attempt to arrange for a mutually agreeable time and place for a meeting. Most often this will be the local offices of FMCS, a neutral site where neither party has the psychological advantage of meeting site ownership.

In the first mediation conference the parties will normally convene jointly to elicit *all* remaining unresolved issues. To facilitate this process, the parties should be prepared to furnish copies of their original proposals, a summary of the outstanding issues including their current positions on them, and a copy of the expiring agreement. During this joint session both parties will have an equal opportunity to express their respective positions and present any pertinent general comments. The supporting arguments for the parties' positions are not generally required at this time.

The importance of bringing *all* issues to light at this time cannot be overemphasized. It must be clear to both parties and to the mediator precisely which issues must be addressed to resolve the dispute. There is nothing more frustrating and potentially disastrous to successful negotiations than for one of the parties to "remember" an important issue at the last moment.

Bringing up late issues not clearly defined at the initial joint mediation conference session can upset the sometimes delicate costing balance of an economic package settlement proposal. There is much give and take in the bargaining process as the parties narrow the issues until the outer limits of the employer's willingness to pay and the union's willingness to settle begin to be discernible to the negotiators. At this point commitments are made, and once made, they are extremely difficult to withdraw for restructuring should the "remembered" issue drive the settlement costs beyond the limits of willingness to pay or settle. If this situation is allowed to develop, the entire basis for tentative agreement may be destroyed, resulting in an unnecessary strike.

SEPARATE CAUCUS

Following the initial joint conference, the mediator will meet separately with the parties to probe in depth each of the issues and the reasons for the parties' respective positions.

From information gathered in joint and separate conferences and the mediator's own knowledge of the issues and the health care industry, the mediator will explore possible solutions and package issues together for resolution. This is commonly done through a series of "what ifs" (If labor does that, will you do this?).

The mediator will constantly evaluate each party's responses, weighing whether or not to keep dialogue open, and deciding if and when the parties should meet jointly, separately, or off the record.

OFF-THE-RECORD MEETINGS

Off-the-record meetings of the principal negotiators are often necessary to find solutions to particularly difficult issues and/or to reinforce a firm stand on a specific issue. The objective is to provide an atmosphere of total and complete candor not subject to misinterpretation. The parties are encouraged to openly discuss what they are willing or unwilling to do to resolve the dispute. If this off-the-record discussion does not resolve the problems, neither party is commited to any suggested or proposed terms discussed at the session.

It should be noted that mediators are subject to a "Code of Confidentiality." The mediator's continued acceptability to the parties depends on his or her keeping confidential what is discussed in private talks. A guarantee of confidentiality aids the mediation process because it encourages free and open discussions in which the mediator can ask questions, draw conclusions, and make suggestions and recommendations that may provide the basis for a mutually acceptable agreement.

One of the major advantages of mediation to both parties is that many options may be explored unofficially with the other team, leaving official positions on the table while facts are being gathered or confirmed. For example, if the issue is scheduling every other weekend off, it may be necessary to investigate changes in recruiting policies and procedures, consider turnover rates based on past experience, the availability of qualified personnel within the labor pool area, policies and procedures defining emergency relief staffing, or the possibility of establishing an employee pool resource. Specific actions will be influenced by the perceived needs of the parties and their willingness to seek compromises that can lead to settlement.

Mediators have no authority to dictate or enforce any of their suggestions or recommendations. Because of their neutrality, mediators can be a valuable resource, exploring, without commitment, the issues at dispute and developing a constructive atmosphere for agreement.

BARGAINING POWER

The mediator must continuously assess each party's relative bargaining power throughout the negotiations to effectively help them look objectively at their positions on the various issues. In determining the relative power of each side, the mediator considers the labor organization's ability and willingness to strike and the employer's preparedness to take a strike or lock out the employees.

Many factors enter into the mediator's determination of relative power. For example, are there questions of corporate or company policy involved? If so, how realistic are they in comparison to other similar institutions? Has the union been successful in obtaining their demands at those other institutions? Are each party's economic resources sufficient to sustain job action over a long enough time period to force the other party to reconsider its position? Which issues are most strongly supported by individuals on the bargaining committees? Why? Will their willingness to strike or take a strike be affected by partial accommodation to their issues? Is this a personal issue or does it truly reflect the demands and attitudes of the people they represent?

There are literally hundreds of such questions, the answers to which will guide the mediator in determining how best to time his or her suggestions and requests for joint, separate, or off-the-record conferences. Each mediator has a particular style of accomplishing the task, as do the negotiators for the parties. Therefore, the successful outcome of the negotiations relies heavily on the abilities and willingness of each of the three parties at the table to listen carefully to one another and be realistic and objective about their positions and the process.

Since the dispute has probably placed both parties under substantial stress, they may sometimes misinterpret the mediator's hard analysis of the factors at play. It is important to remember that the mediator is not there to prolong or disrupt the bargaining, but rather to facilitate agreement. The mediator calls upon an adroit sense of timing, tact, firmness, frankness, perceptiveness, sensitivity, and a solid working knowledge of the group process to create a problem-solving attitude between the parties in place of raw exercise of power and the resistance this engenders.

REACHING AGREEMENT

When tentative agreement is reached, the mediator will request the parties to affirm it in joint session so that both are clear on the settlement terms reached through mediation. It is always a good idea for the parties to write down the agreements in a memo of understanding and initial them at this time to avoid later disputes when definitive contractual language is being developed.

When agreement cannot be reached through mediation, the mediator will, in joint session, review the open issues and the parties' official positions on these issues. Unofficial positions discussed in separate caucuses or in off-the-record meetings are left unofficial and are not noted in joint session.

STRIKE NOTICE REQUIREMENTS

Issues at dispute are sometimes insoluble through the give and take process of negotiations without a test of strength on the picket line. At any health care institution, the law requires that the labor organization notify the institution and the FMCS in writing at least 10 days prior to a strike, picketing, or other concerted refusal to work. The notice must state the date and time that such action will commence. This notice may run concurrently with the last 10 days of the 60-day notice to FMCS except that in the case of bargaining for an initial agreement following certification or recognition, the 10-day notice shall not be given until the expiration of the 30-day notice to FMCS.

If the action does not begin as specified in the 10-day notice, it may still legally commence within the 72-hour period immediately following the time specified in the 10-day notice. However, an additional 12-hour notice to the institution and FMCS must be filed before any action may begin. Should no strike begin during the 72-hour "window" period, another 10-day notice must be filed and the process repeated. It is considered unfair labor practice to repeatedly file this 10-day notice for purposes of harassment.

Mediation will continue during the 10-day notice period in a final effort to avoid disrupting the delivery of health care. If, at the end of the notice period, the parties remain unwilling to accede to or accommodate each other's demands, the mediator will normally return them to joint session and clearly state the issues remaining at dispute and the parties' positions on them. Following this confrontation certain "housekeeping" chores, such as arranging for future meetings and setting up communications procedures to be used during the job action, are addressed and the parties are then free to dispute the issues on the street.

Mediation does not cease with the onset of job action. In fact, mediation activity generally escalates as one or both parties feel the effects of the action. When stark reality begins to alter the convictions of the parties it is usually a propitious time to return to the bargaining table. The mediator can and will assist in preserving some dignity for the parties during the painful withdrawal process. This can be a critical factor affecting the tenor of the parties' relationship for years to come. Remember, revenge is sweet and the balance of power is always subject to change. In any case, the mediator will remain involved until there is a negotiated settlement or job action ceases.

TECHNICAL ASSISTANCE

Mediators also provide assistance in other forms, often helping to prevent problems or disputes between the union and management. Technical assistance includes both teaching and counseling the parties jointly and/or separately during the life of the labor agreement. Mediators often instruct the parties in effective use of the collective bargaining process and grievance procedure through films and programs designed to meet their specific needs.

In counseling the parties, mediators assist labor and management to look objectively at their relationship and to learn techniques for mutually working out their problems. In addition to training supervisors and/or union representatives in the methods of effective grievance handling and human relations, mediators will sometimes recommend establishing labor management committees, chaired by the mediator, that meet on a regular basis during the life of the agreement to discuss and resolve issues of mutual concern, such as productivity, business prospects, and other noncontractual matters. This technique usually follows difficult negotiations or strikes where the mediator recognizes that a poor relationship exists between the parties.

In one such situation hospital management became concerned about the increasingly high labor and equipment maintenance cost in its laundry facilities when they learned that a local linen supply service could supply the hospital for less than one-half the cost of operating their own laundry.

The hospital administrator brought this problem to the labor/management committee for discussion before taking any action on the matter. The laundry was closed, but the four employees affected were retained at their full wages and upgraded to much needed higher skilled jobs in the hospital. Funds for the retraining program were obtained through the mutual effort of the parties to qualify the displaced employees for state and federal programs.

This is a typical example of how cooperative behavior can satisfy both the union's concern about the welfare of its members and the hospital's concern with cost and staff morale.

PUBLIC INFORMATION

FMCS commissioners throughout the country are highly visible in the labor/management community. They play an active role in professional organizations, such as the Industrial Relations Research Association, the Society of Professionals In Dispute Resolution, and the Society of Federal Labor Relations Professionals, that bring labor, management, and third-party neutrals together to further the principles and arts of constructive labor/management relations.

Mediators frequently present basic information about FMCS and the bargaining process at college and university classes, union meetings, service clubs, and occasionally on radio and television talk shows. Some mediators also teach part time in the industrial relations program at local colleges and universities.

CONCLUSION

Mediation is similar to the three-legged stool. Without the concerted and knowledgeable participation of all three parties, the process cannot stand to fulfill its designated purpose, peaceful and speedy resolution of labor disputes.

Just as health care providers must skillfully apply the necessary knowledge and tools for effective patient care, so must nursing administrators in unionized settings understand and use the process and tools of collective bargaining for successful negotiations. Mediation is one such tool and the FMCS is a valuable resource for both the prevention and the resolution of employee-management conflict.

Call the mediator before trouble begins—prevention is the best therapy.

BIBLIOGRAPHY

Health Care Act (Public Law 93–360, 93rd Congress, S.3203. July 26, 1974).

Hohman, J. Taft-Hartley amendments, implications for the health care field. *Labor Relations Journal,* 2(3):256–258, 1978.

Maggiolo, W. A. *Techniques of Mediation in Labor Disputes.* Dobbs Ferry, New York: Oceana Publications, 1971.

Simkin, W. E. *Mediation and the Dynamics of Collective Bargaining.* Washington, D.C.: The Bureau of National Affairs, 1971.

29 Functional Redundancy and the Process of Professionalization

THE CASE OF REGISTERED NURSES IN THE UNITED STATES

Margaret Levi

IN CAPITALIST DEMOCRACIES, an individual has two ways to achieve upward economic and social mobility; through education and personal attainment, an individual project, and through raising the status and salary of the job one holds, a group enterprise. Related to the second strategy are a number of important theoretical questions, such as the conditions under which people choose collective as opposed to individual action, or the implications of the group's success for the allocation of societal resources. The focus of this article will be the constraints on the collective mobility strategy, particularly for registered nurses. Because the research is based on a single case study complemented by an extensive review of the literature, the conclusions are tentative.

Semiprofessionals are distinguished from other wage earners in the United States by the availability of two mechanisms of collective mobility: unionization and professionalization. The power of a union rests on its ability to stop the delivery of services, that of a profession on its monopoly over the access to valued skills and knowledge. In other words, it controls a supply of labor for which there is no legal substitute. When two such powers are combined, the occupation's demands may prove nearly irresistible. Perhaps it is for that very reason that they are seldom combined.

Occupations seeking union or professional recognition must engage in political conflict with employers and, equally importantly, with the state [1]. It is the state that grants collective bargaining and licensure. However, state recognition usually signals the completion of the unionizing project, which is only one of many steps of the professionalization process. Indeed, one way of conceptualizing professionalization is through the identification of a series of necessary historical "events" [2], which include: the performance of full-time work; the formation of a national professional association; the development of a formal code of ethics by which to eliminate the incompetent and unscrupulous; political activity in a state-granted monopoly; and the requirement of an advanced degree, usually at a university. Ultimately, professionalization is ". . . an attempt to translate one order of scarce resources—special knowledge and skills—into another—social and economic rewards" [3]. This usually requires the support of powerful groups within the social structure [4]. More importantly, the group must persuade ". . . the society that no one else can do the job, and that it is dangerous to let anyone else try" [5]. In other words, those demanding professional status must be able to *demonstrate* the importance and nonsubstitutability of the work they do.

Reprinted with permission by *Journal of Health Politics, Policy and Law,* Volume 5, Number 2, Summer 1980. Copyright © 1980 by the Department of Health Administration, Duke University.

In a sense, the best description of a profession is offered by Joseph Schumpeter. Although he claimed to be characterizing social classes, his description fits the meaning of a profession even better [6]:

Every class . . . has a definite function, which it must fulfill according to its whole concept and orientation, and which it actually does discharge as a class and through the class conduct of its members. . . . Moreover, the position of each class in the total national structure, depends, on the one hand, on the significance that is attributed to that function, and, on the other hand, on the degree to which the class successfully performs that function. Changes in relative class position are always explained by changes along these two lines, and in no other way.

To reach the top of the professional hierarchy—and to stay there—requires the *continued* performance of service functions, or an "array of associated roles" [7], generally recognized as socially significant. This in turn depends on two factors: (1) monopolization over the function and, if need be, related functions; and (2) high social status for both the occupation and its members.

Most of the occupations currently engaged in the professionalizing campaign are what T. H. Marshall characterized as semiprofessions [8]:

To put it briefly, scientific methods have been introduced into non-manual routine work. . . . These techniques are not, by older standards, professional. They do not call for creative originality . . . nor must they be linked with sound human judgment and the power to inspire trust in one's character and personality. . . . They demand accuracy and efficiency along established lines. They are, in fact, the mental equivalent of the manual craftmanship of the Middle Ages, and they lend themselves in the same way to the establishment of semiprofessional *(emphasis mine) associations. But in many respects these groups are indistinguishable from the great body of the salaried employees of trade and industry, the white-collared workers of the middle class.*

Technical specialties, particularly in the health field, increasingly are securing licensure requirements and, thus, monopolies over the practice of their jobs. Nonetheless, they lack some of the important attributes of a profession, namely, long training in the body of knowledge on which the technique is based, discretionary authority on the job, and what (to Marshall and many analysts) is the most important element of all, an essential relationship of trust between practitioner and client [9]. Paritally as a result, they also lack high prestige. As Marshall pointed out some forty years ago, they are more like crafts than professions.

However, there are some occupations that have a stronger claim to professional standing. These are what the contemporary literature calls semiprofessions: namely teaching, social work, librarianship, and registered nursing [10]. Nevertheless, their work lacks the prestige of the older professions of law, medicine, and university teaching. Four factors contribute to this situation: First, most semiprofessionals are women; this in itself apparently decreases the likelihood of the attribution of high social significance to the work they perform [11]. Their tasks tend to revolve around nurturant and educational services considered "natural" to women and, therefore, easy to learn and replicate without much training. Second, semiprofessionals tend to work in bureaucratic settings [12]. Although their work requires a certain degree of discretion with regard to patients and clients, they tend to be subject to supervision, time clocks, and routine checks in a way that professionals seldom are. Moreover, the head of the administrative hierarchy in which the semiprofessional works is unlikely to be a colleague, but is rather a person trained in some other profession. At the same time, bureaucraticization leads to an abundance of supervisory and administrative personnel who have been trained in the semiprofession. They usually are excluded from the bargaining unit by law and, thus, are able to perform the tasks of their subordinates during a work stoppage. Third, semiprofessionals have relatively little control over the numbers of people being produced to perform their work or the schools that are producing them. In other words, there is likely to be an oversupply of labor combined with ambiguity about qualifications (beyond the minimal ones confirmed by state examinations). Competition is also beginning to affect lawyers and university professors in the United States today. Although this tends to reduce job possibilities and deflate wage scales, it does not detract from their professional status. Their education remains relatively standardized and, at the same time, it is possible to distinguish among candidates for a position. Grades are the criterion for the lawyer; written materials for the scholar. Semiprofessional applicants, in contrast to the professionals, tend to be diverse as a group and difficult to rank individually. The fourth major obstacle to professionalization is the failure to control the labor supply, which results in a superfluity of credentialed job applicants. Failure to monopolize the tasks leads to the superfluity of the occupation itself, or functional redundancy. In operational terms, this means that (1) there are acceptable substitutes for the service; and (2) the occupation has developed in such a way that its original functions are now performed by a combination of persons above, below, and at the same level in the occupational hierarchy. In other words, the occupation not only lacks an effective monopoly over the service, it could potentially be eliminated altogether. Under such circumstances the occupation has little claim to social significance.

Functional redundancy makes it difficult for some semiprofessionals, particularly social workers and registered nurses, to prove there is no substitute for the services they perform. There is always another occupation that has already established itself as a profession whose members, if need be, can legally perform their work. The semiprofessional is almost defined by his or her lack of ". . . the most highly developed body of knowledge in the relevant field" [13]. At the same time, other related specialists, such as dietitians, operating room technicians, physician's assistants, and psychologists have taken over tasks previously defined as the registered nurse's or social worker's. Finally, orderlies, licensed practical nurses, financial management officers and clerks do their "dirty work" [14]. The fact that such acceptable substitutes exist is only in part a result of the changing division-of-labor. It is also further evidence of the political failure of the semiprofessionals. After all, physicians have no legal substitutes; nor for that matter, do the organized crafts [15].

The rest of this paper will explore the development of registered nursing in the United States in order to illuminate the obstacles to professionalization in a semiprofession. A brief history of the professionalizing project and its difficulties will be followed by a short case study of the RN strike in Seattle in 1976, which demonstrates some of the consequences of failure to control the labor supply or to monopolize essential tasks. Finally, I will attempt to lay out a set of propositions appropriate for comparing the professionalizing project of several occupations.

THE EARLY HISTORY OF NURSING

Since the beginning of history nursing has been one of the roles of women in both the family and the community [16]. In the early nineteenth century, European and North American women became nurses by joining a religious order or by simply deciding to perform that role; they required no training. Hospitals were established mainly for the poor, for prisoners, and for soldiers fighting wars. In most of these institutions, the ambulatory sick had the job of caring for the more acutely ill. Middle and upper class families seldom used hospitals; they hired nurses as they would any other domestic servant. Poor families could not afford such "nurses"; instead, they relied on women from their own communities who had learned the arts of herbal medicine and midwifery, and who had practiced nursing in addition to their daily routines as a service to their neighbors. Occasionally, the poor would also receive aid from rich ladies who engaged in nursing as a form of "Christian service."

In the 1850s, Florence Nightingale changed all that. In her view, good nursing required both theoretical and clinical training. Well aware of recent advances in science, she was eager to apply new sanitary methods and knowledge about disease to the care of the sick. She received her opportunity during the Crimean War: The Minister of War, a friend of Nightingale's, was interested in experimenting with the use of female nurses on the battlefield. In 1854, Nightingale accepted his invitation to organize this effort. By applying her methods, she was able to reduce significantly the mortality rates at Scutari and, later, at other hospitals she supervised or influenced.

Nightingale secularized nursing by giving it an institutional base outside of the religious orders. More importantly, she made of it a socially acceptable livelihood for middle and upper class women, and one that required training and expertise. The contributions and commitment of Florence Nightingale created the possibility of a nursing "profession" and endowed it with some occupational prestige. The efficacy of the Nightingale nurses created a demand for their services. The high social status of these nursing pioneers combined with the Victorian feminist movement [17] to provide further support for the revolution in nursing.

The growth of nursing as a profession in the United States in the second half of the nineteenth century had similar causes. The Civil War, as did the Crimean War before it, provided the opportunity to demonstrate the utility of female nurses using Nightingale's methods. When the war was over, the feminist movement of the time supported the continued participation of women in nursing as a paid and trained occupation. Schools founded in 1872 and 1873 followed the model of the Nightingale Training School in requiring both clinical and classroom work, practice and theory.

The early U.S. schools lacked the generous funding of the Nightingale School, however. In order to pay for their education and board, students had to work as staff nurses in the hospital to which the training school was attached. Graduate nurses who had completed the training tended to be administrators and teachers in the hospitals, private duty nurses, or public health nurses; they were seldom ordinary hospital staff. In fact, the largest proportion were private duty nurses, a situation that continued until the 1930s. These nurses were hired by physicians to provide constant bedside care to their patients. Available nurses were located by means of a registry, as often run by the local pharmacy as by a hospital or professional agency. Occasionally the private duty nurse was hired for special duty in the hospital, but usually she lived with the patient's family and was on duty around the clock. Her importance lay in her skill in monitoring the course of the disease. Until the introduction of antibiotics and sulfa drugs, the ability of the nurse had a great deal to do with the recovery of the patient.

By the turn of the century, new discoveries in science (particularly in bacteriology), and the development of surgery required the nurse to learn new methods and take on new tasks. Training became an absolute prerequisite to good nursing practice. However, training was generally oriented toward the development of technical skills. Only public health nursing (another consequence of advances in bacteriology) required relatively complete understanding of scientific principles. It was the job of the public health nurse to educate the society in proper hygiene, sanitation, and preventive care, as well as to care for the sick. Often this meant direct intervention in schools and homes and considerable autonomy and discretion on the job. Consequently, she usually received training beyond that of other graduate nurses.

Despite these changes, nursing was still not considered a profession [18]. Not only was the normal training short and limited, it tended to take place in a hospital rather than a university setting. Moreover, the availability of nursing as a legitimate occupation for women had encouraged a proliferation of training schools whose students were diverse and often ill-prepared. Consequently, nursing education lacked standardization, a major and necessary aspect of the professionalizing project [19]. Nor is there much evidence that nurses contributed to the development of scientific knowledge—despite claims to the contrary by the nursing leadership of the era. Most graduate nurses were skilled adjuncts to physicians; few were autonomous. Moreover, they suffered from a characterization of their work as an extension of that of domestic servants and ordinary housewives [20]. This sustained the belief that students could staff the hospitals without ill effects, and that almost any well-tempered female could provide adequate bedside care. In other words, graduate nurses had lost the social status of their Victorian forerunners.

However, the most important obstacle to professionalization lay in the nature of nursing duties. From the turn of the century until at least the 1930s, the graduate nurses' functions included: (1) the administration of other nurses; (2) the supervision of laundry, food preparation and other housekeeping tasks; (3) staffing of hospitals; (4) bedside care; (5) the provision of skillful technical assistance to physicians, particularly surgeons and other specialists; (6) immunization programs; and (7) education of the public in proper sanitation and hygiene. Of these functions, only the last comes even close to what is generally considered professional work. Few of these tasks represented socially valued skills or knowledge, and those that did were not monopolized by nurses.

THE PROFESSIONALIZING CAMPAIGN

Graduate nurses were fully aware of the basic inadequacies in both their training and public image. As early as the 1890s, they began to organize to make themselves functionally indispensable in actual fact, as well as in public perception. Between 1893 and 1912, most of the national associations for nursing were established, and the *American Journal of Nursing (AJN)* began publishing. The aim was to develop procedures by which the profession would control education, entry into the job market, and the definition of nursing practice. The rationale was the protection of the public from unqualified and, by implication, dangerous nurses. Hospital administrators and state legislators were the immediate targets of the campaign which took as its model the physician, whose profession had waged just such a campaign in the nineteenth century with considerable success. The concrete goals of the campaign were standardized education, preferably in the university; state registration or licensure on the basis of examinations written, optimally, by the professional association; and state nurse practice acts that explicitly restricted any but professional nurses from performing certain tasks.

Any achievement of such goals required intensive organization and lobbying. By 1919, the American Nurses' Association (ANA) had 38 state affiliates, and 33 of these had already succeeded in securing some sort of nurse practice act. However, few of these laws adequately provided for the supervision or examination of student nurses. Indeed, hospitals and the public initially resisted the registration of graduate nurses; they feared that the price of nursing would skyrocket, particularly if they were forced to use a graduate nurse where previously a student or "untrained" nurse would do.

Further impetus to the campaign came with the onslaught of a depression in nursing employment in the 1920s, caused by what appeared to be an oversupply of trained nurses and the increasing inability of the public to afford private duty nurses. At the same time, there seemed to be a shortage of nurses adequately trained to perform increasingly specialized and technical tasks [21]. These facts permitted graduate nurses to appeal to some powerful allies to win registration and licensure as well as improvements in education. The various national nursing organizations joined with the American Hospital Association (AHA) and private foundations such as Carnegie, Rockefeller, and later Russell Sage to initiate several important studies of nursing [22]. One result was the closure of 219 schools between 1931 and 1934 due to poor training [23]. Perhaps more important, and certainly more controversial, were recommendations for "grades" of nursing. Proposals included distinguishing public health from private duty nurses, who in turn would be distinguished from a subsidiary group of practical nurses. Each grade would receive a different kind of training. Ultimately, this would mean that subsidiary nurses, who were cheaper both to train and hire, could be used for the routine care of convalescents or patients with minor or chronic illnesses. Graduate nurses could then be reserved for the acutely sick.

The establishment of different grades of nursing was probably what finally enabled graduate nurses to win both licensure from recalcitrant states and, more importantly, increased employment in hospitals. In 1946, institutional nurses represented 56 percent of all active nurses; by 1960, the figure was 64 percent; by 1966, 67 percent, and by 1974, it had risen to over 74 percent [24]. However, the nurse/patient ratio went up even higher than the growth in professional nursing in hospitals, which to a large extent can be accounted for by the change in the ratio of nonprofessional to professional nurses, from 1:1 to 3:2 between 1946 and 1966 [25]. The more expensive labor of the RN was to be replaced, where appropriate, with that of practical, auxiliary, and volunteer nurses. The demand for nursing services during the Second World War and the postwar boom in hospital construction encouraged such substitutions. This time the cause seemed to be the shortage amd maldistribution of registered nurses rather than their overproduction [26]. Contemporary concerns with cost have only escalated the trend toward substitution to the point where hospital administrators may be choosing "quantity over quality," despite some resulting losses in productivity [27]. One consequence is that professional nurses are no longer responsible for housekeeping tasks or other "dirty work" in the hospital. However, in exchange for giving up functions lacking in social significance, the registered nurses may have stimulated competition from below.

The postwar period also witnessed the establishment of other health professionals, such as dietitians and psychologists, and of other health specialists, such as hospital social workers, mental hygienists, and various laboratory and operating room technicians. Again, the professional nurse was giving up tasks, this time to occupations in parallel positions in the hospital hierarchy.

Of course, registered nurses are developing significant new specialities of their own [28]. The hospital nurse was a generalist for only a short period in the history of professional nursing [29]. The fundamental work of the RN in the hospital today seems to involve administration or tasks that require advanced training. These functions can be viewed as a return to a position close to that of the original Nightingale nurse [30]. Nonetheless, the result has not been professional status, largely because of a lack of clarity regarding the distinctiveness of the RN's role. There is not even consensus among the RNs themselves: should they concentrate on providing "tender loving care" or adopt a scientific, administrative, or teaching orientation [31]?

The introduction of two new health professions, the nurse practitioner and the physician's assistant, further demonstrates the extent to which registered nurses lack a monopoly over any particular task. Attention has once more turned to the state nurse practice acts, since restrictions on what nurses are legally permitted to do at first hindered the development of these substitutes for the even more expensive and poorly distributed medical labor. Twenty-nine of the state acts are based on the ANA standard [32]:

The term "practice of professional" nursing means the performance, for compensation, of any acts in the observation, care, and counsel of the ill, injured, or infirmed in the maintenance of health or prevention of illness of others, or in the supervision and teaching of other personnel, or the administration of medications and treatments as prescribed by a licensed physician or a licensed dentist; requiring substantial specialized judgment and skill and based on knowledge and application of the principles of biological, physical, and social science. The foregoing shall not be deemed to include acts of diagnosis or prescription of therapeutic or corrective measures. *(emphasis mine)*

This is fairly vague language, clearer in what it prohibits than in what it permits. Indeed, it serves more to distinguish professional nurses from physicians than from nonprofessional nurses. However, as of 1977, numerous amendments and additions to this language have resulted in only twenty-four states explicitly forbidding acts of diagnosis by registered nurses, but among these states the definition of diagnosis varies. The requirements relating to education, supervision, and even the necessity of a license to practice are equally diverse. Language intended to cover the responsibilities of the nurse practitioner is probably the most inconsistent of all [33]. Perusal of the acts confirms that professional nurses continue to have overlapping functions with subsidiary nurses, other health professionals, physicians, and now physician's assistants (generally covered by medical practice acts). Professional as opposed to nonprofessional nursing tasks seem to be those that require direct medical supervision or permission and that bring the RN into conflict with the physician. Whereas the medical practice acts have been standardized by the American Medical Association (AMA) to the point where it is difficult "to choose to be another kind of physician than the AMA normatively defines" [34], the ANA does not even control, let alone standardize, the licensing requirements and examinations in every state [35].

A recent study of women in the health care industry finds that registered nurses not only continue to seek professionalization, they also seek recognition ". . . that their role is different from but equal to that of the physician" [36]. However, the history of their attempts to achieve such standing indicates the persistence of the obstacles outlined at the beginning of this paper. Although nursing is one of the few relatively high status occupations that women dominate [37], this very fact seems to hurt their efforts to secure high prestige. When compared with most other female employees, registered nurses do well, at least in salary. For example, the ratio of nurses' salaries to those of other female "professional, technical, and kindred workers" fluctuated between 0.98 and 0.86 from 1949 to 1967, with an increase to the advantage of the nurses in 1968 and 1969. However, they continue to lag behind teachers [38]. It is assumed they lag even further behind male professions since the studies referred to have chosen as the relevant reference groups "all civilian workers" and various female categories, never the free professions.

Nurses (and teachers) continue to be perceived as transients, ready to leave their jobs for husbands and children [39]. Perhaps this is part of the explanation for their relatively low occupational prestige scores on both the socioeconomic index and the National Opinion Research Center (NORC) scale. Among professional, technical, and kindred workers in 1950, only dancers and dancing teachers, dietitians and nutritionists, and entertainers had lower scores. Physicians and lawyers ranked nearly twice as high; college professors were also much higher. Among the traditional professions, only the clergy had a ranking anywhere approaching that of the professional nurse [40]. There is reason to believe that this situation has not altered very much since the 1950 survey [41].

The second obstacle to professionalization is the work setting, which is increasingly bureaucratic. Registered nurses today are overwhelmingly employed by hospitals. Moreover, while general duty nurses in hospitals increased by 199 percent between 1946 and 1966, head nurses increased by 143 percent, supervisory nurses by 95 percent, and superintendents by 109 percent [42]. As of 1972, the ratio of staff or general duty nurses to all supervisory nurses was 2:1, or approximately the same ratio as that of blue-collar workers to their supervisors [43]. This suggests the lack of one of the central attributes of a profession: relative autonomy on the job.

The third obstacle is the continued lack of control over the labor supply in nursing. Education still remains unstandardized: of the registered nurses who graduated in 1972, 21.3 percent had baccalaureate degrees, 37 percent had associate degrees, and 41.7 percent had diplomas from hospital training schools [44]. The proportions in the employed nurse population for that year were 13.8, 4.5, and 78.6 percent, respectively [45]. Legally, all of these nurses are equally qualified. However, in some locales, the result of these educational disparities has been an overproduction of nurses and, consequently, competition among registered nurses with different levels of training.

Another area of conflict within nursing is between the leadership, i.e. RNs who have gained reputations through administration, teaching, and research, and the hospital staff nurses. Both may share the desire for professional status, but the emphasis of most staff nurses has been on obtaining more control over decisions affecting patient care within the hospital setting, a goal that sometimes brings them into conflict with their nurse administrators. The two segments [46] of registered nursing have also employed different tactics to achieve their ends—although both tend to use the same organization, the ANA. Leadership relies on pressure and lobbying activity. The rank-and-file has increasingly come to rely on collective action, even strikes, to promote their drive for professional recognition.

All of these factors contribute to the failure of registered nurses to achieve professional status. However, the major obstacle remains functional redundancy. There is very little, if anything, that is defined as exclusively the province of the RN. Thus, the RN finds herself in a dilemma: her lack of monopolization at an earlier stage has meant that a changing division of labor now makes it nearly impossible for her ever to attain a monopoly. "Professional" nurses have won registration and licensure, but they have failed to define or monopolize their special contribution to medicine.

THE SEATTLE STRIKE

It should not be surprising, given this history, that registered nursing has failed to win professional stature. What is surprising is the seeming inability of the nurses to recognize their dilemma. The Seattle strike is a case in point [47].

During the summer of 1976, over 2000 staff nurses walked out of fifteen area hospitals for ten weeks, and out of another major local hospital for four. Their principal demands included salary increases, union security through mandatory membership in the Washington State Nurses Association (WSNA), and some control over staffing patterns and patient care policies through the already existent nurse practice committees. This last demand was similar to that of striking RNs in the Bay Area in 1974, and in Los Angeles' Cedars of Lebanon Hospital in 1968 [48]. Indeed, it was this issue that the Seattle strike leaders, at least, claim was the major motivation for their action, for they perceived control of this sort as essential to professional status.

The WSNA is, of course, a professional association as well as a collective bargaining representative. As such, it has actively pressured nursing schools and state legislators in its efforts to achieve professional status for nurses. One important result of the Association's lobbying was the passage of an extensive Nurse Practice Act, which significantly broadens the role of the RN. It may also have been a catalyst to militance by reenforcing the nurse's perception of her importance in the hospital and of WSNA power in the state.

The WSNA began its campaign for a state collective bargaining act in 1957. In 1972, two years before the extension of the National Labor Relations Act to hospital employees, it won the necessary enabling legislation. Thus, the WSNA had already negotiated two contracts before the one that precipitated the strike. Both were with the Seattle Area Hospital Council (SAHC), an organization of management that also negotiates with the Licensed Practical Nurses Association and with the Operating Engineers [49]. However, the WSNA represents by far the largest bargaining unit of health employees in the city, and it is one of the most militant. It had almost called a strike before the two prior contracts.

It is hard to say who "won" the 1976 strike. The SAHC considers itself the victorious party [50]. The WSNA failed to win amnesty for the strikers, full participation in staffing decisions, mandatory membership, or the salary gains it sought. Nonetheless, the hospitals did make concessions: the new contract resulted in some salary increase, maintenance of the "just cause" protection for nurses who are terminated, and response to several of the WSNA's nurse practice concerns [51]. Moreover, the hospital lost income: many potential patients and physicians discovered that care generally given in hospitals could be provided in doctors' offices more quickly and cheaply. Indeed, the census never fully recovered. This has resulted in serious consideration of a reduction in the number of hospital beds and, therefore, of hospitals.

To some extent, the outcome of the strike was the result of good planning by management and bad mistakes by the WSNA and its membership. The hospital administrators were prepared for the strike. They saw to it that the contract expired simultaneously with no other major hospital union contract. Moreover, the strike took place during the summer when the hospital census was down. Equally important, management permitted the Directors of Nursing Service (DNS) to sit in on the collective bargaining sessions as advisors to the management team. This was partly a response to a long-time DNS demand, and partly a self-conscious device for dividing the registered nurses, and for undermining feminist-based militance by putting women on both sides of the table.

At the same time the striking nurses made several strategic errors: they lacked experience in negotiations, and their emphasis on democratization in their bargaining committee made it difficult for them to bargain effectively. Furthermore, the RNs rebuffed possible coalitions with other hospital workers. They felt their professional stature depended on their differentiation from other health care employees. They not only wanted to reject possible comparisons and similarities, they also held themselves superior to everyone else in the hospital—with the obvious exception of the physicians. This is not to claim that the RNs believed they could act without allies. However, they assumed that the public would put pressure on the hospitals to end the strike. This was a serious miscalculation. So many strikes had occurred in so many "essential" services during the past few years in Seattle that the citizens remained disinterested and unexcited by another job action [52].

By far the most interesting aspect of the strike was the ability of the hospitals to maintain service without the absent RNs, albeit with some difficulty. First, management limited admission to critical cases; second, they took advantage of the hospital bureaucracy by having the head nurses (the line supervisors, and other qualified RN administrators) do staff work [53]; third, Seattle turns out to be an area with an overabundance of registered nurses (thus, management was able to hire approximately 1000 scabs); and fourth, it turned out that other hospital employees could do much of the necessary work without ever doing tasks proscribed by law. LPNs took on much of the direct nursing. Pharmacists, physicians, supervisory RNs, and—in at least one hospital—LPNs passed medications to patients. Operating room technicians made RNs unnecessary in surgery. In other words, when possible, hospital management took advantage of the functional redundancy of the RN.

By the end of the strike, the RNs' confidence was severely undermined. The striking nurses ended up fighting among themselves. Some blamed their paid negotiator for the outcome; others blamed the WSNA and advocated affiliation with another bargaining representative, possibly the Teamsters. However, most of the rank-and-file staff nurses simply felt discouraged. It is unlikely they will engage in a strike again in the near future [54]. They had hoped, through the strike, to demonstrate their functional indispensability. Instead, they became painfully aware of their substitutability and functional redundancy; and so did the hospitals. At least one of the institutions affected by the strike used the opportunity to reduce the ratio of RNs to LPNs. The strike also indicated to the state rate commission that much of what goes on in hospitals is unnecessary or too expensive. Consequently, the commission has begun to advocate a reduction in beds and services, that is nurses, in Seattle.

Conflict is the only way an occupation is able to win professional standing, but conflict can also hurt the professional cause [55]—as the Seattle strike indicates. Accusations of "nonprofessional" behavior were trivial compared to the other costs of the action. The strike demonstrated that registered nurses had neither powerful allies nor clout, the two prerequisites of achieving their professional goals. The physicians and public may have expressed some discomfort as a result of the strike, but they exerted little pressure on behalf of the RNs' demands. Moreover, those who might have given the staff nurses the most help were not supportive. Supervisory RNs were restricted by law from striking, but often they actively allied with management or with an image of professionalism that excluded job actions. Other hospital employees, another potential source of alliance, are also the registered nurses' greatest rivals, the very persons engaging in work that makes their own redundant. Many of the LPNs and technicians actually enjoyed the absence of the RNs, for it increased their own importance. Moreover, this rivalry was reinforced by the RNs themselves, whose claims to professional standing often rest on invidious comparisons with other hospital employees. Nor have the RNs demonstrated eagerness to ally with other health care unions.

It is not even clear that the achievement of the RNs' goal of meaningful participation in decisions about staffing patterns and patient care policy would have aided their professionalizing campaign. Had they won this demand, the nurses might have achieved more power in the hospital. However, they still would have lacked the criterion of a profession, namely control over the access to valued skills and knowledge.

Perhaps most important, the strike clarified the dispensability of the strikers. The RNs failed to provide evidence that they monopolize a socially significant service or, indeed, any service at all. This is attributable partially to the labor supply in Seattle, and partially to the presence of so much supervisory personnel. However, the work stoppage also provides further evidence of the increasing functional redundancy of the RN.

CONCLUSIONS

This study of registered nursing in the United States, and of the 1976 strike by the Seattle WSNA, illustrates the nature of the obstacles that confront the professionalizing project. Registering nurses—and by implication, other semiprofessionals—is handicapped by the identification of their work with female roles and bureaucratic settings. Further, their lack of status within the university contributes to their lack of status in the occupational structure. However, two other obstacles are of equal or even greater importance. First, registered nurses do not control the labor supply. Consequently, registered nurses can be subject to intense competition from others with presumably the same credentials. Second, registered nurses have failed to secure a monopoly over any set of socially significant, or even insignificant, roles. Without a monopoly, they are subject to competition from others whose training and skills overlap. In other words, they can become functionally redundant.

Nursing leadership has given considerable attention to the first problem. Currently nurses are lobbying for increased university training, research, and technical sophistication among RNs. Most importantly, they advocate increased stratification in nursing. Their campaigns include: (1) raising the educational requirements of the "professional" nurse to a baccalaureate degree; and (2) giving registered nurses more discretion and prestige through the creation of nurse practitioners dedicated to the "total care" of the patient and to the provision of services that fit into the grey area between medical and routine care [56].

However, there has been little appreciation of monopoly. Discussions of manpower substitution seldom address the implications for professionalism or job actions. Yet, functional redundancy is a testable concept, with relevance for all emerging professions [57]. The documentation of its existence should help explain difficulties experienced, not only by registered nurses and other semiprofessionals, but also by accountants and architects (traditionally male occupations).

Control over the labor supply coupled with monopolization of a socially significant function seems to be the *sine qua non* of a professional [58]. But whether or not a group already possesses control and monopoly determines the kind of conflict in which it has the highest probability of success. Interns may use a strike successfully to win "professional" demands, such as participation in hospital policymaking. It is not clear that registered nurses can.

Any group attempting to professionalize, then, must try to remove the possibility of functional redundancy. This is certainly a major problem confronting nursing today. At least one employment projection predicts an increase of RNs by 40 percent between 1972 and 1985, and of LPNs by 96 percent during the same period [59]. Physician's assistants and other health professionals also are projected to increase proportionately. Moreover, as part of attempts to prevent the creation of exclusively RN collective bargaining units, hospitals are beginning to claim that there is little distinctive about the RN role [60]. In other words, the nursing leadership might be advised to augment their stress on education to a stress on the legal definition of RN work that restricts others from performing certain key tasks.

A second possible RN strategy is to make manpower substitution unattractive. This can be done only by providing evidence that it is more efficient to use a highly productive, if more highly paid, registered nurse than several less well-trained or more specialized employees. Finally, and this is true for all emerging professions, strikes are unlikely to assist in the attainment of *professional* goals unless a monopoly over a crucial service already exists [61]. Otherwise, the strikers may serve to discredit their claims and perhaps themselves.

Such strategies and concerns make sense only as long as the semiprofessionals wish to gain professional stature. Indeed, there is a very real question about whether registered nurses, or other semiprofessionals, can ever achieve professional standing. Most nurses, social workers, teachers, and librarians work in hierarchies in which access to valued skills and knowledge is controlled by another group. Nonetheless, it is possible, if improbable, that semiprofessionals may yet gain a monopoly over an important function. However, this will not necessarily make them professionals in the public's eye. Unless the monopolized function has high social significance, the occupational group will be more like a craft—or the semiprofessional of Marshall's terminology—than a profession. The emergence of a new profession probably requires the emergence of a new occupation as the result of a major breakthrough in scientific or other knowledge, as the example of the engineer demonstrates.

Professionalization is not the only route to group mobility, however. Unionization is an alternative process, although its emphasis is on economic rather than status goals. If semiprofessionals gave up the professional model, they might more readily accept that of the industrial union. This implies alliances with all other employees in the institution and the possibility of a total shutdown during a work stoppage. In such a circumstance, functional redundancy is irrelevant.

REFERENCES

1. This is well documented in the literature on professionalism. See, for example, Rue Bucher and Anselm Strauss, "Professions in Process," *American Journal of Sociology (AJS)* 66 (January 1961): 325–334; William J. Goode, "Encroachment, Charlatanism, and the Emerging Profession," *American Sociological Review (ASR)* 25 (December 1960): 902–914; Margali Sarfatti Larson, *The Rise of Professionalism* (Berkeley: University of California Press, 1977); and Harold L. Wilensky, "The Professionalization of Everyone?" *(AJS)* 70 (September 1964): 137–158.
2. See, particularly, Wilensky, "The Professionalization of Everyone?"; William J. Goode, "The Theoretical Limits of Professionalism," *The Semi-Professions and Their Organization,* ed. Amitai Etzioni (New York: The Free Press, 1969); and Wilburt E. Moore, *The Professions* (New York: Russell Sage Foundation, 1970).
3. Larson, *Professionalism,* p. xviii. Robert K. Merton, "The Functions of the Professional Association," *American Journal of Nursing* 58 (January 1958), makes a similar point, p. 53.
4. See, for example, Eliot Freidson, *Profession of Medicine* (New York: Dodd and Mead, 1970), pp. 71–72; Larson, *Professionalism;* and Talcott Parsons, "The Professions in the Social Structure," in *Essays in Sociological Theory* (New York: The Free Press, 1954), pp. 34–39.
5. Goode, "Theoretical Limits," p. 279.
6. "Social Classes in an Ethnically Homogenous Environment," *Social Classes/Imperialism* (Cleveland: Meridian Books, 1955), p. 137; also see pp. 159–160.
7. Robert K. Merton, "Continuities in the Theory of Reference Groups and Social Structure," *Social Theory and Social Structure* (New York: The Free Press, 1957), p. 369.
8. "The Recent History of Professionalism in Relation to Social Structure and Social Policy," *Canadian Journal of Economics and Political Science* 5 (August 1939): 338.
9. See Everett C. Hughes, et al., *Twenty Thousand Nurses Tell Their Story* (Philadelphia: J.P. Lippincott Company, 1958), p. 762; and Goode, "Theoretical Limits," pp. 291–296.

10. See, particularly, Etzioni, *Semi-Professions.*
11. This is discussed by James W. Grimm, "Women in Female-Dominated Professions," *Women Working,* eds. Ann H. Stromberg and Shirley Harkness (Palo Alto: Mayfield Publishing Company, 1978), pp. 293–315; Hughes, *Twenty Thousand Nurses,* p. 228; and Richard L. Simpson and Ida Harper Simpson, "Women and Bureaucracy in the Semi-Professions," *Semi-Professions,* pp. 196–265. Also see Cynthia Fuchs Epstein, *Woman's Place* (Berkeley: University of California Press, 1970) for information on women in the traditional professions. Beverly Duncan and Otis Dudley Duncan, *Sex Typing and Social Roles* (New York: Academic Press, 1978) offer the most complete survey of changing attitudes towards working women.
12. See Goode, "Theoretical Limits," pp. 294–295; and Simpson and Simpson, "Women and Bureaucracy," *passim;* and W. Richard Scott, "Professional Employees in a Bureau-cratic Structure," *Semi-Professions,* pp. 82–140.
13. Goode, "Theoretical Limits," p. 287; also see pp. 277–278 and 281–289.
14. Everett C. Hughes, "Personality Types and the Division of Labor," *AJS* 33 (1928): 754–768.
15. A hospital stands in sharp contrast to a construction site. In the first, many different people engage in overlapping tasks. In the second, each craft controls its own labor supply, and the law restricts anyone else from performing that work.
16. The sections on the history of nursing are based on extensive reading in the literature. The most important sources are: Joanne Ashley, *Hospitals, Paternalism and the Role of the Nurse* (New York: Teachers College Press, 1976); Gerald Bowman, *The Lamp and the Book* (London: The Queen Anne Press, 1967); Edward Cook, *The Life of Florence Nightingale* (2 vols) (London: Macmillan, 1913); Vicki Cooper, "The Lady's Not for Burning," *Health/PAC Bulletin* (March 1970), pp. 2–6; Lydia Flanagan, *One Strong Voice* (Kansas City, Missouri: The American Nurses' Association, 1976); Elizabeth M. Jamieson and Mary F. Sewall, *Trends in Nursing History* (Philadelphia: W.B. Saunders Company, 1954); Deborah MacLurg Jensen, *History and Trends of Professional Nursing* (St. Louis: The C. V. Mosby Company, 1959); M. Adelaide Nutting and Lavinia L. Dock, *A History of Nursing* (New York: The Knickerbocker Press, 1907); Susan Reverby, "The Search for the Hospital Yardstick: Nursing and the Rationalization of Hospital Work," *Health Care in America,* eds. Susan Reverby and David Rosner (Philadelphia: Temple University Press, 1979); Mary M. Roberts, *American Nursing* (New York: The Macmillan Company, 1954); and Lucy Ridgely Seymer, *A General History of Nursing* (New York: The Macmillan Company, 1956).
17. Lee Holcombe, *Victorian Ladies at Work* (Hamden, Conn.: Archon Books, 1973).
18. In 1915, at the National Conference of Charities and Correction, Dr. Abraham Flexner spoke to the question of whether or not social work constituted a profession. Judging by the number of references in the nursing literature to this talk, graduate nurses accepted his criteria. He concluded that nursing could not be considered a profession.
19. See Larson, *Professionalism,* esp. Ch. 4. As Roberts, *American Nursing,* p. 61, notes, "no other profession has been developed on the assumption that an education be secured in exchange for service. . . ." Ashley, *Paternalism,* also discusses the use of students in the hospitals in Chs. 3 and 4.
20. Ashley, *Paternalism,* Ch. 4; and Roberts, *American Nursing,* pp. 20–22.
21. May Ayres Burgess, *Nurses, Patients, and Pocketbooks* (New York: Committee on the Grading of Nursing Schools, 1928) is the basic statistical source on the position of the nurses at this time.
22. Burgess' *Patients and Pocketbooks* was one of these as was Esther Lucille Brown, *Nursing as a Profession* (New York: Russell Sage Foundation, 1936); and Josephine Gold-mark, *Nursing and Nursing Education in the United States* (New York: The Macmillan Company, 1923).

23. Donald E. Yett, *An Economic Analysis of the Nursing Shortage* (Lexington, Mass.: Lexington Books, 1975), p. 4.
24. These figures are from Yett, *An Economic Analysis,* pp. 82–83; and the American Nurses' Association, *1976–77 Facts About Nursing* (Kansas City, Mo.: American Nurses' Association, 1977), "Table I-A-3. Estimated Number of Employed Registered Nurses, by Field of Employment, Selected Years, 1960–72," p. 5.
25. Yett, *An Economic Analysis,* p. 97.
26. The most extensive discussion of the nursing shortage, the extent to which it has actually existed, and its policy implications, is in Yett, *An Economic Analysis;* but also see D. C. Jones, et al., *Trends in RN Supply* (Bethesda, Md.: U.S. Department of Health, Education, and Welfare, 1976); and Frank A. Sloan, ed., *The Geographic Distribution of Nurses and Public Policy* (Bethesda, Md.: U.S. Department of Health, Education, and Welfare, 1975). Important post-War advocates of the use of subsidiary nurses, "team nursing," and various other ways to both differentiate and more efficiently use nurses included The Committee on the Function of Nursing (formed by the Division of Nursing Education, Teacher's College, Columbia University), *A Program for the Nursing Profession* (New York: The Macmillan Company, 1948), esp. Ch. III; and the Russell Sage Foundation through Esther Lucille Brown, *Nursing for the Future* (New York: Russell Sage Foundation, 1948), esp. pp. 57–72.
27. Myron D. Fottler, "Manpower Substitution in the Hospital Industry: Some Causes and Implications," *Hospital Administration* 17 (Summer, 1972): 27.
28. See Bonnie Bullough and Vern Bullough, eds., *New Directions for Nurses* (New York: Springer Publishing Company, 1971); Esther Lucille Brown, *Nursing Reconsidered* (Philadelphia: J.B. Lippincott Company, 1970); Hughes, *Twenty Thousand Nurses,* pp. 125–176; and Susan Reverby, "Health: Women's Work" (A Health/PAC reprint, 1972), pp. 11–12.
29. By 1958, according to a study done for the ANA by several eminent sociologists: "Nursing today is not the diffuse and generalized business it was until not many years ago. In the large hospitals, the graduate nurse is likely to be, first of all, an administrator and a teacher. She will direct a team of student nurses, practical nurses, and aides. Not only has her work become managerial on ward and floor, but also that part which is strictly nursing has become specialized. In large hospitals, the general duty nurse is on the way to becoming a specialist by default. Like the general practitioner among physicians, she is a residuary legatee, and her inheritance is the nursing which is left over from the operating room nurse, the obstetric nurse, the nurse in pediatrics, in psychiatry, and so on; and she is growing more specialized as the specialities keep breaking away." Hughes, et al., *Twenty Thousand Nurses,* pp. 32–33.
30. Harry Braverman, *Labor and Monopoly Capital* (New York: Monthly Review Press, 1974), has written of the proletarianization of white collar work in contemporary capitalism, given the increasing division of labor into specialized routine tasks. Without doubt, registered nurses are affected by changes in the division of labor. Although there has been some routinization, degradation of the work—in the Braverman sense—has not clearly occurred. Indeed, the history indicates that the RN has regained at least some of the stature she may have lost in the first half of this century. Thus, my argument contrasts with that of Reverby, "The Search for the Hospital Yardstick."
31. Rose Laub Coser, *Life in the Ward* (East Lansing, Michigan: Michigan State University Press, 1962); Robert W. Habenstein and Edwin A. Christ, *Professionalizer, Traditionalizer, and Utilizer* (Columbia, Missouri: University of Missouri Press, 1955); Fred E. Katz, "Nurses," *Semi-Professions,* pp. 54–81; and Isidor Thorner, "Nursing: The Functional Significance of an Institutional Pattern," *ASR* 20 (1955): 531–538 are among the studies that describe this confusion.
32. Quoted in Mary W. Cazalas, *Nursing and the Law* (Germantown, Md.: Aspen Systems Corporation, 1978), p. 86. The information about the number of states using such a

definition is from the U.S. Department of Health, Education, and Welfare, and Byrne, Inc., *Review and Analysis of State Legislation and Reimbursement Practices of Physician's Assistants and Nurse Practitioners* (Washington, D.C.: U.S. Government Printing Office, 1978), p. 34.

33. These findings are based on Cazalas, *Nursing and the Law,* "Appendix D: State-by-State Summary of Nurse Practice Acts," pp. 223–230. A more complete discussion of the acts, particularly as they relate to nurse practitioners, can be found in DHEW, *Review and Analysis,* esp. Ch. II; and Virginia C. Hall, "Summary of Statutory Provisions Governing Legal Scope of Nursing Practice in Various States," *The New Health Professionals,* eds. Ann Bliss and Eva Cohen (Germantown, Md.: Aspen Systems Corporation, 1977).

34. Arthur L. Stinchcombe, "Merton's Theory of Social Structure," *The Idea of Social Structure,* ed. A. Cosner (New York: Harcourt Brace Jovanovich, 1975), p. 16. Stinchcombe makes this point as part of a discussion of Merton's notions of the relationship between the completeness of a group and its social standing. See Merton, "Continuities in the Theory," particularly p. 314, where he contrasts the ANA and the AMA.

35. ANA, *76–77 Facts About Nursing,* "Table 1-G-10. Responsibilities for Selected Functions Relating to Registered Nurse Licensure, 1975," p. 68; and Cazalas, *Nursing and Law,* pp. 79–84.

36. U.S. Department of Health, Education, and Welfare, *A Study of the Participation of Women in the Health Care Industry Labor Force: Executive Summary* (Bethesda, Md.: U.S. Department of Health, Education, and Welfare, 1977), esp. pp. 3 and 4.

37. Women have represented 93 to 98 percent of professional nursing since 1900. In librarianship, they have represented 79 to 91 percent and in social work from 52 to 68 percent. The figures for 1960 were 97, 85, and 57 percent for nurses, librarians, and social workers, respectively. Richard H. Hall, *Occupations and the Social Structure* (Englewood Cliffs, N.J.: Prentice-Hall, 1969), "Table 10.5. Women As Percent of All Workers in Selected Occupations, U.S.A. (1900–1960)," p. 334.

38. Yett, *An Economic Analysis,* "Table 4.2. Year-Round Full-Time Professional Nurse Salaries Relative to Comparable Wages and Salaries of All Workers, Female Workers, and Teachers," p. 160. Also, see pp. 159 and 161. Also, see Jones, *Trends,* "Table 45. Relative Earnings of Registered Nurses Relative to Public School Teachers (W), 1956–57 through 1964–65," p. 96.

39. Yett, *An Economic Analysis,* writes, "popular opinion to the contrary, job changes in nursing are not abnormally numerous," p. 147. He proceeds to marshall considerable evidence to make his case. Also, see DHEW, *Participation of Women,* pp. 4–5. For a different viewpoint, see Jones, *Trends,* esp. pp. 18–21, p. 30, and Ch. V.

40. Hall, *Occupations,* "Table 9.3. Socio-Economic Index for Occupations in the Detailed Classification of the Bureau of the Census: 1950," pp. 275–276.

41. Robert W. Hodge, et al., "Occupational Prestige in the United States, 1923–63," *AJS* (1964): 296–302, discover a remarkable continuity in prestige rankings during these years. However, they do not discuss nursing.

42. Yett, *An Economic Analysis,* pp. 82–132. In particular, see "Figure 3.1. Estimated Number of Professional Nurses by Field of Nursing," p. 83; and "Figure 3.3. Hospital-Employed Professional Nurses in Selected Positions," p. 89.

43. I determined this ratio on the basis of figures in ANA, *76–77 Facts About Nursing,* "Table A-6. Employed Registered Nurses by Field of Employment and Type of Position, 1972," p. 8. For figures on blue-collar employment, see Erik Olin Wright, "The Class Structure of Advanced Capitalism," in his *Class, Crisis, and the State* (London: New Left Books, 1978), pp. 30–110, esp. p. 86.

44. Health Manpower References, *Report to the Congress: Nurse Training Act of 1974* (Bethesda, Md.: U.S. Department of Health, Education, and Welfare, 1974), "Table 4. Percentage Distribution of Nursing Student Data for 1962, 1967, and 1972," p. 17.

45. ANA, *76–77 Facts About Nursing,* "Table I-A-1. Estimated Number of Employed Registered Nurses, by Educational Preparation, Selected Years, 1964–1974," p. 4.

46. Bucher and Strauss, "Professions in Process."

47. My knowledge of this strike is based primarily on approximately sixty interviews with hospital administrators, labor negotiators, union representatives, and mediators who were involved. These interviews were carried out under the grant from the National Center for Health Services Research.

48. Cooper, "Lady's," p. 3; and David Gaynor, et al., "RN's Strike: Between the Lines," *Health/ PAC Bulletin,* no. 60 (September/October 1974), pp. 1–6.

49. A fuller discussion of the SAHC appears in Peter Feuille, et al., "Determinants of Multi-Employer Bargaining in Metropolitan Hospitals," *Employee Relations Law Journal* 4 (Summer, 1978): 96–115.

50. David L. Roach, et al., "Hospitals Stand Firm, Ensure Care in Lengthy Areawide Nurses' Strike," *Hospitals* 51 (August 1977): 49–51.

51. *The Seattle Nurse* (June 1979): 5.

52. Former Mayor Wes Uhlman recognized this fact in an earlier strike by City Light Employees. He received public support for waiting out the strikers rather than ending the strike at any cost. Consequently, he succeeded in breaking the strike. It would not be surprising if SAHC shared his strategic perception, uttered both in speeches and in print.

53. First line supervisors, that is head nurses, were removed from the bargaining unit at the beginning of the negotiations. This was in keeping with current labor relations practices, but it certainly affected the outcome of the strike on behalf of the management.

54. In the spring of 1979, when the contract came up for renegotiation, the WSNA was faced with the problem of motivating, let alone mobilizing, its membership. But despite the apathy of the general membership, the elected representatives were as active and more sophisticated than their predecessors. At the same time, the hospitals were more conciliatory than in the 1976 negotiations. The result was a relatively good contract from the RNs' point of view and one that was ratified by approximately 99 percent of those voting.

55. This important perception is elaborated by Edward Gross, "When Occupations Meet: Professions in Trouble," *Hospital Administration* 12 (Summer, 1967): 40–59.

56. See Glenn Jenkins, "1985: Closing the Door on Nurses, New York Style." *Health/PAC Bulletin, no. 78* (September/October 1977), pp. 1–7; Brown, *Nursing Reconsidered,* pp. 29–30; Bullough and Bullough, *New Directions,* Part I; and Reverby, "Women's Work," p. 11.

57. Fottler, "Manpower Substitution," cites a study that uses job family and level of content to document substitution. This method may also be applicable to functional redundancy. See Jeffrey Weiss, "The Changing Job Structure of Health Manpower," unpublished Ph.D. dissertation, Department of Economics, Harvard University, 1966.

58. Thus, my case study seems to document the arguments of Larson, *Professionalism.*

59. U.S. Department of Labor, Women's Bureau, *1975 Handbook on Women Workers, Bulletin 297* (Washington D.C.: U.S. Government Printing Office, 1975), p. 266. For other projections, which to some extent contradict those cited, see Health Manpower References, *Nurse Training Act of 1975; First Report to the Congress* (Hyattsville, Md.: U.S. Department of Health, Education, and Welfare, 1979), esp. Table 2, p. 111.

60. See *National Labor Relations Board v. St. Francis Hospital of Lynwood,* No. 78–1048, United States Court of Appeals for the Ninth Circuit, July 18, 1979, for a recent NLRB case in which a hospital argued that RNs are too diverse in their duties to constitute a "community of interest", the basis on which they have traditionally been granted a separate unit. Also see the hospital's brief, pp. 35–36, where it is asserted that LPNs can assume all the duties of the RN; and the transcript of the proceedings, pp. 169–170 and 174–176, where the argument is made that other hospital professionals have tasks that overlap with those of the RN. The American Hospital Association, it should be noted,

submitted an *amicus curiae* brief on behalf of St. Francis. The decision denied the appropriateness of a separate RN unit *per se* and permitted the possibility of an all-professional unit that includes the RNs.

61. Another example of this dilemma comes from the social work literature. Chicago case workers went on strike and discovered the clients were happy to have them gone. The checks simply came in the mail. See Arnold R. Weber, "Paradise Lost: Or Whatever Happened to the Chicago Social Workers?," *Collective Bargaining in Government,* eds. Joseph Loewenberg and Michael Moskow (Engelwood Cliffs, N.J.: Prentice-Hall, Inc., 1972), pp. 163–177.

Section 7
Change

30 Planned Change in Nursing

THE THEORY

Lynne Brodie Welch

PLANNED CHANGE requires a well-thought-out effort on the part of an individual or organization to make something happen. Planned change involves problem-solving and decision-making skills as well as interpersonal competence—the ability to work well with other groups and on a one-to-one basis [7]. Planned change is initiated and carried out by a *change agent* who is skilled in the theory and practice of planned change. Planned change has a specific client system—which can be an individual, group, or institution—who is the focus for the change.

The ability to identify and carry out planned change is an integral part of the role of the professional nurse. Since planned change is part of the leadership role of the nurse, many professional nursing programs have included change theory in their curricula. Some initial research on the ability of graduate nurses to initiate and carry out change is being done by Kramer and Schmalenberg [3]. Their research may give nursing additional insight into the nurse as an agent of change.

This article gives the nurse a general introduction to change theory as it has evolved to date. It is designed to give the nurse a basic understanding of the process of planned change: how it is diagnosed, implemented, and maintained.

LEWIN'S THEORY OF CHANGE

Classical change theory has its origins in the works of Kurt Lewin, who saw the process of change as having three basic steps: the stage of unfreezing, the stage of moving (the change), and the stage of refreezing (Fig. 30-1) [4].

STAGE OF UNFREEZING

In Lewin's first stage of change, the *unfreezing,* the motivation to create some sort of change occurs. It is in this stage that the client system becomes aware that there is a need for a change. The client system recognizes that there is a problem or a better way of accomplishing a task. This first stage is a mental (cognitive) one in which the individual is exposed to the idea that change needs to occur. The individual then needs to decide just what is wrong; that is, to diagnose the problem. Once the problem is identified, a solution that best suits the situation is selected from a group of alternatives. According to Lewin, the initial impetus to

Welch, Lynne Brodie, "Planned Change in Nursing: The Theory," *Nursing Clinics of North America,* Volume 14, Number 2, June 1979, pp. 307–321, ©1979. Reprinted with permission of W. B. Saunders Company.

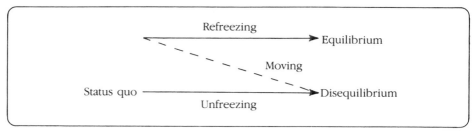

Figure 30-1. Lewin's phases of change.

create change occurs through three possible mechanisms: lack of confirmation or disconfirmation, induction of guilt-anxiety, or creation of psychologic safety. That is, the individual becomes aware of the need for change because: his expectations have not been met (lack of confirmation); he feels uncomfortable about some action or lack of action (guilt-anxiety); or a former obstacle to the change has been removed (psychologic safety).

STAGE OF MOVING

In Lewin's second stage of change, the actual changing or *moving,* new responses are developed based on collected information. This information has been sought by the individual to clarify and identify the problem. The information can be gathered from a single source or a variety of sources. Lewin believes that cognitive redefinition (looking at the problem from a new perspective) occurs through either identification or scanning. In the process of *identification,* particularly knowledgeable, respected, or powerful peer or superior influences the decision of the change agent with regard to the possible avenues for solving the problem. This approach would tend to limit the number of alternative solutions, but it might insure the success of the change project if the individual were powerful in the environment where the change would take place.

In the process of *scanning,* the same kind of information is sought from a variety of sources. This gives the change agent more solutions from which to choose but might increase the time it takes to make a decision about the best possible solution to the problem.

In Lewin's second stage of planned change, the change itself is planned out in detail and then initiated. Additional details about and strategies for this particular aspect of planned change are discussed later.

STAGE OF REFREEZING

Lewin's third stage of change is that of *refreezing*, in which the new changes are integrated and stabilized. In this stage, the individual(s) involved in the change integrate the idea into their own value system. The idea is perpetuated because it is now part of the value system in which they operate.

Another of Lewin's theories about change includes the notion that there are forces at work that facilitate or impede the process of change. The facilitating forces he calls *driving forces,* and the impeding forces he calls *restraining factors* (Fig. 30-2). It is important to identify the driving forces in a change project so that they can work for one and one can consciously capitalize on them. It is equally important to identify the restraining forces so that they can be avoided or modified so as not to interfere with the planned change. Many

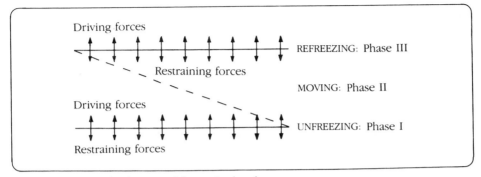

Figure 30-2. Lewin's phases and forces in the change process.

excellent planned change projects have failed because restraining forces were not identified. Brown's article gives an excellent example of negative forces that came as a surprise to the change agent, who was not equipped to deal with them [p. 365]. Preferably, restraining forces should be a known obstacle which can be taken into account during the planning and implementation of the change project.

APPLICATION OF LEWIN'S THEORY

The following situation is an example of planned change using Lewin's framework.

A new medication system was introduced into a community hospital. The change was planned by the pharmacy committee, on which several nurses served as nursing service representatives. The actual change was initiated and presented to the nursing staff by the doctor of inservice education.

UNFREEZING. All nursing personnel were introduced to the new medication system shortly before its initiation, through a filmstrip presentation. The inservice education director was available at this time to answer any questions.

MOVING. A time schedule was set up so that only two patient care units per week started using the new medication system. Again, the inservice education director was on hand to answer any questions. Eventually, the entire hospital adopted the new system for administration and charting of medications.

REFREEZING. On many of the patient care units, this author has noticed a general confusion about how to use the new medication system. The behavior of medication nurses ranged from compliance to the new system to omitting one or more crucial steps, or circumventing it entirely and using the old system. Several loopholes turned up because certain things had not been adequately understood by the medication nurse.

EVALUATION. Briefly, the driving and restraining forces can be summarized as follows.

Driving forces:
1. Approval by the hospital pharmacy was obtained;
2. Approval by the director of nursing service was given;

3. Unit dose medication system was already in effect;
4. It had been made a policy by nursing service;
5. It was anticipated to reduce cost, error, and nursing time.

Restraining forces:
1. There was an inadequate trial period;
2. It was explained immediately before it was put into effect;
3. Potential problem areas were inadequately identified;
4. The nurses who would actually use the change did not all have input;
5. Channels for feedback did not exist;
6. Staff nurses in general were not unhappy with the old system.

This author believes that the medication system as initiated will have difficulty succeeding owing to the strength of the restraining forces.

ADAPTATIONS OF LEWIN'S THEORY

Planned change theory can be seen from a variety of perspectives, all of which have their foundations in the works of Kurt Lewin. Some theorists take a behavioral or developmental view of change and see it as taking place primarily within and between individuals. Other change theorists take a systems or organizational view of change and see the change as being due to interactions within a particular system or group of intermeshed systems. Others see a model for change as a combination of the first two approaches [1]. A brief presentation of several important adaptations of Lewin's change theory follows.

ROGERS' THEORY

Everett Rogers saw the process of change as having antecedents that included the background of the individuals involved in the change as well as the environment in which the change took place. Rogers identified five phases in what he called the adoption of the process of change. The five phases that he identified were: awareness, interest, evaluation, trial, and adoption (Fig. 30-3) [8]. Rogers' stage of "awareness" corresponds to Lewin's first stage of "unfreezing." His stages of "evaluation," "trial," and "adoption" expand Lewin's second stage of "moving." Rogers' final stage of "adoption" amplifies Lewin's third stage—that of "refreezing."

In this amplified stage of adoption, Rogers identified two different outcomes which resulted from the adoption of a change. First, the adoption could be accepted. If accepted, then the adoption could be either continued or subsequently dropped, which is called "discontinuance." Second, the change could be rejected. If the change was rejected, it could either remain rejected or be adopted later in a different form. Central to Rogers' theory of change is the need for the individual to (1) be interested in the innovation (the change) and (2) be committed to making the change occur. Interest and support, particularly on the part of key people of the policy makers, are essential to the execution of successful planned change.

FACTORS IN SUCCESS OF PLANNED CHANGE. According to Rogers, the characteristics that are associated with successful planned change are: relative advantage, compatibility, complexity, divisibility, and communicability [8]. *Relative advantage* occurs when the change is perceived by the client system as being better. Whether or not it is an actual improvement is not significant; what is important is that the change is thought to be better than what preceded it.

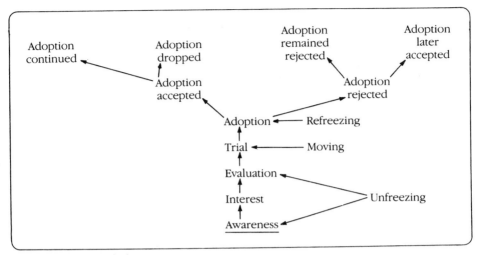

Figure 30-3. Rogers' phases.

Second, the change must be *compatible* with the existing values of the client system. It must take into account the existing norms, organizational structure, rules, and regulations.

Increasing difficulty, particularly of a mechanical nature *(complexity)*, makes the change less likely to be adopted. Simple techniques seem to be adopted more readily. Ideas in general are difficult to spread, possibly because they are less tangible. However, in a recent Rand study on planned change in education, it was shown that more complex ideas, once diffused, persisted where simple ones did not [6]. The researchers theorized that the change needed to be complex enough to survive the adaptations made at each level of the hierarchy that dealt with the change. Simple changes either were lost or were so modified that they no longer contained the original change. (It may be that this applies only to cognitive [thought] and not psychomotor [skill] changes.)

If the change is *divisible,* that is, if it can be tried out on a small scale first, it has more chance of succeeding. A trial also gives the change agent an opportunity to work out any unanticipated bugs or blocks.

The easier something is to describe—i.e., if it has *communicability*—the more likely it is to spread. This may have something to do with the complexity of thought needed to grasp something abstract as opposed to something more concrete in nature.

Rogers goes on to point out that different types of diffusion techniques are appropriate at different stages in the process of change. For instance, in the initial stage of awareness, mass media techniques such as pamphlets or radio broadcasts work well. In the adoption stage of change, however, face-to-face communication with someone who has used the change successfully is most effective.

HAVELOCK'S THEORY

Havelock also modified Lewin's theories about planned change. He described six elements in the process of planned change: building a relationship, diagnosing the problem, acquiring the relevant resources, choosing the solution, gaining acceptance, and stabilization and self-

Table 30-1. Havelock's Phases: An Expansion of Lewin's Theory

UNFREEZING
1. Building a relationship
2. Diagnosing the problem
3. Acquiring the relevant resources
MOVING
4. Choosing the solution
5. Gaining acceptance
REFREEZING
6. Stabilization and self-renewal

Table 30-2. Lippitt's Stages of Change: An Expansion of Lewin's Theory

UNFREEZING
1. Diagnosis of the problem
2. Assessment of the motivation and capacity for change
3. Assessment of the change agent's motivation and resources
MOVING
4. Selecting progressive change objectives
5. Choosing the appropriate role of the change agent
REFREEZING
6. Maintenance of the change once it has been started
7. Termination of a helping relationship

renewal (Table 30-1) [2]. Havelock's emphasis is on the planning stages of the change process, which take the most time and are where the significant change occurs. He correctly saw that the actual implementation of the change was usually less time-consuming than its planning.

LIPPITT'S THEORY

Another view of planned change is that of Lippitt, who identified seven phases in the change process: diagnosis of the problem; assessment of the motivation and the capacity for change; assessment of the change agent's motivation and resources; selecting progressive change objectives; choosing the appropriate role for the change agent; maintenance of the change once it has been started; and termination of a helping relationship (Table 30-2) [5]. Lippitt emphasized problem-solving as well as the interpersonal aspects of the change process.

With all these various views of change, it is important to bear in mind that none of these stages or phases are rigid. The change process may flow back and forth between the stages or phases, or it may move rapidly through one stage and then get stuck at another for quite some time.

Since this author believes that Lippitt's seven stages in the change process represent a well-rounded view of change, his stages are used as a framework for the rest of this article.

THE PROCESS OF CHANGE

STAGE ONE: DIAGNOSING THE PROBLEM

Once the nurse has discovered a problem or a general problem area, she has already begun the initial step of the process of change. Proper diagnosis of the problem is extremely important. If the problem is not accurately identified, the nurse will not obtain the desired results from the change. The following questions should be answered by those involved in initiating a change project: (1) What are all the possble ramifications of the proposed change? (2) Who else will be affected by the change, either directly or indirectly?

Everyone who will be affected by the change should know of the proposed change before it actually occurs. Ideally, they should all have an opportunity to participate in identifying the problem. All who will be involved in the change process or who will be affected by the change will need time to integrate the new idea or behavior into their repertoire of responses. Group meetings with those involved in the change project, which allow them to share ideas and help to shape the process of the change, are vital to the success of the change project. Commitment to an idea, an ideal, or a project is usually derived from personal involvement with it.

Key people—those who make policy decisions or who have important political connections—need to be involved in the change project as early as possible. Unless these key individuals are involved and are committed to the change, they can create obstacles such as noncompliance or setting up objections or roadblocks. Many change projects have failed because key people did not give the necessary help or sanction. Such key individuals may be directors of nursing, members of the board of directors of a hospital or an agency, or influential physicians.

For example, a head nurse and her nursing staff wished to institute primary nursing on their oncology unit. This change from team nursing to primary nursing was accepted by the director of nursing service. However, the change could never be implemented because the number of staff nurses was inadequate. Not only were several of the staff nurse positions unfilled, but also whenever there were more than three R.N.'s on the day shift, one of them was "floated" to another patient care unit. Such noncompliant behavior on the part of nursing service made it impossible for the head nurse and her staff to implement primary nursing.

STAGE TWO: ASSESSMENT OF THE MOTIVATION AND CAPACITY FOR CHANGE

An accurate assessment of the people involved and the environment in which the change is to take place is important to the success of the change project. It is in this stage that planning should begin to take place. The following questions need to be answered by the nurse:

1. What are the possible solutions to the problem?
2. What are the pro's and con's of each possible solution?
3. How would each of these solutions be implemented?
4. What are possible roadblocks to the completion of the change project within the framework of each possible solution?
5. What are the factors that are motivating people to participate in the change project?
6. How can these driving forces be capitalized on for each participant?

7. What are the limiting factors—restraining forces—in the environment that will inhibit the implementation of the change project?
8. What are the factors or forces that would facilitate the implementation of each possible solution?

Such factors as organizational structure, rules and regulations, cultural taboos and prohibitions, individual personalities, power, authority, the nature of the organization, and the credibility of those initiating the change should be carefully evaluated. Crucial to much change is the financial aspect, which often acts as a restraining force. The lack of identification of or planning for financial aspects may have been one of the restraining factors in the previous example concerning primary nursing.

As many people as possible should have some input into the planning stages. Meetings with small groups of people conducted in a democratic manner are felt to be the most effective in producing a successful change project. A group of more than five to seven individuals should be broken down into smaller groups, and occasionally representatives of each group should come together to share ideas. Ideally, those involved in each of the small groups should be peers to facilitate a give-and-take and democratic type of relationship.

STAGE THREE: ASSESSMENT OF THE CHANGE AGENT'S MOTIVATION AND RESOURCES

Obviously, the ability of the nurse to motivate others, guide the change project, and utilize available resources effectively is critical to the success of the change project. A change agent may be internal or external to the client system that he is trying to change. Whether it is better to have an insider or an outsider as the change agent generally depends on the identified problem and the type of environment in which the change is to take place. External change agents are often able to take a more unbiased view of the problems and possible solutions. However, the external change agent may experience more resistance from the client system because she is new or an unknown element, or because it is perceived that she does not really understand their unique situation. To be accepted, the external change agent must come with credentials and expertise compatible with and acceptable to the client system. She needs to be able to speak their language as well as be looked upon as an expert.

A nurse who is part of the client system knows it quite well. She usually knows the key people whose approval is needed to back the change project. The nurse's role and participation in the organization may, however, blind her to possible solutions and hamper her in her ability to get things done.

Sometimes the combination of both an external and an internal change agent—as co-agents—can be effective, since this utilizes the special insights and abilities of both. An example of the effectiveness of this approach is given in Miller's article. When more than one change agent is responsible for a change, it is important that they both view the problem and solutions in similar ways. They should also have similar leadership styles and should be able to get along well with each other. In-fighting among the change agents will frequently result in an unsuccessful change project.

The motivation of the nurse—her reasons for wanting to initiate the change—may affect the focus for possible solutions to the problem, the diligence with which she follows through with the change, and her overall commitment to the change. The following questions may be helpful for the nurse to ask herself or for client systems to ask of the prospective change agent(s):

1. Does the motivation stem from a genuine desire to improve something?
2. Does her motivation stem from a personal desire for power or recognition?
3. Does she want to change simply for change's sake; that is, to keep things constantly moving?
4. What is the orientation of the change agent: behaviorist or systems theorist?
5. Does the situation call for an interpersonal or an organizational approach, or both?
6. How much experience has the change agent had with this particular type of problem?
7. What are the credentials for the change agent? Do these credentials define an expert, according to the key people in your situation?
8. Is the personality of the change agent suitable to the particular situation?

In looking at the nurse as change agent, some attempt should be made to project the effect of her personality, behavior, and leadership on the client system. Most change agents believe that a group-oriented approach utilizing a democratic style of leadership is most conducive to effective change. The nurse, while very much a part of the process, must be able to divorce herself from it far enough to spot problems and guide it to successful resolution. The nurse should be flexible enough to see when modifications of the project are needed and to make the appropriate adjustments. The nurse agent should have the credentials, knowledge, and abilities necessary to be accepted by *all* those involved or potentially involved in the change project.

STAGE FOUR: SELECTING PROGRESSIVE CHANGE OBJECTIVES

Once a decision has been made about the role of the change agent, the change process moves into Lippitt's fourth stage, that of selecting progressive change objectives. It is at this point that the specific planning begins to identify exactly how the change is going to occur. The individuals involved in the change need to identify the steps in carrying out their change and the measures that they plan to use to achieve it. This stage of the planning needs to be quite specific, with timetables included. Deadlines are very helpful in moving the group toward decision-making. Plans should include the "where" of the initiation of the change as well as the "how" of it.

It may be helpful for the nurse to set a definite trial period in which to try out the innovation. At the end of the trial period, a decision can be made regarding whether to continue or terminate the change project. Lilla Dean in her article points out the effectiveness of such a trial period. Setting up a definite time to re-evaluate the change project may encourage some of the less involved people to go along with the change project. This will give the nurse more time to involve them in the project.

Specific goals can be re-evaluated in light of the actual trial experience. Modifications can be made that may improve the change project. The nurse needs to be sure that everyone involved knows her role, her responsibilities, and the deadlines that have been set.

STAGE FIVE: CHOOSING THE APPROPRIATE ROLE OF THE CHANGE AGENT

In most cases, the nurse will have a relatively active role in the implementation of the change project. She may serve as the expert for the client system, gathering and providing information. She may also teach the client system how to obtain their own information, or her function might be to make new connections within or between organizations. The nurse might be called upon to reorganize old connections within the client system to facilitate this particular change. In most instances, the nurse's role will also be to facilitate the work of the client system and the decision-making process.

The manner in which the nurse and the client system view the change agent's role may be very different. It is important that both the client system and the nurse clarify the role that the change agent is to play. This will help prevent unrealistic expectations on the part of both the client system and the change agent. The client system may, for instance, view the change agent as an expert whose only function is to provide information. If the nurse views her role as that of helping the system to obtain its own information, however, conflict will result. Frequent communication between the two to clarify information will prevent misunderstandings and speed the process of planned change. In her article, Olson deals in depth with strategies that can be used by the nurse to deal with conflict and confrontation.

STAGE SIX: MAINTENANCE OF THE CHANGE

The key to keeping the change project going, once it has been initiated, is to keep lines of communication open. Frequent feedback to the policy-makers and all those involved in the change project will serve to keep participants informed and sustain their interest. Memos, on-the-spot observation by key people, and group meetings for participants on a regular basis are all helpful methods of feedback. Photographs of "before" and "after," if appropriate, can be very effective in maintaining an interest in the change project.

Once the planned change has taken place, plans should be made for its spread or diffusion. If the project was run on a small scale first, then those who are next in line to experience the change can be sensitized to it through direct observation and communication with those who have already experienced it. It may be spread simply by work of mouth among peers and may not be a conscious effort. One change frequently triggers off a chain of changes that are related in some manner to the original planned change.

Everyone involved in the change should be encouraged to be as innovative and flexible as possible in their dealings with the change project. All changes must be adapted to the environment or to the personalities of those involved in the project. The nurse must make sure that the general direction and intent of the change project are not obscured by these adaptations. Since change often leads to more change, the change agent must be careful not to alter too much at one time. Care should also be taken to undertake only small changes, since they have a better chance of succeeding. Large changes are usually doomed to failure, since it is difficult to monitor and plan for all the ramifications of the change. If the client system desires a sweeping change, then it may be best to introduce a totally new power structure or to plan the change in a series of small steps.

STAGE SEVEN: TERMINATION OF THE HELPING RELATIONSHIP

In the last of Lippitt's stages, the change agent withdraws from the situation, leaving the client system alone to maintain the change. This too must be a planned effort. The goal of the nurse in this stage is to have the client system gradually take over the functions of the change agent. This is necessary to ensure perpetuation of the change. Certain individuals within the client system should be identified as those who will maintain the change. It is important that these people have some power and authority within the client system of either a formal or an informal nature. They should be involved with the change project from the beginning and should be committed to the change. Obviously, the more people within the client system committed to the change, the more likely it is to survive. Development of a written procedure or policy concerning the change will help to ensure its perpetuation.

The client system should know when their relationship with the nurse will be terminated and what their role will be subsequently. A definite date for termination should be set up to facilitate the leave-taking process. It may be helpful to the client system if the nurse is available to them for advice and to reinforce the change. She may be better able to evaluate her effectiveness as a change agent if she views the effects of the change over time.

SUMMARY

In the final analysis, whether the change is adopted or rejected will depend upon the accurate diagnosis of the problem, finding an appropriate solution to the problem, the extent of involvement of the client system, and the skill of the change agent. If the change is adopted, the change agent should focus her energy on maintaining or modifying it so that it lasts. If the change is rejected, the change agent should try to identify the restraining factors. Sometimes it is possible to rediagnose the problem in light of new information and to formulate a new solution. Not all change projects are successful, due to the complexity of the change process.

Planned change is part of today's nurses' leadership role. The ability of each nurse to identify and effect change is vitally important in meeting the needs of her clients. Implementation of change is a natural part of the action phase of the nursing process. Thoughtful use of planned change on the part of nurses does and will continue to promote quality nursing care based on the identified needs of health care consumers.

REFERENCES

1. Chin, R.: The Utility of System Models and Developmental Models for Practitioners. *In* Bennis, W. G., et al. (Eds.): The Planning of Change: Readings in the Applied Behavioral Sciences. 2nd Ed. New York, Holt, Rinehart and Winston, 1969, pp. 297–312.
2. Havelock, R.: The Change Agent's Guide to Innovation in Education. New Jersey, Educational Technology Publications, 1973.
3. Kramer, Marlene, and Schmalenberg, Claudia: Bicultural training and new graduate role transformation. Nursing Digest, 78:1–48, Winter, 1978.
4. Lewin, K.: Group Decision and Social Change. *In* Maccoby, E. (Ed.): Readings in Social Psychology. 3rd Ed. New York, Holt, Rinehart and Winston, 1958.
5. Lippitt, G.: Visualizing Change: Model Building and the Change Process. La Jolla, Calif., University Associates, Inc., 1973.
6. McLaughlin, Milbrey Wallin: Implementation as mutual adaption: Change in classroom organization. Teachers College Record, 77(3):339–350, February, 1976.
7. Rodgers, Jenet: Theoretical considerations involved in the process of change. Nursing Forum, 12(2):161–174, 1973.
8. Rogers, E.: Diffusion of Innovations. New York, The Free Press of Glenco, 1962.

SELECTED READINGS

1. Baldridge, J. V., and Deal, T.: Managing Change in Educational Organizations. Berkeley, Calif., McCutchan Publishing Corporation, 1975.

2. Barnett, H. G.: Innovation: The Basis of Cultural Change. New York, McGraw-Hill, 1953.
3. Bennis, K., Benne, K., and Chin, R.: The Planning of Change. 2nd Ed. New York, Holt, Rinehart and Winston, 1969.
4. Brooten, Dorothy, Hayman, Laura, and Naylor, Mary: Leadership for Change: A Guide for the Frustrated Nurse. Philadelphia, J. B. Lippincott Co., 1978.
5. Carver, F., and Sergiovanni, T.: Organizations and Human Behavior: Focus on Schools. New York, McGraw Hill, 1969.
6. Etzioni, A., and Etzioni, Eva: Social Change. New York, Basic Books, Inc., 1964.
7. Goodlad, J.: The Dynamics of Educational Change. New York, McGraw-Hill, 1975.
8. Havelock, R.: The Change Agent's Guide to Innovation in Education. Englewood Cliffs, New Jersey, Educational Technology Publications, 1973.
9. Lewin, K.: Field Theory in Social Science. New York, Harper and Row, Publishers, 1951.
10. Lippitt, R., Watson, Jeanne, and Westley, B.: The Dynamics of Planned Change. New York: Harcourt, Brace and World, Inc., 1958.
11. Schaller, L.: The Change Agent. New York, Abington Press, 1972.
12. Steward, J.: Theory of Culture Change: The Methodology of Multilinear Evolution. Urbana, Illinois, University of Illinois Press, 1973.
13. Western Interstate Commission for Higher Education: Models for Cultural Diversity in Nursing: A Process for Change—Final Report. Boulder, Colorado, WICHE, July, 1978.

31 Guidelines for Introducing Change

J. Randolph New and Nancy A. Couillard

WHENEVER CHANGES OCCUR in the health care system, they must ultimately be dealt with by nursing administrators. To be successful in managing any change requires an understanding of the basic nature of change, why people resist change, techniques for dealing with resistance, and how situational variables influence the effectiveness of various change techniques.

Whatever the nature of the change, or the impetus for making it, change ultimately requires altering the attitudes and behaviors of *individuals*. But, such attempts often encounter difficulty, or fail, because individuals often resist change, expressing their resistance in counterproductive behavior such as apathy, hostility, absenteeism, or a decline in job performance. It is important to nursing administrators to understand why this resistance occurs, and more important, how to deal with it.

RESISTANCE TO CHANGE

Individuals resist change for any one or more of five basic reasons; threatened self-interest, inaccurate perception of the intended change, objective disagreement with the change, psychological reactance, and low tolerance for change.

THREATENED SELF-INTEREST

Perhaps the major reason individuals resist change is their perception that the personal costs of the change are greater than the personal benefits. Depending on the particular change, personal costs may include loss of money or status, a belief that more effort or work will be required, or a belief that valued social relationships will be disrupted.

For example, a large hospital in the southwest set up large centralized nursing stations (each serving 120 beds) to improve the coordination of nursing services, particularly during the off-shifts and weekends when staffing is a major problem. The physicians resisted the new arrangement, contending that patients farthest from the station received less prompt and adequate care. However, further questioning revealed that the real reason some physicians disliked the new arrangement was that they perceived a decrease in personal services provided them by the nursing staff. When individuals resist change due to threatened self-interest, they tend to propose "other reasons" why the change should not be made.

Reprinted by permission from "Guidelines for Introducing Change" by J. Randolph New and Nancy A. Couillard, *Journal of Nursing Administration*, Volume 11, Number 3, 1981.

INACCURATE PERCEPTIONS

Individuals who do not understand the nature or implications of a change may erroneously believe it is not beneficial. A medium-size hospital revealed plans to begin using a computer for scheduling personnel. Opposition by nurses and other staff members was based on the perception that computerization would reduce their freedom in choosing working hours and days off. Actually, the new scheduling process was easier and less time-consuming for the head nurse doing the scheduling, allowing more time for consideration of individual requests.

OBJECTIVE DISAGREEMENT

In some circumstances individuals place the organization's interest above their own, but offer resistance because they feel the change will not benefit the organization. Such resistance occurred when one hospital introduced a new performance evaluation program, following the advice of many management experts by focusing on behavioral performance criteria (for example, repositioning a comatose patient in correct body alignment). Implementation of the system was resisted by head nurses, who felt behaviorally oriented evaluations would force them to evaluate personnel on easily defined criteria that would not be appropriate for certain jobs. They believed such a system would not accurately measure an individual's contribution to the organization, and that it might be detrimental to patient care.

Objective disagreement often results when change agents and resistors have different information available to them. When the resistors' judgment is based on more complete and accurate information, such resistance can be beneficial to the organization. This possibility is often overlooked by change agents.

PSYCHOLOGICAL REACTANCE

Individuals, perceiving that their freedom to engage in particular behaviors has been threatened or eliminated, will be motivationally aroused. This arousal, called psychological reactance [1], manifests itself in several ways. The threatened or eliminated behaviors may become more desirable and important. Or, there may be direct attempts to reestablish behaviors that have been eliminated. Thus reactance theory offers a general explanation of why people resist change: they perceive that it threatens or eliminates their freedom to engage in alternative behaviors.

An example of resistance that may have been due to psychological reactance is provided by a change introduced in a large hospital in the southeast. A cart was designed and produced for the critical-care nursing staff to use when assisting in the insertion of a right-heart catheter. The cart had materials contained in six drawers which were arranged in the order normally used in such an insertion. Although the cart was generally acknowledged as an important contribution to patient service (the designer received commendation) several nurses refused to use it and could not offer objective reasons for their behavior. Psychological resistance offers a plausible explanation.

LOW TOLERANCE FOR CHANGE

Many organizational changes require rapid attitudinal and behavioral changes. While affected individuals may intellectually understand the change, they may be emotionally unable to make the required transition. Some individuals have more difficulty dealing emotionally with change than others, due to low self-confidence, aversion to risk, or low tolerance for uncertainty.

For example, at a medium-size southeastern hospital, management determined that critical care nursing service would be improved if the critical care department was decentralized into four specialized critical care units (medical, surgical, trauma, coronary). An excellent assistant-head nurse (under the old arrangement) was offered a promotion to head nurse in the new medical intensive care unit. She then began to express considerable doubt about the efficacy of the proposed reorganization. When she was questioned it became apparent that her opposition was the result of fear of failure in her new role.

TECHNIQUES FOR DEALING WITH RESISTANCE

There are a number of techniques for dealing with resistance to change. While each approach may be useful in certain situations, no single approach will always be successful. The eight techniques to be discussed here are participation, coercion, manipulation, education, use of an external agent, incentives, supportive behavior, and gradual introduction.

PARTICIPATION

Involving those who will be affected by a change in its design and implementation is one way of dealing with resistance. It has been suggested that, with mature individuals, participation offers a panacea for effective introduction of change [2]. Unfortunately, such a prescription is simplistic, overlooking some important situational requirements.

There are two important assumptions underlying the use of participation as a change technique. The first is that those affected by the change actually desire to participate before the change is made. This is not always the case. Some individuals may view the cost of participation (for example, time) to be too high when compared with the potential benefits (for example, influencing the change process). Interestingly, individuals who decide not to participate in planning a change may be less likely to offer resistance once the change is made than if they had not been asked.

A second assumption underlying the use of participation is that those who are asked to participate in planning and implementing change have something beneficial to contribute. Unless this is true, the time and effort expended on participation is unlikely to be productive. In addition, the input of uninformed participants is likely to be ignored in the change decision, causing more resentment than if they had not been asked to participate.

Even when individuals affected by change have relevant information that they desire to contribute, there are still difficulties associated with the use of participation. First, it is a time-consuming process, and some decisions must be made quickly. Secondly, some participants will believe their input has been ignored in the final decision, and may become resentful. Finally, if the environment is characterized by mistrust, it is quite possible that attempts to generate participation will be viewed as manipulation.

COERCION

Coercion involves implicitly or explicitly threatening individuals in order to force them to accept a change. Authoritarian persons often resort to formal positional authority when resistance to change is either anticipated or actually encountered. But individuals often resent having change forced on them, and this resentment may increase their resistance. If the change agent has too little power to enforce threats, the result may be refusal to accept the change.

In spite of the severe limitations, there are circumstances in which coercion may be useful; for example, where the change agent has sufficient power, the willingness to enforce the threats, and where it is essential that the change be made quickly [3]. Alternative change techniques are likely to be no more effective, and may be less efficient.

MANIPULATION

It is manipulation when a change agent deviously structures the context in which the change will occur to increase the likelihood the change will be accepted. Manipulation frequently involves distorting information or using it in a selective fashion, causing affected individuals to view the change as less costly or more beneficial than it actually is.

Manipulation tends to be time and cost efficient; generally quicker than participation or education, and less expensive than incentives.

Ignoring the question of ethics, the major difficulty associated with the use of manipulation is that it may be detected by the individuals being manipulated. Whether individuals sense the manipulation as it occurs or recognize it only after the change process is complete, they are likely to respond negatively. The distrust created will generally add to the difficulty of future change efforts.

EDUCATION

As a change technique, education is the process of providing individuals with information intended to help them see the need for the logic of the change. A combination of verbal and written methods may be used.

Education is the change technique most frequently reported in the health-care literature [4]. It is particularly valuable in situations where resistance is due to incomplete or inaccurate information. However, it can be expensive in terms of time and effort, especially if many individuals are involved. Also, at least a moderately trusting relationship must exist between the initiators and potential resistors for this approach to be successful [5]. Otherwise, the resisting individuals may not believe the information. Such an education effort may even increase resistance, particularly if the effort is perceived as a "hard-sell."

EXTERNAL AGENTS

An external agent used to help introduce a change may be anyone who is normally not involved in the relationship. The agent could be someone who is part of the organization, such as a staff specialist, or someone from outside the organization. An external agent may be particularly useful in two situations; (a) where the unit lacks knowledge, either about the change process or about the specific change itself (for example, computer usage in a new area), and (b) where there is a lack of trust between the initiator of the change and the affected individuals.

One difficulty with using an external agent is the extra expense that almost always is involved. Another problem is location of a suitable agent. This third party not only must possess the necessary knowledge, skill, and ability, but must be perceived as trustworthy, a particularly difficult requirement when the initiator of the change (and sponsor of the external agent) is not trusted.

INCENTIVES

Incentives can overcome resistance, particularly when the resistance is the result of threatened self-interest. Incentives may be anything that resisting individuals value; extra pay, status symbols, desired work activities, and so forth. To increase commitment to the change, incentives may be tied to the benefits that the organization expects to derive from the change.

Incentives can be expensive, particularly if other members of the organization discover their use. However, in situations when resisting parties are powerful and clearly have something to lose as a result of the change, incentives may be useful.

SUPPORTIVE BEHAVIOR

If resistance is expected from individuals due to their low tolerance for change, offering them support during the change process may help. Support may include special counseling services, training in new skills, and generally considerate treatment. When used in appropriate circumstances offering support may reduce resistance, but it may also be time-consuming and expensive. When individuals have an extremely low tolerance for change, offering support may be minimally helpful at best. Where apprehension about the change is not the major reason for resistance, offering support is not likely to be beneficial.

GRADUAL INTRODUCTION

Introducing change gradually may reduce resistance [6]. This may involve making a series of minor changes that, taken together, constitute the complete intended change, or it may consist of demonstrating the feasibility of the change in one segment of the organization before introducing it to the extent ultimately desired. An example of the first situation is where decentralization is introduced by gradually giving select subordinates more decision making authority. The second situation is exemplified where new patient monitoring equipment is tested in the surgical intensive care unit before being incorporated in all critical care units.

Both approaches are useful when affected individuals are having difficulty envisioning the intended benefits of the change. In select situations, actual demonstration is the best solution. But the gradual approach may be time consuming and expensive, particularly in situations where major benefits can be achieved through rapid or large scale introduction of the change.

CHOICE OF CHANGE TECHNIQUES

Most nursing administrators are aware of the change techniques that have been discussed. Yet most can cite personal experiences with severe resistance to change and its accompanying problems. In most cases, resistance can be reduced if change is introduced skillfully. To develop the skills required for the successful introduction of change, the nursing administrator must learn first to avoid the mistakes commonly made when introducing change and then to assess situational factors that determine the appropriate change technique.

COMMON MISTAKES

The first common mistake is to plan and implement change with only vague or ambiguous objectives in mind. Often the change is introduced with the only objective being "to improve things." Unless objectives are stated precisely, it is difficult to select the appropriate change technique and to evaluate its degree of success.

A second mistake is to approach change without a clearly considered strategy [7]. Although such a problem is frequently related to poorly defined objectives this is not always the case. The initiators may have a clear vision of their intended outcome, without having thought through either the alternative ways of reaching that outcome or the different ways of introducing the alternative selected. While time-pressures and the "action orientation" of administrators may help explain why change is undertaken in a disjointed fashion, such excuses do not lessen the long-run costs of proceeding in such a manner.

A third mistake is to rely on a limited set of change techniques regardless of the situation. The authoritarian personality typically resorts to coercion, the considerate supervisor constantly tries to involve and support subordinates, and the rational administrator relies heavily on education and information [8]. Each approach has its strengths and weaknesses, and the particular change situation must be assessed to determine the technique that "fits."

ASSESSING THE SITUATION

When initiating change, the chance of success can be improved through careful assessment of the particular situation before choosing a change technique. Many factors have already been examined. The major questions to be answered include the following:

1. Which individuals will be affected by the change? The analysis should include the number of individuals, their power in the organization, and their willingness and ability to contribute to the change effort. Generally, if large numbers of people are involved, only key individuals and group characteristics can be examined.
2. Who is likely to offer resistance, and why? Attempts to overcome or reduce resistance are likely to be successful only if they address the underlying reason for the resistance.
3. How much time is available for the introduction of the change? There are major differences in time required for effective utilization of the various change techniques, and these differences should be explicitly considered before change is undertaken.
4. How important to the organization is the planned change? The more important the change, the more important it is to develop a strategy to deal with potential resistance.
5. To what degree is the organization characterized by mutual trust and cooperation between members? Without trust and cooperation, some change techniques will almost certainly fail to reduce resistance.

These questions are designed to assist in developing a change strategy, and their usefulness will be undermined if they are not answered realistically. If, for example, the organization is characterized by a lack of trust and cooperation, this problem must be acknowledged and considered in developing an effective change strategy.

SUMMARY

A major task facing the nursing administrator is to plan and implement changes in the organization. To increase the likelihood of successful change, the nursing administrator must understand the basic change process, the reasons people resist change, and the techniques for dealing with this resistance. In addition, she must have the skill to correctly diagnose her situation in order to develop the appropriate change strategy.

REFERENCES

1. Brehm, J. *Responses to Loss of Freedom: A Theory of Psychological Reactance.* Morristown, N.J.: General Learning Press, 1972, p. 1.
2. Hersey, P., and Blanchard, K. *Management of Organizational Behavior.* Englewood Cliffs, N.J.: Prentice-Hall, 1972, p. 159.
3. Kotter, J.P. Power, dependence, and effective management. *Harv. Bus. Rev.* 55(4):125, 1977.
4. Lang, N.M. A Model for Quality Assurance in Nursing. In Davidson, S. (Ed.). *PSRO Utilization and Audit in Patient Care.* St. Louis: C. V. Mosby, 1976, p. 24.
5. Kotter, J.P., and Schlesinger, L.A. Choosing strategies for change. *Harv. Bus. Rev.* 57(3):106, 1979.
6. Hillriegal, D., and Slocum, J.W., Jr. *Organizational Behavior.* St. Paul: West Publishing, 1979, p. 562.
7. Kotter, J.P., and Schlesinger, L.A., 1979, p. 112.
8. Kotter, J.P., and Schlesinger, L.A., 1979, p. 112.

32 Primary Nursing and Change

A CASE STUDY

Claire Manfredi

THE FACT that primary nursing has appeared in a number of hospitals throughout the country in the last few years is certainly not unusual. In many respects, it appears to be a response to the need for continuity, coordination and accountability in nursing service departments today. With the reported success of primary nursing to date, it is conceivable that more hospitals will attempt to implement primary nursing in the future. Manthey et al. [1] and Marram et al. [2] suggest the need for further research in the area of primary nursing. Manthey advocates the repeated implementation of the concept and the evaluation of the system in order to develop a design of care which is more nearly comprehensive [2]. Implementation must precede evaluation; thus the successful implementation of primary nursing must be achieved in order that the effects of the system upon patient care and personnel can be effectively evaluated and additional research can be conducted.

Since the implementation of primary nursing is considered to be a planned change, the use of a change model in bringing about this change is most appropriate.

Lippitt lists three purposes of a change model as:

1. To display abstractly the nature of a system or situation.
2. To illustrate the interrelationships of various parts of the situation or system.
3. To provide the basis for predicting what damage might occur in one part of the situation or system when a change is made in another part. [3]

For the change agent in nursing the availability of a model for the implementation of primary nursing will prove to be extremely valuable. The model can aid the change agent in achieving a smooth transition to primary nursing, thus providing opportunities for further research and evaluation of primary nursing as a nursing care delivery system.

CHANGE MODELS

Although there are a number of change models available for use today, the models of Kurt Lewin and Edgar Schein were utilized by the writer in the implementation of primary nursing.

Lewin identified three stages in the change process and described them in the following manner:

Reprinted with permission by Charles B. Slack, Inc., from *Nursing Leadership*, Volume 3, Number 3, September 1980.

1. Unfreezing: involves problem awareness and the desire for change.
2. Moving: concerns the change itself; moving to a new level.
3. Freezing: concerns stabilization of the change and refreezing group life on the new level. [4]

Lewin looks upon human behavior in an institutional setting as a dynamic balance of forces working in opposite directions within the socio-psychological space of the institution. Group life in an organization can be viewed as a social field consisting of the group and the setting. According to Lewin:

One of the fundamental characteristics of this field is the relative position of the entities which are parts of the fields. . . . What happens within such a field depends upon the distribution of forces through the field. [4]

There are two basic methods of changing levels of conduct. One can either increase the driving forces or diminish the resisting forces. Change occurs when there is an imbalance between the driving forces and the restraining forces. The resultant disequilibrium serves to unfreeze the group and move the group to a new level of equilibrium.

Lewin's model is based upon the use of the group in the decision-making process. According to Lewin, it is much more difficult to change individuals than it is to change a group. Individuals belong to a group because they adhere to the norms or standards of that group. An individual would risk ejection from the group should he/she display conflicting attitudes or values. Consequently, effective change is dependent upon change in attitudes and values or norms of the group.

Schein took Lewin's model and developed mechanisms for each of Lewin's stages of change [5].

UNFREEZING

Schein identifies three mechanisms in the unfreezing stage. The first is the lack of confirmation or disconfirmation which creates a disequilibrium in the change target and establishes the conditions necessary for change. The second is the induction of guilt-anxiety, which is a reaction to the disconfirmation. The change target responds with feelings of inadequacy or failure. The third mechanism is the creation of psychological safety by the reduction of threats or the removal of barriers. Schein suggests that the change agent provide support and reassurance during this stage.

CHANGE

According to Schein, the change occurs through one of two mechanisms: identification or scanning. Identification involves identifying or emulating another person who holds certain attributes or values. Scanning involves surveying the environment for a whole range of ideas and combining them into a format that will fit into the system to be changed and thus facilitate refreezing. Schein refers to scanning as a means of producing change through internalization. Internalization occurs when an individual learns new attitudes by being placed in a situation where new attitudes are demanded as a way of solving problems.

REFREEZING

This stage concerns the process of stabilizing and integrating the changes, and involves integrating new responses into the personality and significant ongoing relationships. It would be difficult for an individual to support a change that fits into the culture of which he/she is a member but is inconsistent with the individual's personality. Likewise, it is difficult for an individual to sustain a change that suits her/his personality but is inconsistent with the culture.

THE CASE STUDY

This is a case study in which the writer, utilizing a change model approach, acted as change agent in the implementation of primary nursing. The hospital was a 350-bed community teaching hospital utilizing team nursing as the nursing care delivery system. The change agent was invited by the director of nursing service to develop a plan for the implementation of primary nursing on one unit within the hospital. Although the director of nursing service had been in the position for a short period of time, she was not new to the institution and was well liked and respected by the staff. She was interested in exploring various methods of delivering care to patients and was most interested in the primary nursing concept. The director had explored the possibility of the project during meetings with the nursing service administrative staff.

In preparation for the project, the change agent developed an introductory audiovisual program on primary nursing; drafted a proposal utilizing Lewin's and Schein's change models; and developed criteria for the selection of a nursing unit, based upon information in the literature. The criteria included size of the nursing unit, nurse/patient ratio and interest of the nursing staff. The change agent then met with the director of nursing to discuss the project.

Since administrative support and commitment are essential in order to institute and maintain a change to primary nursing, the change agent met with the hospital administrator and the administrative council. They responded favorably to the proposal and raised questions concerning the staffing and budgetary considerations; reactions of patients, physicians, and staff; utilization of nonprofessional personnel; and the potential for implementation on other units within the hospital. The council agreed to provide the facilities for the project and pledged their support.

The change agent then met with the nursing service administrative staff. They raised questions concerning the nurse/patient ratio, the use of nonprofessional personnel, and the implications for other units within the hospital. They were most receptive to the proposal, and several patient care coordinators offered suggestions for nursing units that would meet the established criteria. Since the nursing process forms the basis for primary nursing practice, the inservice staff agreed to present programs on the nursing process to assist in preparing the staff for the change.

Subsequently, the change agent met with the chief of staff, director of cardiology, director of medical education, and selected department heads. The physicians appeared interested and agreed to support the project. The director of medical education volunteered to arrange a meeting of the active members of the medical staff to provide the change agent with the opportunity to explain the system and elicit their support. The department heads appeared most interested in the concept. They explained that the system appeared to be an improvement over the existing system since few staff members really knew the patients on the nursing units.

In conjunction with the director of nursing service and members of the nursing service administrative staff, the change agent selected a unit as a possible project unit. This was a 20-bed post-coronary unit that had been in operation approximately one year. The staff consisted of diploma, associate degree and baccalaureate degree nurses; two licensed practical nurses; and a team leader in charge of the nursing unit.

The change agent decided to meet first with the team leader and then with the entire nursing staff. If the nursing staff decided against participation in the project, the change agent was prepared to explore other units within the hospital. The change agent met with the team leader to review the proposed project. The team leader was receptive to the idea but not extremely enthusiastic. When the investigator explored with the team leader her feelings concerning participation in the project, she admitted she had heard about the project from one of the enthusiastic physicians on the staff. She stated she was concerned about her position, fearing that someone from outside the institution would be taking control of her nursing unit. She admitted she had shared these fears with several of the patient care coordinators and that they had assured her that the change agent would work cooperatively with her. Upon hearing this, the change agent assured the team leader she was under no obligation to participate in the project. The team leader said she believed she could work cooperatively with the change agent and was interested in becoming involved in the project.

The change agent then met with the nursing staff. Their response was most encouraging. They raised questions concerning their own role and the role of the team leader. They were impressed with the idea that they would be involved as a group in the decision-making process. They stated they felt bored, unchallenged, and in need of a change, and this appeared to be a solution to their problems. The investigator proceeded to arrange a meeting plan with the team leader and staff, to begin discussing details concerning the project and the stages of change. The staff requested that all meetings be taped so that those who were unable to attend a meeting would be kept informed.

IDENTIFICATION OF DRIVING AND RESTRAINING FORCES

If one conceives of the hospital nursing unit as an environment consisting of driving and restraining forces which maintain the established nursing care delivery system on the unit, the first step in the change process is directed toward identification of the driving and restraining forces, and the design of strategies to alter these forces in order to bring about change.

For the next few weeks the change agent spent a great deal of time observing on the nursing unit. Numerous meetings were held with the nursing staff to discuss the project and provide them with opportunities to express their thoughts and feelings concerning the change. They voiced their concerns regarding their ability to accomplish the change, the threat of the change itself, their need for additional information on the primary nursing, and the fact that the proposed system required more work than the existing system. They also discussed their need for stimulation and their desire to participate in decisions that directly affected their performance.

Given Lewin's force field analysis as a diagnostic tool [4], the change agent proceeded to postulate the driving and restraining forces on the nursing unit in order to develop strategies for the unfreezing stage:

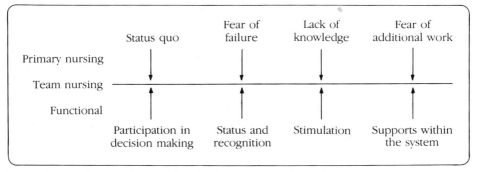

Figure 32-1. Driving and restraining forces on the nursing unit.

1. Restraining Forces:
   a. The need to maintain the status quo on the nursing unit.
   b. Fear of failure.
   c. Lack of information on primary nursing.
   d. Fear of additional work.
2. Driving Forces:
   a. Desire to participate in decision making.
   b. Need for status and recognition.
   c. Need for stimulation.
   d. Individuals supportive of primary nursing.

Figure 32-1 is an illustration of the dynamic balance of driving and restraining forces on the nursing unit.

UNFREEZING STAGE

When one is bringing about change, generally it is wiser to work on reducing the restraining forces. To increase the driving forces may result in the creation of more tension than one wishes to precipitate during the change process. Consequently, the change agent decided to approach the unfreezing stage by designing strategies that would reduce the restraining forces on the nursing unit. This approach consisted of exposing the staff to literature on primary nursing, arranging for the staff to visit institutions utilizing the primary nursing concept, and conducting group discussions on primary nursing. This approach was designed to encompass Schein's three mechanisms for unfreezing in the following manner.

LACK OF CONFIRMATION OR DISCONFIRMATION

The literature and group discussions would create disconfirmation by focusing on the advantages of primary nursing and the disadvantages of team nursing. The visits would demonstrate that team nursing is not a preferred system for delivering care to patients. During the visits staff would be exposed to nurses who verbalized the disadvantages of the traditional nursing care delivery systems.

CREATION OF GUILT-ANXIETY

The literature and group discussions would focus on the disadvantages of team nursing, thus inducing guilt-anxiety in those nurses interested in delivering quality care to patients. Visits to other institutions, providing opportunities for discussions with patients and personnel in these settings, would create dissatisfaction in those nurses interested in functioning on a higher level.

PSYCHOLOGICAL SAFETY

The field visits would demonstrate that primary nursing is possible, and many nurses function in this capacity, thus reducing the fear of failure. The group discussions would provide reassurance through peer support. Finally, reassurance by the change agent that staff would participate in decisions and determine their own readiness to move to the next stage would reduce anxiety and provide psychological safety.

The unfreezing stage occurred over a period of two months. During this time each staff member visited at least one institution in which primary nursing was practiced.

Following the visits, the change agent met with the staff to discuss their observations and reactions to the visits. They reported they had talked with patients, nurses and physicians in these settings and had been impressed with their comments regarding primary nursing. They also reported they had obtained copies of assessment and nursing history forms in use in these settings. The enthusiasm of the staff became obvious as the change agent listened to comments such as: "When we start primary nursing, we are going to have a much better system than the one at the hospital we just visited."

Group meetings were conducted twice weekly to discuss the literature on primary nursing and provide opportunities for the staff to share their thoughts and feelings concerning the content of the literature. Gradually, their comments began to indicate they were undergoing cognitive dissonance. They appeared to identify with the primary nursing concept and discard their feelings concerning team nursing. According to Festinger, the theory of dissonance predicts that once an individual makes a decision he will attempt to convince himself that the chosen alternative is even more attractive, relative to the unchosen one, than he had previously thought [6]. This dissonance was evident in comments such as the following: "When we begin primary nursing, we will know our patients a lot better and give them much better care. You just can't do this with team nursing." Other comments included: "Team nursing is a terrible system. Primary nursing is so much more patient-oriented."

Toward the end of the second month the staff began to verbalize their interest in moving to the next stage in the change process. During staff meetings they would volunteer such comments as: "We're ready to start primary nursing." "I think we're all unfrozen. We should begin to move to the next stage." The change agent was seeking evidence of guilt-anxiety, which as yet had not been manifested. However, just at the end of the second month it became very obvious during one of the staff meetings. Gradually, the staff began to verbalize their feelings of inadequacy. One nurse commented:

I think people are not too happy with the way we are functioning on this unit. I am sure the doctors are disappointed in us. I think they expected that we would be doing much more patient teaching.

Another nurse commented:

It makes you sad to know that you could be doing more for your patients and you really are not doing enough.

Still another nurse commented:

We knew we were not functioning the way we should, but we never did anything about it.

The team leader commented:

I've been unhappy about not being able to spend more time with patients. I know I should have more contact with the patients, but somehow I just have not been able to do this.

The change agent now believed the staff was ready to move to the next stage. An informal questionnaire given to the staff at this time indicated that they believed they had been well prepared for the change; they felt comfortable and confident and were anxious to move to the next stage.

CHANGE STAGE

Since the title "team leader" is inconsistent with the concept of primary nursing, the first step in the change stage was to change the title of the team leader. The change agent met with the team leader and offered several suggestions for titles that might be appropriate. The team leader selected the title "primary nursing leader." She felt she would be comfortable with this title, and it would not set her apart from her peer group.

The change agent, desiring to produce change through internalization, selected scanning as the change strategy. Each staff member was given literature describing the primary nursing models. The change agent then arranged a workshop designed to assist the staff in comparing and contrasting the models. The staff made selections from each of the models which could be incorporated into the model designed for their own nursing unit. During the workshop the following decisions were made by the staff:

1. The geographic assignment plan would not be utilized in this model. The assignments would be individualized, based upon the interests and abilities of the primary nurses and the needs of patients, regardless of the patient's location on the nursing unit.
2. The practical nurses would function as associate nurses.
3. All of the reports would be taped and the staff would develop guidelines for taping the report.
4. Three staff groups would be organized. One group would collaborate on the development of an assessment form, a second group would plan a patient teaching project, and the third group would develop a transfer form to provide continuity of care when patients were transferred from the post-coronary unit to other units within the hospital.
5. Since the existing assignment form was designed for team nursing, the change agent would work with the primary nursing leader to develop an assignment form.
6. The staff would collaborate with the change agent in the development of a philosophy and objectives of primary nursing and in determining the roles of the primary and associate nurses.

7. The primary nursing leader would work collaboratively with the change agent in developing the role of the primary nursing leader.
8. The introduction of primary nursing would begin with the assignment of each nurse to a group of patients. Each primary nurse would have approximately three primary patients and would serve as associate nurse for one or two patients. Each associate nurse would care for approximately four patients whose primary nurses were off duty. A target date for implementation was selected by the group.

When the target date arrived, there was much enthusiasm on the part of the nursing staff. Several of the nurses arrived on the unit at 6 A.M. to begin to plan and organize the care for their patients. The nurses visited their patients and discussed the change with them. The patients appeared to be as enthusiastic as the nurses. Several patients sought out the change agent to discuss the concept and explain the advantages. One patient stated:

You know, the part I like best is the idea that I will have the same nurse every day.

Another patient commented:

Why didn't someone think of this system before? I've been a patient in a number of hospitals, and I always knew there was a better way.

By the end of the first month of the change stage the philosophy, objectives and roles had been developed. The primary nurses gave total care to a group of patients for the entire time they remained on the nursing unit. The associate nurses relieved the primary nurses when the primary nurses were off duty. On each tour of duty, nurses taped the report on their patients and communicated verbally with the oncoming nurses as well.

By the beginning of the second month of the change stage the three groups were developing and designing their projects. The group responsible for the assessment form had reviewed literature on assessment, examined forms from other institutions, and developed a form for use on the nursing unit. The group responsible for the transfer form had accomplished their goal. Both the assessment form and the transfer form were reviewed with the staff. The nurses offered suggestions and additions and approved the forms for use. The forms were given to the printing department and were available for use within a few days.

The group responsible for the patient teaching project had visited the local chapter of the American Heart Association and secured literature for patient teaching. Literature racks were placed on the nursing unit in selected areas, and pamphlets dealing with hypertension, heart disease, and smoking were placed in the racks. A rack was placed in the conference room containing literature to be used by the primary nurses for patient teaching.

By the beginning of the third month of the change stage each patient was assigned a primary nurse on admission. The primary nurse performed an initial assessment and developed a nursing care plan. Nurses were involved in patient and family teaching, and patients and family members were observed removing literature from the racks on the nursing unit. When a patient was transferred from the nursing unit, the primary nurse completed the transfer form and accompanied the patient to the nursing unit. All staff members attended the report, and the primary nurses taped a report on their patients. In addition, staff members communicated verbally with the oncoming nursing staff.

By the end of the third month of the change stage the primary nursing leader was conducting daily nursing rounds and was frequently observed referring physicians to the primary nurses. She had developed an assignment board listing the names of the patients and the primary and associate nurses. The primary nurses were conferring with physicians and other disciplines. Physicians were observed seeking out primary nurses and sharing information with them.

REFREEZING STAGE

Lippitt, Watson, and Westley maintain that change becomes stabilized when it spreads to other areas within the system [7]. The change agent's approach throughout the stages of change was directed toward the refreezing or stabilization of the change. Each month the change agent prepared a bulletin entitled the "Primary Nursing Newsletter," which contained information regarding the project and the progress of the staff. The Newsletter was distributed to the administrative council, nursing service administrative staff, full-time physicians, department heads and nursing staff. The purpose of the Newsletter was to provide information on the primary nursing project and stimulate interest in primary nursing on other units within the hospital.

During the change stage the intensive care and coronary care staffs requested permission to use the assessment forms. As a result, frequently assessments were initiated in the critical care areas and then continued when the patient was transferred to the project unit.

When patients were transferred from the project unit to other nursing units, the assessment and transfer forms became part of the patients' records. These forms stimulated interest in staff members on other nursing units. On several occasions, staff members contacted the change agent to comment on the forms and voice their approval.

During the unfreezing stage the change agent was requested by the patient care coordinator to present several programs on primary nursing to the medical, surgical and coronary care unit staffs. The purpose of these programs was to stimulate interest and assist the nurses with plans for the implementation of primary nursing in the future.

During the change stage the patient care coordinator established a patient teaching committee, composed of staff members from medical intensive care, coronary care and the project unit. The purpose of this committee was to develop specific teaching programs for cardiac patients.

Toward the end of the change stage the change agent was invited to present several programs on primary nursing to the baccalaureate nursing students affiliating at the hospital, since a number of students would be assigned to the project unit in the future.

In an effort to encourage the spread of the change to other units, the change agent spent a great deal of time with the inservice staff, the patient care coordinators and the director of nursing service, to discuss the change and offer suggestions for implementation in other areas.

Following the implementation of primary nursing, the change agent met with the hospital administrative council and nursing service administrative staff to review the model that had been developed and implemented on the project unit. The change agent suggested that the unit serve as a model unit, and that the primary nursing leader and the primary nurses teach the primary nursing concept to other staff members within the hospital.

The change agent remained in the setting four months following the implementation of primary nursing. At that time the staff appeared enthusiastic and secure in their own roles. The primary nursing leader felt she was able to make rounds, spend more time with patients, and be available to the primary and associate nurses. The primary and associate nurses felt they were functioning on a higher level and giving better care to patients.

The change agent conducted a final interview with each staff member and their comments were most revealing. Several of these comments are listed below:

Before primary nursing I did nothing but make beds and give baths. I never really knew the patients. Now I know my patients quite well and I am able to do a great deal more for them.

Whenever my patients are transferred or discharged, I can state with confidence that they have been well prepared for the move. I could never say that before.

I know I am giving better care to my patients, and that my patients are better off because of this. I feel I know my patients well and have greater insight into their needs.

The system has helped me make better use of my skills. In many respects I am a better nurse because of it. I think the doctors have greater respect for our knowledge and I believe that the communication between medicine and nursing has improved.

You become so much more involved with your patients. Before primary nursing, I would make notations on the care plan and assume someone else would handle the problems. Now I know that I am responsible and accountable for the patient.

Finally, one nurse summarized her feelings in these words: "For the first time since I graduated, I feel like a nurse."

Follow-up visits conducted one and two years following implementation revealed that primary nursing was still being practiced in the setting. All of the nursing staff agreed that they would never return to team nursing.

ROLE OF THE CHANGE AGENT

Throughout the change, the change agent utilized a nonthreatening approach with the staff. At times the agent offered advice and solutions to problems. Other times, the change agent encouraged the staff to seek their own solutions to problems. During staff meetings the change agent attempted to create a climate conducive to the open exchange of ideas and communication on the part of the staff. The change agent conveyed the impression that she had no intention of ridiculing, belittling, or embarrassing any staff member at any time. Encouragement and support were offered by the change agent throughout the change.

Finally, from the very beginning, the change agent conveyed to the staff her confidence in their ability and her belief in their capacity to accomplish the change. The staff responded by bringing about the change.

CHANGE: PLANNED VS SPONTANEOUS

In nursing today we find ourselves well beyond the point of debate over whether or not change is inevitable. Our current predicament revolves around the question of how one becomes involved in the process of change. In many respects we find we are faced with two alternatives: we can either utilize models that have been specifically designed to aid in the implementation of planned change or we can let change occur spontaneously without attempting to control the process or the outcome. The advantages of the former alternative are obvious: one is able to control the change and predict with accuracy the outcome. Perhaps the disadvantages of the latter can best be illustrated in the following example:

At exactly 5:13 A.M. the 18th of April, 1906, a cow was standing somewhere between the main barn and the milking shed on the old Shafter Ranch in California, minding her own business. Suddenly, the earth shook, the skies trembled, and when it was all over, there was nothing showing of the cow above ground but a bit of her tail sticking up. [8]

The moral of this story is quite clear. The cow stood quietly enough, thinking such gentle thoughts as cows are likely to have, while huge forces built up around her and suddenly a great movement occurred that changed the configuration of the earth, destroyed a city, and swallowed her up [8]. Unfortunately, we are faced with this same possibility in nursing for, if we do not learn how to become involved in the process of change, we may find ourselves, like the Shafter cow, engulfed in chaos, quite early some morning.

REFERENCES

1. Manthey M, Ciske K, Robertson P, et al: Primary nursing: A return to the concept of "my nurse" and "my patient." *Nurs Forum* 9:81-83, 1970.
2. Marram GD, Schlegel MW, Bevis EO: *Primary Nursing: A Model for Individualized Care.* St Louis, CV Mosby Co, 1974, p 157.
3. Lippitt GL: *Visualizing Change.* Fairfax, Virginia, NTL-Learning Resources Corporation, 1973, p 86.
4. Lewin K: Frontiers in group dynamics, in Cartwright D (ed): *Field Theory in Social Science.* New York, Harper & Row, 1951, pp 200-202, 228.
5. Schein EH: *Professional Education.* New York, McGraw-Hill Book Co, 1972, p 76.
6. Festinger L, Aronson E: The arousal and reduction of dissonance in social contexts, in Cartwright D, Zander A (eds): *Group Dynamics: Research and Theory.* New York, Harper & Row, 1953, pp 214-215.
7. Lippitt R, Watson J, Westley B: *The Dynamics of Planned Change.* New York, Harcourt, Brace and Co, 1958, p 140.
8. Fabun D: *The Dynamics of Change.* Englewood Cliffs, New Jersey, Prentice-Hall, Inc, p 1.

Section 8
Conflict Resolution

33 Conflict Resolution

Ann Marriner

SOME COMMON APPROACHES to handling conflict are withdrawing, smoothing, compromising, confronting, and forcing. Withdrawing from the conflict does not resolve it, and the individual who retreats frequently harbors a gnawing anger over a situation which drains off energy needed for more constructive purposes. By complimenting one's opponent, accentuating points of agreement, and underplaying their differences, one may smooth out an agreement on minor issues, but you still must deal with the real problems. Both parties in a compromise make concessions and neither party wins. This solution satisfies no one. *Forcing* the resolution of a conflict gets quick action but usually without the necessary accompanying commitment. A superior can always fall back on his authority and give orders to a subordinate, but because the resolution is forced, it almost frequently will be unsatisfactory. Confrontation is generally the most effective method of conflict resolution.

A foundation of mutual trust must underlie any attempt to understand alternative views and to actively seek solutions which will allow each party to achieve its goals. This trust creates an atmosphere conducive to successful conflict resolution.

STRATEGIES FOR CONFLICT RESOLUTION

There are three ways of dealing with conflict: the win-lose, lose-lose, and win-win strategies. *Win-lose* methods include the use of position power, mental or physical power, failure to respond, majority rule, and railroading a minority position over the majority. *Lose-lose* strategies include compromise, bribes for accomplishing disagreeable tasks, arbitration by a neutral third party, and resort to the use of general rules instead of considering the merits of individual cases. In win-lose and lose-lose strategies, the parties often personalize the issues by focusing on each other instead of on the problem. Intent on their personal differences, they avoid the more important matter of how to mutually solve their problem. Solutions are emphasized instead of goals and values. Rather than identifying mutual needs, planning activities for resolution, and solving the problem, each party looks at the issue from his own point of view and strives for total victory.

By contrast, *win-win* strategies focus on goals. They emphasize concensus and integrative approaches to decision making. The consensus process demands a focus on the problems (instead of on each other), on collecting of facts, on accepting the useful aspects of conflict, and on avoiding averaging and self-oriented behavior. The group decision is thus often better than the best individual decision.

Problem solving strategies include identifying both the problem and each party's needs,

Reprinted with permission by *Supervisor Nurse: The Journal for Nursing Leadership and Management*, May 1979.

exploring alternatives, choosing the most acceptable alternative, planning, defining roles, implementing, and evaluating the decision.

INTERPERSONAL CONFLICT

Interpersonal conflict is inevitable, but the supervisor can lessen its impact by coaching subordinates in assertive communication and fair fighting. Engaging in a fair fight demands that the individual with a complaint first ask his opponent for a meeting. Once a time and place are agreed upon, both parties should determine whether or not their supervisor should be present. Moreover, a fair fight demands that both parties know the purpose of the meeting so neither will be caught off guard—each can be prepared. The encounter should begin with a statement of the problem. If the supervisor is present she should act as mediator, asking the complainant to explain the perceived problem to the opponent. The opponent then should relate his understanding of how the complainant perceives the problem. After each has spoken, each can clarify any differences over the statement of the problem. Next the opponent describes his own perception of the problem which then should be followed by the complainant repeating his understanding of how the opponent perceives the problem. Again, there is a pause for clarification.

A clear statement of the problem helps to shed light on the negative effects of each person's behavior. This feedback process, which requires each party to repeat what the other just said, forces each to listen carefully. Were it not for such interaction, both parties might be so busy thinking of *what they are going to say next* that they fail to hear what is being said. Feedback does not imply parroting: understanding of meaning is more important than memorization of words. Differences often begin to disappear when both parties really hear each other for the first time.

Through exploring the alternatives to the problem and the ramifications of their options, the parties can identify and request changes in each other's behavior—and respond to the other's request. The discussion should close with an agreement on whether or not to change and the establishment of the accompanying conditions. A follow up engagement should be set to discuss the success or failure of the agreement.

GROUP CONFLICT

Team development can help prevent and resolve conflict. Planning, goal setting, and prioritizing goals comprise the first step in team development. The statement of the core mission of the team develops from brainstorming and sharing individual mission statements. The nominal group technique, an effective method of group problem solving, can be used to develop and prioritize team performance goals. First, the individual group members write down on paper what he thinks should be the team performance goals. During a round robin session, each person in turn states one of his team performance goals which is then written on a chalk board. The process continues until all of the team performance goals have been stated. The group clarifies the goals during a discussion period and selects a specific number of goals. Each group member prioritizes the goals and writes each goal on a separate card and rank orders the cards. After the cards have been collected and the votes counted, the group discusses them and the top priority items are selected for a final vote. The voting process is repeated with the appropriate number of priorities written onto separate cards and then ranked. These votes are then counted and rank weighting is determined. An item selected less often than others may receive a higher priority because it was given a higher rank more often than a more popular item.

Role negotiations, the process of preventing role conflicts, role ambiguities, and role overload, become important once priorities have been set. During this process, group members clarify each individual's role on the team and help to resolve any disagreements over the team members' roles. Each member initially sends one written message to every other team member indicating that for him to act, he needs the other team member to do more, less, or to continue his previous performance. *To whom* and *from whom* are essential parts of the message. The number of role messages sent to any one individual should be limited to prevent an information overload. The message must clearly state how the sender wants the receiver to behave and how a change will help the sender.

The receiver responds, indicating what he can or cannot do, explaining why, and offering alternative solutions, e.g., "I can't do X, but I can do Y, which should help solve your problem," or "If I do X, I would like you to do Y." The receiver analyzes the role messages he received in "do more, do less, and do the same" categories, and according to who sent the message, and his response to that message. Does he know what is expected of him? Do different people want him to do more *and* less of the same activity at the same time? Does the receiver have time to meet all the demands made of him? Role definition helps identify role ambiguity, role conflicts, and role overload. After roles are negotiated, a contract is written which defines the problem, indicates what each involved person will do, and sets a date for a follow up check.

The next major phase of team development is concerned with who should be involved in decision making and with the nature of that involvement. To determine who should be involved, one should assess who has the information necessary to make a sound decision and who is responsible for implementing that decision. The latter needs to understand the decision and be committed to it.

People can be involved in decision making in a variety of ways. Some are directly involved because they have the necessary information or are responsible for implementing the decision. The involvement of some may be limited to input or consultation. Others need to be informed about the decision, and someone must be responsible for managing the overall decision making process.

A decision chart helps visualize the decision making process. Decisions to be made are listed down the side of the page and the involved people across the top in a grid pattern: Placing an *M* in a square indicates who manages the process; *D* indicates who is directly involved; *C* indicates who should be consulted; and *I* indicates who should be informed. Anyone who is expected to implement the decision must obviously be informed.

Group process is critical for team development. How the group functions, communicates and sets and achieves objectives are all related to group dynamics. Both task oriented behavior and maintenance oriented behavior are necessary for adequate team development.

People who assume group task roles coordinate and facilitate the group's efforts to identify the problem, explore alternative options, identify the ramifications of the options, choose the most viable option, and implement and evaluate the plan. There are numerous group task roles, and any member of the group may fulfill a number of these roles in successive participation.

The *initiator-contributor* proposes new ideas or different ways of approaching a problem. His task is to identify the problem, clarify the objectives, offer solutions, suggest agenda items, and set time limits. The *information seeker* searches for factual information about the problem while the *opinion seeker* clarifies values pertinent to the problem and its solution. Unlike the information seeker, the *information giver* identifies facts, shares his experiences, and makes generalizations. The *opinion giver* states his beliefs and indicates what he thinks the group should value. His focus is on values rather than on facts. The *elaborator* develops suggestions, illustrates points, and predicts outcomes. Relationships are clarified by the *coordinator*. The *orienter* summarizes the discussion, activities, and points of departure to provide perspective on the group's progress toward its goal. Evaluation of the problem, content, and process is done by the *critic* who may contrast the group's achievement against a set of standards. The *energizer* stimulates the group to increase the quantity and quality of their work. The *procedural technician* facilitates group action by arranging the room for the meeting, distributing the materials, working the audio-visual equipment, and generally functioning as the "gofor"—the person who goes for what is needed. An account of the discussion, suggestions, and decisions is kept by the *recorder*.

The roles of group building and group maintenance focus on how people treat each other while accomplishing a task. The *gatekeeper* regulates communication and takes actions to assure everyone an opportunity to be heard. The *encourager* radiates warmth and approval. He offers commendation, praise, and indicates acceptance and understanding of others' ideas and values. The *harmonizer* creates and maintains group cohesion, relieving tension through his sense of humor and helping others reconcile their disagreements. The *compromiser* promotes group process by yielding status, admitting mistakes, modifying his ideas for the sake of group cohesiveness, maintaining self-control for group harmony, or by generally making compromises to keep the group action oriented. The *follower*, acting as a passive audience, goes along with the group. The *group observer* keeps records of the group process and gives interpretations for evaluation of the proceedings. The quality of the group process is compared to standards by the *standard setter*.

Some members of the group may try to satisfy their individual needs irrespective of the group tasks or maintenance roles. For example: (1) The *aggressor* meets his needs at the expense of others by disapproving of others and deflating their status. (2) The *dominator* asserts authority or superiority through flattery, interrupting others, and by giving directions authoritatively. (3) The *recognition seeker* calls attention to himself by boasting and acting in unusual ways. (4) The *special interest pleader* speaks for an interest group and addresses issues which best meet that need. (5) The *blocker* is negative, resistant, and disagreeable without apparent reason and brings issues back to the floor that the group has rejected. (6) The *self-confessor* uses the group to express personal feelings while (7) the *help-seeker* expresses depreciation, insecurity, and personal confusion which elicits sympathy responses. (8) The *playboy* has a lack of involvement in the group process and appears nonchalant. A high incidence of individual roles in a group requires self-diagnosis to suggest what group training efforts are needed.

INTERGROUP CONFLICT

Intergroup conflict is common and can be dysfunctional. As with interpersonal conflict, intergroup resistance may result from low trust, poor communications, and false assumptions. People resist what they perceive as threatening. Intergroup actions may threaten territorial rights and contribute to role overload and conflict. Avoiding win-lose situations, emphasizing organizational goals and effectiveness, rotating personnel among groups to facilitate understanding, and increasing interaction and communication between groups help reduce intergroup conflict.

When a group recognizes its need to solve some intergroup conflict, it must first decide how to begin. A study of the organizational chart will determine who should be involved. Who should represent the group, a person or a committee? someone who already is friendly with members of the other group? someone with strong or moderate feelings about the position? What is the group's position and how much negotiation is acceptable? It helps to emphasize common goals and discuss constraints. The same process used in interpersonal conflict should be used in group conflict situations: setting and prioritizing goals, negotiating roles and making decisions.

ORGANIZATIONAL CONFLICT

Organizations in conflict display the collective symptoms expressed by their members, and the symptoms can be numerous. Personnel feel pain and frustration at work. If they don't think their skills are being used, they experience a loss of self-esteem and a sense of impotence, both of which lead to withdrawal from the situation instead of an attempt to solve the problems. Group members may also engage in backbiting, and blame others for the problems. Subgroup formations are common. Organizational members identify the same task and group maintenance problems, but act contrary to the information thereby increasing their frustrations or exhibit the same dysfunctional behaviors outside the organization.

Consultation may be sought to deal with organizational conflict. The consultant must analyze the organizational structure, the leadership and authority of the institution, the communication patterns, the amount of intergroup cooperation or competition, the group's norms and goals, the group's problem solving and decision making processes and various individual roles and functions within the group. Organizational research can help to provide the information necessary to solve the problem.

After data have been collected and analyzed, the consultant offers feedback about the themes and supporting data. Organizational members can publicly note whether or not they agree with the consultant's views. A public vote facilitates ownership of ideas. If there is disagreement, the consultant helps the group clarify the reasons for the difference and modifies the statement until it reflects the group's thinking.

The consultant then asks each member to write a few sentences about the way he contributes to the situation so that each can recognize his own part in the problem. Individuals are likely to try to maintain the status quo for fear of serious consequences if they confront the issues. The consultant shares his theory with the group, helps develop an awareness of dysfunctional behavior, helps individuals cope with their feelings, encourages fantasy and reality testing, and coaches group members toward new behaviors.

PREVENTION OF CONFLICT

Careful development of an organizational structure, strategic and comprehensive planning, management and organizational development, and careful selection and placement of personnel help prevent organizational conflict. The same strategies also prevent intergroup, group, and interpersonal conflict.

BIBLIOGRAPHY

Bach, George R., and Herb Goldberg. *Creative Aggression: The Art of Assertive Living.* New York: Avon Books, 1974.

Bonner, Herbert. *Group Dynamics: Principles and Applications.* New York: The Ronald Press Company, 1959.

Bradford, Leland P. *Group Development.* La Jolla, California: University Associates, Inc., 1974.

Burke, R.J., "Methods of Resolving Superior-Subordinate Conflict: The Constructive Use of Subordinate Differences and Disagreements," *Organizational Behavior and Human Performance,* 5 (1970), 393-411.

Burke, W. Warner, ed. *New Technologies in Organizational Development.* La Jolla, California: University Associates, Inc., 1972.

Burke, W. Warner, and Harvey A. Hornstein. *The Social Technology of Organization Development.* La Jolla, California: University Associates, Inc., 1972.

Carey, Marcia C., "Staff Disunity: A Destructive Force," *American Journal of Nursing,* 69 (November 1969), 2375-2377.

Claus, Karen E., and June T. Bailey. *Power and Influence in Health Care: A New Approach to Leadership.* St. Louis: The C.V. Mosby Company, 1977.

Delbecq, Andre L., Andrew H. Van de Ven, and David H. Gustafson. *Group Techniques for Program Planning: A Guide to Nominal Group and Delphi Processes.* Glenview, Illinois: Scott, Foresman, and Company, 1975.

de Lodzia, George, and Leonard Greenhalgh, "Creative Conflict Management in a Nursing Environment," *Supervisor Nurse,* 4 (July 1973), 33-41.

Donovan, Helen M. *Nursing Service Administration: Managing the Enterprise.* St. Louis: The C.V. Mosby Company, 1975.

Filley, Alan C. *Interpersonal Conflict Resolution.* Glenview, Illinois: Scott, Foresman, and Company, 1975.

Ganong, Warren L., and Joan Mary Ganong, "Reducing Organizational Conflict Through Working Committees," *Journal of Nursing Administration,* 40 (November-December 1974), 50-57.

House, Robert J., "Role Conflict and Multiple Authority in Complex Organizations," *California Management Review,* 12 (Summer 1970), 53-60.

Jandt, Fred E. *Conflict Resolution Through Communication.* New York: Harper & Row, Publishers, 1973.

Kast, Fremont E., and James E. Rosenzweig. *Organization and Management: A Systems Approach.* New York: McGraw-Hill Book Company, 1974.

Koontz, Harold, and Cyril O'Donnell. *Principles of Management: An Analysis of Managerial Functions.* New York: McGraw-Hill Book Company, 1972.

Lewis, Joyce H., "Conflict Management," *Journal of Nursing Administration,* 6 (December 1976), 18-22.

Likert, Rensis, and Jane Gibson Likert. *New Ways of Managing Conflict.* New York: McGraw-Hill Book Company, 1976.

Margulies, Newton, and John Wallace. *Organizational Change: Techniques and Applications.* Glenview, Illinois: Scott, Foresman, and Company, 1973.

Rizzo, John R., Robert J. House, and Sidney I. Lirtzman, "Role Conflict and Ambiguity in Complex Organizations," *Administrative Science Quarterly,* 15 (June 1970), 150-163.

Rubin, Irwin M., Mark S. Plovnick, and Ronald E. Fry. *Improving the Coordination of Care: A Program for Health Team Development.* Cambridge, Massachusetts: Ballinger Publishing Company, 1975.

Rubin, Irwin M., Mark S. Plovnick, and Ronald E. Fry. *Managing Human Resources in Health Care Organizations: An Applied Approach.* Reston, Virginia: Reston Publishing Company, Inc., 1978.

Schein, Edgar H. *Process Consultation: Its Role in Organizational Development.* Reading, Massachusetts: Addison-Wesley Publishing Co., 1969.

Veninga, Robert, "The Management of Conflict," *Journal of Nursing Administration,* 3 (July-August 1973), 12-16.

Walton, Richard E. *Interpersonal Peacemaking: Confrontations and Third-Party Consultation.* Reading, Massachusetts: Addison-Wesley Publishing Co., 1969.

Walton, Richard E., and John M. Dutton, "The Management of Interdepartmental Conflict: A Model and Review," *Administrative Science Quarterly,* 14 (March 1969), 73-83.

Zand, D.E., "Trust and Managerial Problem Solving," *Administrative Science Quarterly,* 17 (1972), 229-239.

34 Organizational Conflict

A CREATIVE OR DESTRUCTIVE FORCE

Dorothy L. Sexton

PREFACE

Conflict is numbered among the major characteristics of our society. It has become the order of the day. We can't escape it. For too long now society has termed conflict bad, while looking upon adjustment with favor. Society has suppressed [healthy] conflict and felt its costs. Society needs conflict; it cannot progress without it. Conflict must be seen as a creative force. When conflict is managed appropriately, the parties can "ride the curve," so to speak, to fruitful and creative ends.

Early American sociologists (Ross, 1920; Small, 1905; Cooley, 1909) (who were reformers at heart) viewed conflict as a fundamental and constructive part of social organization [1]. That is, conflict was an inherent element in social structure. This feeling is evident in folk language, which is easily recognized—"divide and conquer," "even up the score," "offense is the best defense," "playing the ends against the middle."

A change is noted toward the early part of the twentieth century, when sociologists tended to center attention on problems of adjustment, rather than conflict. That is to say, their focus was social statics as opposed to dynamics. For example, Parsons was concerned with those elements in social structures that assure their maintenance. He viewed conflict as dysfunctional and disruptive. Mayo favored the avoidance of conflict and the promotion of equilibrium. In short, sociologists (Parsons, Lundberg, Warner) favored adjustment of the individual to given structures rather than the need for structural change [1].

For a long time the general value in society has been that adjustment is good and conflict is bad. The cultural hush-hush re conflict is reflected in the sayings—"let sleeping dogs lie," "let's not stir up trouble," and "let's not make an issue of it."

In our turbulent environment, conflict has become the order of the day. New conflicts continually arise as changing conditions produce new challenges. While a society can survive without violence and war, it cannot progress without a good deal of both competition and conflict. Conflict must be seen as an important creative force in today's society.

Kahn states that "conflict and ambiguity are among the major characteristics of our society, and . . . are among the unintended consequences of . . . the growth of large scale organizations" [3]. However, in most modern organizations conflict is not formally recognized. Since it is not formally accepted, it is forced into hiding.

Kelly informs us that in recent years some managerial meetings have been the occasion for the emergence of naked conflict. That is to say, conflict that is common and visible has

Reprinted with permission by Charles B. Slack, Inc., from *Nursing Leadership,* Volume 3, Number 3, September 1980.

emerged. "Let's go for confrontation" and "let's introduce a little uncertainty into the situation" are examples of the argot of those who engage in conflict [4].

CONFLICT

Conflict is the gadfly of thought. It stirs us to observation and memory. It instigates to invention. It shocks us out of sheeplike passivity, and sets us at noting and contriving . . . conflict is a sine qua non *of reflection and ingenuity. [5]*

The definition of conflict, commonly accepted in conflict literature is: conflict exists when two parties (belonging to the same organization) exhange behaviors that symbolize opposition [6, 7]. Boulding is more explicit. "Conflict may be defined as a situation of competition in which the parties are *aware* of the incompatibility of potential future positions and in which each party wishes to occupy a position that is incompatible with the wishes of the other" [8]. In actual conflict situations there must be the element of awareness and also the incompatible wishes.

Boulding suggests that:

The evaluation of conflict has two aspects: quantitative and qualitative. In a given situation, we may have too much or too little conflict, or the amount may be just right. In a given situation, we may also have the wrong kind of conflict. There is no simple operational definition, but common speech has words that describe these qualitative differences: conflicts may be bitter and destructive, or they may be fruitful and constructive. [8]

Conflicts which arise from frustration of specific demands within the relationship and from estimates of gains of the participants, and which are directed at the presumed frustrating object, can be called rational conflicts. Nonrational conflicts . . . *still involving interactions between two or more persons, are not occasioned by the rival ends of the antagonists—but by the need for tension release of at least one of them. [1]*

The conflicts with which this paper will be concerned are those which may obtain between individuals or groups.

FUNCTION OF CONFLICT

For some, conflict is motivating and arouses energies that would not otherwise be available for task accomplishment; for others, conflict is a major threat.

The position that conflict is always bad warrants a closer examination, for, as Kelly notes, "perfect organizational health is not freedom from conflict" [4]. Conflict behavior may contribute to a system of checks and balances. The expression of conflict allows divergent interests and beliefs to emerge. Confrontation of the divergent views may lead to a synthesis with adjustment of the organizational system to the real situation, and organizational peace. Nash suggests that "differences among men should be regarded as potentially creative rather than potentially threatening" [9]. Skolik reports that "dynamic and lasting contributions seem to come when the differences between workers are creatively focused on . . ." [10]. In short, the function of conflict is to defend conflicting but valued principles and to effect a creative synthesis.

To echo Shakespeare's *King John,* "So foul a sky clears not without a storm" [1]. "Institutions that merely serve a reaction of feelings of hostility—thus leaving the terms of the relationship unchanged, may function as lightning rods but they cannot prevent a regathering of clouds (i.e., new accumulation of tension)" [1].

When conflict is not recognized it tends to go underground. Then it becomes less direct but more destructive and eventually becomes more difficult to confront and to resolve. In such an atmosphere, in which divergent ideas are avoided, new ideas tend to appear with less frequency, and old ideas are more likely to go unexplored [11].

As Seiler counsels, it is therefore important that we "isolate those aspects [of conflict] which are harmful to productivity and those which represent stimulating and productive competition" [12].

A moderate level of interpersonal conflict may have the following constructive consequences:

1. It may increase the motivation and energy available to do tasks required by the social system.
2. Conflict may increase the innovativeness of individuals and the system because of the greater diversity of the viewpoints and a heightened sense of necessity.
3. Each person may develop increased understanding of his own position, because the conflict forces him to articulate his views and to bring forth all supporting arguments.
4. Each party may achieve greater awareness of his own identity. [13]

CONDITIONS FOR CONFLICT

In today's turbulent environment the rate of change inevitably outstrips the rate of change in the organization. Thus, the organization is kept in a maladapted state. One of the changes we have been witness to in recent years is a change in the labor force. Not only have new occupations emerged, but an increased number of occupations have attempted to professionalize. Work has tended to become increasingly organizationally based. Organizations have increasingly sought to include professionals (lawyers, engineers, researchers) among their members.

Corwin points out that specialization accentuates the differences between individuals. "Specialists have vested interests and monopolistic claims over certain spheres of work, which they defend from encroachment" [14]. Specialist groups are linked together through interdependent needs and requirements. This complex maze of intricate group relations makes interpersonal conflicts inevitable. Task interdependence can be an incentive for collaboration or an occasion for conflict. Harmony and conflict ebb and flow throughout the organization.

A heterogeneous work group increases the likelihood that there will be a representation of differentiated latent roles as well as skills. While social and cultural distinctions may be thought to be irrelevant to an official role, they may "spill over" into it [7].

In summary, intergroup conflict is no stranger to complex organizational life. More than ever, we are seeing greater task interdependence. "This interdependence can help . . . in the accomplishment of mutual goals, or it can breed hostile and disruptive conflicts. Once [hostile] conflict *erupts,* it is difficult to control. It can consume everything and everyone it touches" [15].

In Figure 34-1, I have attempted to depict degrees of conflict on a continuum.

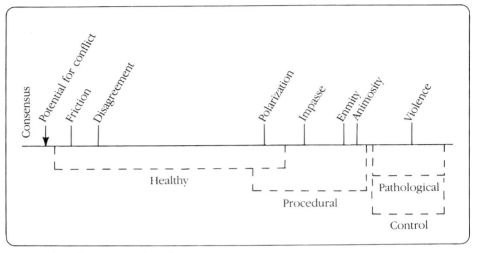

Figure 34-1. Continuum of conflict.

EFFECTS OF CONFLICT

"The systems concept of management teaches . . . that if one of the interlocking elements in the network is changed, then some or all of the other elements will be affected" [4]. It is inevitable for change to be resisted and conflict generated. Conflict has an effect upon both the psychological health of persons and the efficiency of organizational performance. [Unhealthy] conflict relationships tend to involve feelings of low trust and low respect. Such attitudes are reflected in the performance. For example, low trust limits the flow of relevant task information and inhibits coordinative interactions.

If conflict is not expressed directly, it will be expressed indirectly and often in ways that create new conflict or incur other substantial costs [13].

Figure 34-2 depicts the cyclical nature that conflict may assume. It takes emotional energy to totally suppress conflict and it may even take more emotional energy to confront it. Therefore, the parties frequently elect to handle the conflict in an indirect manner. This method usually costs less energy—in the short run. "Indirect conflicts, however, have the longest life expectancy, and have the most costs that cannot be charged back against the original conflict" [13]. In indirect conflict one does not have to expose his feelings.

Repression almost always costs something. Feelings surrounding covert conflict can act as forces siphoning energy away from productive work. For example, if some members' energies are consumed by plans for counter strategies little time will be left for devotion to more fruitful business. As Kluckholn has said, even "witchcraft has its costs . . ." [1].

Pondy points out that the success of an organization hinges on its ability to set up and operate appropriate machinery for dealing with conflict phenomena [16]. A flexible organization reaps the benefits from conflict behavior, which creates and modifies norms and thereby assures its continuance under changed conditions. A rigid organization, however, by not recognizing conflict will experience an impediment to adjustments and will maximize the danger of a breakdown [1].

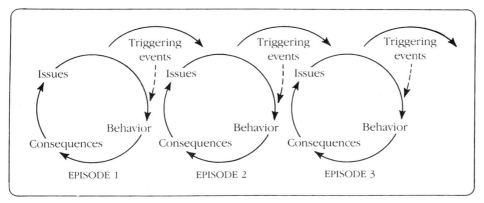

Figure 34-2. A cyclical model of interpersonal conflict.

MANAGEMENT OF CONFLICT

The important questions are: *What* are your conflicts? *How* do you deal with them? [17].

Blake reports that "ignoring, accommodating or suppressing conflict are prevalent dysfunctional actions of many managements . . ." [15]. It is not uncommon for patchwork methods to only touch the symptomatic manifestations of hostility. Hostility may be compared to an iceberg, which hides much of its content below the surface of (consciousness). When dysfunctional methods are employed, an appearance of harmony may be maintained, but when the pressure of covert hostility becomes too great, the situation flares up [8].

Argyris has suggested that in an effective system problems are solved with minimal energy; they stay solved; and the problem-solving mechanisms used are not weakened, but maintained and strengthened [18].

The mechanisms that are chosen to deal with conflict will be influenced by the parties' assumptions about conflict. Figure 34-3 depicts three basic assumptions about interpersonal conflict. Table 34-1 compares the old view and the new view of conflict.

Boulding and Blake include the following as procedures for managing conflict:

Reconciliation—conversation, argument, discussion, debate.
Compromise—bargaining (mediation, conciliation).
Award—arbitration or legal trial. [15]

Studies suggest that organizations are more effective if they *"confront and problem-solve conflicts"* in contrast with "smoothing" or "forcing" them [8, 11]. Blake reports that in his experience "only under conditions of genuine joint efforts of problem-solving between contending groups is an effective, long-term relief of conflict possible" [15].

The problem-solving method incorporates the view that "conflicting images can be eventually understood as special cases of a larger synthesis. The search for such a synthesis is the main *purpose of argument*" [8]. *The focus is a common search for truth, not a struggle for power.* In Blake's experience, a number of solutions arrived at via this method were regarded as unique and original [15].

Benne suggests that:

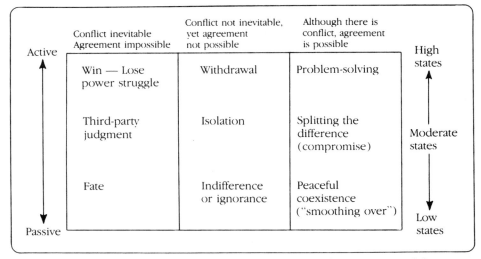

Figure 34-3. The three basic assumptions toward intergroup disagreement and their management. (Source: R. R. Blake et al. *Managing Conflict in Industry.* Houston, Texas: Gulf Publishing Company, 1964.)

The method of learning from conflict must be broadly dialogic—a method in which the status and prestige of parties to the conflict are equalized; in which trusted bridging persons, not involved as partisans in the conflict, are available to encourage and support listening across lines of cleavage between the partisans. . . . [19]

In confrontation the parties directly engage each other and focus on the conflict between them. At times this is difficult and the parties may initially confront on the symptomatic issues. This approach sometimes decreases the costs of conflict, and may create a climate favorable for confrontation on more basic issues [13]. It is this movement of conflict toward some kind of resolution which gives it meaning and makes it good.

Walton identifies two phases of effective conflict dialogue—a differentiation phase and an integration phase. The *differentiation phase* is that period of time during which the parties in conflict describe the issues that divide them and ventilate their feelings about each other. In the *integration phase* the parties appreciate their similarities, acknowledge their common goals, . . . and engage in positive actions to manage their conflict [13].

A third party may be invited in when the two disagreeing parties have come to an impasse, and assume that no further interaction will effect a change. Boulding describes the role of mediator as a "complex one with a whole spectrum of possible degrees of intervention . . ." [8]. The mediator can contribute to the reliability of communication by translating and articulating for the parties, and by developing a common language for the dialogue. This is an important intervention because, as Boulding points out, "messages between the parties have to pass through an intense emotional field in which they are likely to be distorted . . ." [8]. The mediator also acts to rid the situation of nonrational elements and, therefore, permit the parties to deal rationally with the divergent issues.

Table 34-1. Human Relations and Realistic Models of Conflict

Old View	New Look
Conflict is by definition avoidable	Conflict is inevitable
Conflict is caused by trouble-makers, boat rockers and prima donnas	Conflict is determined by structural factors such as the physical shape of a building, the design of a career structure, or the nature of a class system
Legalistic forms of authority such as "going through channels" are emphasized	Conflict is integral to the nature of change
Scapegoats are accepted as inevitable	A minimal level of conflict is optimal

Kelly, J. Make conflict work for you. *Harvard Business Review,* 48(4), July-August.

Walton describes the general operational objective as being one that "interrupts a self-maintaining or escalating*—malevolent cycle in one way or another and to initiate a deescalating†—benevolent cycle" [13].

IMPLICATIONS FOR THE FUTURE

One important skill in organizations today is the ability to successfully manage conflicts between groups which must work together. Yet our knowledge of the dynamics of conflict processes is still primitive at best. Boulding, who is associated with the Center for Research in Conflict Resolution, makes a plea for "improvement of human skills in the conduct of conflict" [20]. There is a need to learn to manage conflict so that we minimize the cost and increase the benefits. We need to determine the boundaries in which conflict can fruitfully operate. We need to learn how to detect situations that are in the early phase of a process that may lead to destructive conflict if it is not checked. Boulding quotes a poem about the two cats at Kilkenny:

There once were two cats of Kilkenny;
Each thought there was one cat too many,
* So they fought and they fit*
* And they scratched and they bit*
'Til instead of two cats, there weren't any! [8]

The idea of conflict management is a new one (although politicians have been masters at it for years). There is a need for those involved in conflict management to become sensitive to triggering events that may be capable of precipitating a conflict cycle. Likewise it is necessary to know about those barriers that prevent a party from initiating or reacting to conflict behavior. Then, if the situation is appropriate for constructive dialogue, or if the situation calls for the prevention of manifest conflict, the mediator can take steps to bolster or overcome barriers, or can head off or encourage triggering events [13].

* Escalation: a tendency for the relationship to become more conflictful [13].
† Deescalation: a trend toward less conflict [13].

REFERENCES

1. Coser LA: *The Functions of Social Conflict.* New York, The Free Press, 1956.
2. Parsons T: *The Structure of Social Action.* Glencoe, Illinois, The Free Press, 1949.
3. Kahn RL, et al: *Organizations and Stress.* New York, John Wiley & Co, 1964.
4. Kelly J: Make conflict work for you. *Harvard Business Review* 48(4): July-August 1970.
5. Dewey J: *Morals and Conduct.*
6. Beals AR, Siegel BJ: *Divisiveness and Social Conflict.* California, Stanford University Press, 1966.
7. Thompson JD: Organizational management of conflict. *Admin Sci Q,* IV, March 1960.
8. Boulding KF: *Conflict and Defense.* New York, Harper & Brothers, 1962.
9. Nash P: *Authority and Freedom in Education.* New York, John Wiley & Co, 1966.
10. Skolik SL: *The Personnel Process.* Pennsylvania, International Textbook Company, 1970.
11. Schmidt WH, Tannenbaum R: Management of differences. *Harvard Business Review,* 38: November-December 1960.
12. Seiler JA: Diagnosing interdepartmental conflict. *Harvard Business Review,* September-October 1963.
13. Walton RE: *Interpersonal Peacemaking: Confrontations and Third-Party Consultation.* Reading, Massachusetts, Addison Wesley Co, 1970.
14. Corwin RG: Patterns of organizational conflict. *Admin Sci Q,* XIV, December 1969.
15. Blake RR, et al: *Managing Conflict in Industry.* Houston, Texas, Gulf Publishing Co, 1964.
16. Pondy LR: Organizational conflict: Concepts and models. *Admin Sci Q,* XII, September 1967.
17. Follett MP: Constuctive conflict, in Netzer, Lanore, et al: *Interdisciplinary Foundations of Supervision.* Boston, Allyn & Bacon, 1970.
18. Argyris C: *Integrating the Individual and the Organization.* New York, John Wiley & Co, 1964.
19. Benne KD: Authority in education. *Harvard Educational Review,* XL, August 1970.
20. Boulding KE: Editorial. *Journal Conflict Resolution,* XII, December 1968.

Questions to Part III

Assertiveness
1. In what situations do you consider yourself assertive? With co-workers? With patients/ families? With other health care facility personnel? With physicians?
2. What do you think about Ujhely's premise that assertiveness is one way we are our brother's keeper?
3. Identify the members of your group that you consider: assertive, aggressive, passive. Upon what specific behaviors did you base your decision? Tone of voice? Statements? Posture?
4. Are you "rewarded" in your health care facility for being assertive? How?

Advocacy
1. Is advocacy an appropriate behavior for nurses? Why?
2. Are advocacy and control synonymous terms and behaviors?
3. Can you identify advocate behaviors of your co-workers? Have you engaged in the advocate role for patients? Describe your behavior. What was the effect?

Mentoring
1. Do you have a mentor? If so, what qualities in your mentor are particularly valuable?
2. What factors interfere with mentoring among nurses?
3. Is mentoring an elitist relationship or a democratic relationship?
4. Why don't women and nurses have a rich history of mentorships?
5. Is it possible for women to be mentors?
6. What is the difference between a true mentor and a reluctant mentor?
7. Differentiate between a role model and a mentor.
8. What are the stages of the mentoring process?

Power
1. Who among your peer group or co-workers has the most power?
2. What makes the laws of power essential knowledge for professional nurses?

Politics
1. What misogynies of power do you see in your practice?
2. Should nurses/nursing participate actively in politics and legislation? Individually? Collectively?
3. Do you know the nurses at your health care facility who are politically active? Do they disseminate and gather information?
4. Do you know what state legislation is being proposed that would affect your nursing practice? Where it is at present in the legislative process? When are hearings to be held, or when were they held?
5. How do you communicate your beliefs regarding prospective legislation? To whom? Is your communication effective? Is it "after the fact" and reactive?
6. To paraphrase what John F. Kennedy once said, "Ask not what your profession can do for you, but what you can do for your profession." When is the last time you did something for your profession in the political sphere?

Collective Action

1. Is professional nursing functionally redundant?
2. What, to you, are the basic conflicts nurses have about collective bargaining?
3. "There is power in unity." Discuss how this can be achieved through collective bargaining. Discuss how this can be achieved without collective bargaining.

Change

1. Discuss this statement: "To change is to grow and to grow is to have changed much."
2. What are some of the common problems you have experienced in trying to effect change?

Conflict Resolution

1. What is the difference you see between friction and violence?
2. What are your usual patterns of dealing with conflict? In what way do they resolve the conflict?
3. What are the worst fears you have about engaging in conflict resolution?
4. Is conflict the same as confrontation?

IV The Organizational Setting

Leadership behaviors do not take place in a vacuum; they require a setting. Although the physical dimensions of each setting may differ, they have one thing in common: they represent a lifeline, one that enables both nurse and patient to interact and work together for the achievement of health care goals.

To the professional nurse entering a health care facility for the first time, any organizational setting must seem like an endless maze diabolically constructed to confound even the most seasoned professional nurse. Its varied structure, endless rules, elaborate communication channels, and layers of authority become obstacles designed to ensnare those who travel through its convoluted paths. While organizational settings may indeed resemble a maze on an organizational chart, their various structures and components all function to deliver health care efficiently and safely.

The degree to which an organizational setting represents a lifeline depends upon how well that organization implements its goals and brings together the necessary people to assist in meeting those goals. This is not an easy task. Organizational goals and values, however relevant they may be to the needs of society, may not be those of the people it has chosen to bring into its setting. Thus the stage is set for conflict that pits those with one set of goals and values against those with another set of goals and values.

Whether entering a health care facility for the first time or working within it for any period of time, each nurse needs to analyze the components of a particular organizational setting in order to determine the degree of congruency between its goals and values and her own. Furthermore, nurses need to appraise the components of an organizational setting to become more knowledgeable about its functions and, together with their leadership behaviors, use it effectively for the welfare of patients. The readings in this part provide that opportunity.

35 The Nurse in the Corporate World

Roxane Spitzer

SIXTY-FIVE PERCENT of all nurses are employed in a hospital setting [1], *i.e.,* the hospital still is the primary area of business employment for nurses. Because there are more similarities between a hospital and a corporate entity than there are dissimilarities, nurses must perceive themselves as people who hold positions in a corporate structure. Unfortunately, many nurses are ill-prepared to deal with the complexities of this corporate structure. However, individuals are placed in status positions based upon their ability to achieve in a corporate environment. Therefore, it is logical to assume that a vital way to improve nursing's image to the public and to achieve success for patients and ourselves depends upon our ability to achieve in the hospital setting. It may be possible that at least some of the "burn out" experienced by nurses at all levels is the result of a failure to prepare nurses to function in a complex, competitive corporate structure.

SIMILARITIES BETWEEN HOSPITALS AND BUSINESSES

That the hospital is a complex, competitive corporate setting is obvious when one considers the following:

1. Although the outcome or product of a hospital is service, it is goal directed and can no more afford to operate in the *red* than can a business.
2. A hospital has a traditional, organizational hierarchical structure that outlines the pyramid of formal power and decision-making and it also has an informal power and decision-making structure.
3. A hospital has a board to which administration is accountable (business administrators are responsible to stockholders).
4. A hospital has planners, organizers and doers.
5. Management for performance outcomes is as critical in hospitals as it is in business enterprises.
6. The mode of payment suggests that the customer can choose where and what services he wants. As hospitals become more competitive, the patient has more choices as to where he wishes to spend health care dollars.
7. Last, but not least, in this era of cost containment, management performance is affected heavily by effective use of the budgets based on such concepts as cost benefit ratios.

If a hospital is a business, then nursing must be examined in terms of the business world. Business enterprises are created and managed by people and not forces. Hospitals, too, are systems designed and implemented by people to meet organizational demands as estab-

Reprinted with permission by *Supervisor Nurse: The Journal for Nursing Leadership and Management,* April, 1981.

lished by the hierarchy. Often the public's health needs are determined by organizational goals rather than by the forces of society. (This is not a comment of good or bad, but rather an observation.)

Peter Drucker in his book *Management, Task, Responsibilities and Practice* has indicated that the hospital is an institution and, as such, *management* must perform for it to continue to function [2]. The term "management" includes both a function and the people who perform that function. In nursing, the people who perform that function often have been ill-prepared to assume such a role. Bedside nurses must be as adept in the management process as is the nursing administrator. The bedside nurse must work in a complex setting to achieve goals for patients and herself in order to obtain the positive feedback necessary to succeed and to *want* to remain in that environment. More aptly stated, without institutions there is no management, but without management there is no institution. To summarize: a hospital needs management, and its management structure parallels the corporate structure of a business enterprise.

HISTORICAL PERSPECTIVE

Our history has worked against the socialization of us as women and nurses in a competing modality. Therefore, most nurses *are not* prepared to compete effectively in these settings. A brief review of the origins of nursing describes our development along a path that differs significantly from management models. Formalized nursing evolved from two completely different sources: the religious, in which devotion to God through service required at all times a sacrifice of the highest order, and the secular that historically was composed of prostitutes and other females without homes or identification. Therefore, subservience and servitude were seen as key values to be maximized among nurses. As nursing developed and gained respectability, the concept of mother and nurse became synonymous. In fact, the generic meaning of the word "nursing" is the suckling of an infant. Mothers traditionally have been seen as capable of assuming responsibility for the day-to-day running of a household, but often were viewed as incapable of even simple financial transactions such as paying the phone bill. Although this view is one of the past, the mother image continues to exemplify nursing's image among the lay public and even among our colleagues—social workers, physicians, administrators and so forth.

Other historical patterns that continue to have an impact on our image and ability to compete include nursing's tendency toward isolationism. Nurses tend to group together rather than mix heterogeneously with other groups—and this is particularly apparent among nurses who have come up the hierarchical ladder in the work setting. Nursing administrators, particularly the ones who have risen from the ranks, are more comfortable with groups of nursing peers and they frequently do not mix socially or informally with peers who are executives in other departments or areas. Nursing will not become more positive visually or change its traditional image as long as nurses continue to cling to traditional patterns in a variety of settings.

NURSING'S QUEEN BEES

Nursing cannot escape the labels placed upon us both as women and nurses. As women these labels include terms such as caring, helpful, obedient, less intelligent, followers not leaders, lack of political awareness or astuteness, dependent, submissive, occupying a role secondary to that of a male and peripheral and passive spectators. As nurses, we have even greater labels placed on us. For example, nurses are accused of suffering from ambivalence: "Take care of me" versus " I am independent." Obviously, if we don't know our own minds—how can we convince others of our worth or our ability to achieve for ourselves and for patients. Another label also attached to nurses in general is a lack of career commitment, *i.e.,* the common belief among our colleagues (and often parents of a former generation) is that nursing is "a great job to fall back on" if a women is divorced, widowed or in need of a supplemental income to provide family necessities or tuition for a college student. Such an attitude is devastating to our image as professionals committed to their careers and willing to take the risks inherent in the work world.

In addition, nursing in the past has been characterized by what has come to be known as the Queen Bee Syndrome. The term "The Queen Bee Syndrome" was coined by Spengler in 1976 to describe anti-feminist behaviors in women who successfully had secured positions in management and other traditionally male dominated career worlds. A Queen Bee exhibits characteristics traditionally ascribed to women and to contemporary professional males. There is a group of anti-feminist women among nurses who exemplify the Queen Bee syndrome. Their counter-militancy has its roots in their personal success within the estab- lished system: professional success (a high status job with good pay) and social success (popularity with men, attractiveness, a good marriage). The true Queen Bee has made it in a "man's world" and holds the opinion that "If I can do it without a whole movement to help me, so can all these other women." Successful people in general, and Queen Bees in particular, tend to be counter-militant for several reasons, each of which has to do with self- interest [3].

Nursing's Queen Bees are characterized by a number of behaviors. They tend to exhibit a high level of motivation and achievement. They are talented individuals who excel in their chosen area of interest and they view themselves as successful. They also think of themselves as different from other nurses and do not want to associate closely with their own group. They identify up, not down. Therefore, they identify with people outside of nursing—very often, with men—and they maintain an allegiance to these men and to the system. Queen Bees in nursing usually hold higher-paying and more prestigious positions in nursing. They do not necessarily hold positions that are as well-paying and prestigious as those held by men in the same system. Because Queen Bees enjoy a privileged position (especially for a nurse), they are not necessarily concerned about making changes in the system [4].

A statistical study that was done in Massachusetts indicated that many nurses who hold high positions are Queen Bees. The prevalence of the Queen Bee Syndrome interferes with the advancement of the professional nurse in an institutional setting. The symptoms of the Queen Bee Syndrome can be summarized succinctly as follows:

1. Identification with those in higher hierarchical positions.
2. Alignment with the establishment and resistance to change.
3. Projection of anti-feminist beliefs about *other* women.
4. A need to "run the show" at the expense of other competent women.
5. A desire to work independently of other nurses as a decision-maker and to avoid group work and group solutions.
6. Unqualified support for the system in which she works because it has recognized and rewarded her special qualities [5].

It is difficult and frustrating to work with a Queen Bee. If she is in a position of authority, she demands personal allegiance rather than loyalty to an ideal, a program or even the profession. If she has special skills, she will not teach other nurses those skills: she keeps them to herself. If a Queen Bee is in clinical practice, she will not recognize the special needs of patients that she cannot meet and she will not refer the patient to a nursing colleague. She may refer to someone else if she can be brought to recognize her own limits, but that someone else will not be a nurse. Some Queen Bees will work with groups of nurses, but only on certain levels. They either must be the star attraction who receives special treatment or recognition or they must be in charge. The decision to get involved with other nurses is made on the basis of how it will benefit the Queen Bee—not how others might benefit [6].

The development of the Queen Bee Syndrome in our male dominated system easily can be understood if not justified. Early twentieth century business texts cite the *Maxims of Napoleon* as a guide for shaping industrial organizations, and Peter Drucker acknowledges the debt organizations owe to the military [7]. Women never have been prepard for or with this military mentality. Betty Lehan Harrigan in *Games Mother Never Taught You* states that she didn't understand how profoundly female ignorance of and indifference to military protocol interfered with the business judgment of intelligent, alert women [8]. Recognition of the fact that nurses indeed are alert, intelligent women may be the first step in overcoming this lack of preparation for the real world. Part of the military mentality so adhered to by men is the establishment of a team network. Although competition is encouraged in the male dominated world, the team concept is recognized as a primary value in the achievement of goals. Team play starts early with males and the ability to engage in effective teamwork is synonymous with success.

WHAT NEXT

To overcome such socialization is not an easy task. To do so, women and nurses must realize that image, successful competition and the acquisition of power are inter-related and pro-portionately developed. As the ability to compete effectively develops, position image increases and the power to determine our own destinies emerges. The ability to gain both an improved image and to acquire power depends on multiple factors. These include:

1. *Reversing the Tendency Toward Isolationism:* It is imperative for nurses to become involved in interdepartmental matters and in community projects. Nurses must be perceived as well prepared professionals who recognize organizational goals as well as personal goals, but to be so perceived, they must be seen. Nurses at all levels must contribute to efforts in a variety of areas—whether the project is an art festival or a health care meeting within the hospital setting. "Business" lunches with people in other departments can be arranged to accomplish a patient goal with a social worker, dietitian, physician or housekeeper.

2. *Teamwork:* Teamwork must become a byword in our profession. Nurses in the past have not trusted their colleagues enough to incorporate them in a group to achieve power and control. Teamwork is essential for our growth, success and survival as a profession.

3. *Management Concepts:* Nurses must have an accurate grasp of management concepts and organizational goals. It must be understood that complete autonomy cannot exist when one is dependent upon an organization for salary and fringe benefits. Only the self-employed can be completely autonomous. However, successful people in the corporate world recognize the formal and informal power structures and work from within to modify this structure. They must learn to be politically astute to achieve the goals that will provide for more autonomy in nursing care.

Corporate successes know that their personal goals must be consistent with the *re-organizational* goals for successful enterprise to occur. Nurses must examine their work setting to ensure that organizational objectives and goals are something that they can accept and modify from within. The environment must be believed to be conducive to this modification. At the time of employment nurses *must* review an organization's philosophy, objectives, and structure to determine its potential for her as a practitioner.

4. *Nursing Leadership:* Nurses in leadership positions must promote an organizational structure and environment that negates the Queen Bee image. Structure must be provided to encourage staff nurse input at all levels in the organization. This includes interdepartmental committees, avenues for upper management decision-making and input into departmental and organizational policies. However, all nurses must help develop and support nursing leaders. Kalisch and Kalisch, in an article entitled, "A Discourse on the Politics of Nursing," stated that "The future for women and nursing will be significantly influenced if nurse leaders can gain support of their constituency and if nurses can look to these leaders for direction" [9]. In the past, the profession has stifled initiative by rewarding subservience. The need for effective leadership is paramount, and recognition must be given to the legitimacy of nurses in leadership roles seeking the power, prestige and status essential to the successful fulfillment of such roles.

Consistently throughout this paper, nurses have been referred to as women. This was intentional for two reasons: the profession of nursing is still predominantly a female dominated profession; and it simply is not appropriate for nurses continually to say, "If we had more men in our profession, things would be different." That is an excuse. It is not that we do not welcome our male counterparts with an open mind and heart, but rather that we must recognize that it is incumbent upon the women in nursing (the majority) to achieve professional and personal success in the corporate structure.

SUMMARY

Not all nurses want to be or are conditioned to be the leaders in corporate management. Their ability, however, to practice *professionally* depends upon the development of the ability to work in a business environment and to utilize the corporate structure and political dynamics to support those nurses who compete well and who will promote the growth of nursing, nursing practice, and the image of the nurse as a capable, alert, intelligent member of a profession designed to provide the best care for the public we serve.

REFERENCES

1. *The American Nurse,* Vol. 12, No. 9, October, 1981, p. 6.
2. Drucker, Peter F. *Management, Tasks, Responsibilities, Practice.* Harper & Row, New York, 1973.
3. Halsey, Suzanne. "The Queen Bee Syndrome." In *Role Theory: Perspectives for Health Care Professionals.* Appleton-Century-Crofts, New York, 1978, p. 233.
4. *Ibid.,* p. 233.
5. *Ibid.,* p. 234.
6. *Ibid.,* p. 235.
7. Harrigan, Betty Lehan. *Games Mothers Never Taught You.*
8. *Ibid.*
9. Kalisch and Kalisch, "A Discourse on the Politics of Nursing," *Journal of Nursing Administration,* 1976.

36 Assessing Organizational Structure

Eleanor C. Hein and M. Jean Nicholson

IN THE LIFE of every organization, two forms of structures coexist: formal and informal. Each has a life and function of its own and each in its way contributes, both separately and in tandem, to the overall goals of the organization. Therefore, each element of both forms of structure must be understood in terms of the part each plays in enhancing or inhibiting organizational goals. The degree to which nurses become functionally successful in a health care delivery system depends on how well they understand that system, its structure, and its day-to-day operation. Although nurses know that a health care delivery system is the setting for the provision of nursing care, what they need to do is to become familiar with how to use the system more knowledgeably and more effectively. To do that, the various elements of both formal and informal organizational structure need to be identified and analyzed in terms of their overall impact on professional nurses and the subsequent effect on nursing practice.

CATEGORIES OF ASSESSMENT IN FORMAL ORGANIZATIONAL STRUCTURES

A health care facility, whether a hospital or a community agency, is a formal organization whose structures are clearly defined and whose existence provides a framework for the working relationships of its staff. Formal organizations systematically and clearly arrange their practices, procedures, and task responsibilities so that they can achieve organizational goals. This clarity and systematic arrangement are best illustrated through a chart that visually represents the organization's structure.

The structure of an organization depends on its concentration of authority. In organizations with a centralized concentration of authority, control is direct and extends into every aspect of organizational life. Decisions affecting the majority of the staff are made and monitored by a relatively small but select group of people through a clearly outlined chain of command. Chains of command are people, human links positioned between those who make decisions and those who carry them out. As such, they hold positional authority, that is, they have the right to act by virtue of the position given them by the organization. They also hold legitimate power in that they have been given the authority and responsibility to exert direct influence in monitoring the implementation of organizational decisions. Because the organization gives them legitimate power, people who comprise the chain of command are accountable to the organization for the way that power is used. Using legitimate power involves the right to use both reward power and coercive power; that is, people with legitimate power have the ability to reward or punish a staff member for failure to comply with organizational directives.

In decentralized organizations, the concentration of authority extends decision-making from "the few" to "the many." While a chain of command continues to be evident, the individual accountability of each staff member is a primary concern of decentralized organizations. Overall governance continues to be within an organization's domain, but more flexibility in task performance is given to its staff members. Input with respect to ideas and suggestions for changes in procedures, task performance, and policies is encouraged and valued, which, in turn, contributes to the increased motivation and job satisfaction of the staff. Assessment questions to consider are:

Does your health care facility have a centralized or decentralized concentration of authority?
Have you reviewed the organizational chart of your health care facility? Has it been modified or altered to reflect changes in structure? Are various professional groups or departments identified in the chart?
Is the concentration of authority used in your health care facility an efficient one? Is it effective? Which is more valued by your health care facility, efficiency or effectiveness? Is there duplication of efforts between departments?
How long does it take to change a policy or procedure in your health care facility? Is your health care facility responsive to change?
Does everyone you work with know who comprises the chains of command to the director of nursing service and to the chief administrator? Do they use them or do they circumvent them?
Is the chain of command used by members of the nursing staff to implement change?
What kinds of decisions are made by nurses in positional authority in your health care facility? How are these decisions made? By whom?
How are new policies and procedures monitored in your health care facility?
Does everyone you work with know to whom they are accountable?
How are conflicts resolved in your health care facility? By whom?
How do nurses in your health care facility contribute to the decision-making process?
Who holds legitimate power in your health care facility?

PHYSICAL ENVIRONMENT

The physical environment of a health care facility greatly influences the physical and mental health of all those who are in that facility. The environment is the place in which both the nurse and the patient work together to achieve health care goals. Factors within the environment that contribute to or interfere with health care goals need to be determined so that health care goals can be fully realized. Unfortunately, many of these factors are overlooked. The design of a unit, its location and accessibility to equipment and supplies, is one factor that easily slips notice. Factors such as lighting, seating, and the space allotted for a nursing station, all seemingly small concerns, play an important part in how nurses deliver health care. Similarly, a patient's well-being is influenced by the location, accessibility, and design of lounge areas, hallways, and individual patient rooms. Noise levels, the degree of privacy, the use of color within the environment, and the resulting emotional stress involved in given or receiving health care are equally important to consider. Each of these factors has a direct relationship to the mental and physical health of both the nurse and the patient. Assessment questions to consider are:

How much physical energy is used to obtain supplies and equipment?
What provisions are made for a patient's privacy?
Are the color schemes used in your health care facility cheerful? Nondescript?
Is there a quiet place for the nursing staff to use for relaxation, other than the cafeteria?

How convenient is the nursing station in your health care facility? Is there ample seating? Room to chart? Is there a great deal of noisy activity at the nurses' station?
Is the area for the preparation of medications and intravenous fluids quiet and convenient? Is there a special place allotted for the preparation of medications?
What is the overall noise level in your health care facility?
Are the patients' rooms designed for *their* comfort and convenience? Are they convenient for the nurses to give care in?
Are the patient lounge areas used by the patients? Where are they located?
What provisions are made to relieve high levels of stress in nurses who work in intensive care units?

ROLE EXPECTATIONS

Role expectations are specific standards or rules of practice assigned to a position that identify the attitudes, behaviors, and knowledge required and anticipated of the person who assumes that role [3]. In formal organizations, role expectations take the form of job descriptions. Each position assumed within a health care facility, for example, should have a corresponding job description that outlines standards of practice, specific professional behaviors, and tasks expected of the person assuming a particular position.

Accountability is a basic component of a job description. In nursing, job descriptions outline the specific responsibilities of the nurse, as well as the person or persons to whom he or she is responsible. By including the process of answerability in a job description, quality of care can be appraised in a realistic manner. Job descriptions serve other practical purposes: they are used to determine how well a nurse is performing the job expected by the health care facility; they are used to determine salary structure; they clarify relationships between jobs, thus avoiding omissions in and duplications of responsibility and individual accountability; they help a nurse to analyze all the duties assigned to a particular position and clarify what the position involves; and they serve as an excellent resource for evaluating an expected level of performance [5]. When these purposes are addressed fully, then role expectations for every nurse will assist a health care facility in meeting its goals and objectives. Assessment questions to consider are:

Is there a job description for your position available? Is it clear? Is it concise?
Does your job description contain performance standards?
What functions or specifications are included in your job description?
Are the criteria for performance standards included in your job description?
Are special demands, whether physical or mental, that are made of you included in your job description?
Does your job description reflect the philosophy of nursing in your health care facility?
Is your job description one that duplicates another title or function?
Does your job description specify the frequency and number of performance evaluations, and by whom they are given?

TYPES OF COMMUNICATION

Three types of communication channels are common to formal organizations: downward, upward, and lateral [2].

Downward communication flows from top to bottom in a health care facility, as from a director of nursing service to the nursing staff. This downward flow serves to inform, to establish limits on the nursing staff's use of power, to instruct them in the performance of their job, and to exert influence. When the physical distance between a director of nursing service and the nursing staff is great, distortions in downward communication result. Common forms of downward communication used in health care facilities include written memos, procedure manuals, and performance appraisal interviews. Although typical, these forms of downward communication may lend themselves to psychological distancing and psychological differences between those in positions of authority and those who are not.

Conversely, communication that is directed from the bottom to the top—from nursing staff to the director of nursing service—is called upward communication. It is this type of communication that a director of nursing service relies upon the most, for it serves as the data base from which decisions are made about the working environment and the future goals and objectives of the health care facility. In other words, upward communication represents a reporting system used by the nursing staff to inform the director of nursing service as to what is happening within the health care facility. The information gleaned from this type of communication can provide answers to such areas of concern as staffing patterns, orientation of new nurses, and the implementation of new procedures. Upward communication is particularly vulnerable when the nursing staff do not consider their information worth communicating, feel they have no access to or are misunderstood by the director of nursing service, and choose to withhold communication altogether. Upward communication may include such items as written progress reports, one-to-one discussions, nursing staff meetings, and grievance procedures.

Lateral communication occurs among members of the nursing staff in order to facilitate the achievement of the health care facility's goals. As such, lateral communication serves as a basis for teamwork in coordinating the efforts of various groups and individuals within the health care facility. Problems in lateral communication are likely to occur when nursing team members or one professional group feels superior to another. Exchanges of lateral communication commonly occur at the end of shift report, at nursing staff meetings, and at interdepartmental meetings.

Irrespective of the type of communication used within a particular health care facility, breakdowns and distortions will occur when the communication exchange is not clear, is selectively heard, or when nonverbal cues go unnoticed or are misinterpreted, and also when the evident emotion accompanying a message is not understood. These factors are all the more reason to assess how communicaton is used in a health care facility and with what effect. Assessment questions to consider are:

What are the formal channels of communication used in your health care facility?

What forms does your health care facility's administration use to communicate its rules, policies, and procedures?

Does your health care facility have a way on checking on whether staff members have read its directives?

What forms of upward communication are used by the nursing staff in your health care facility? Are the channels of upward communication used regularly by the nursing staff? Is information volunteered or requested?

Does the nursing staff withhold information from the people in the chain of command? What do you think are the reasons for this?

What are the common forms of lateral communication used in your health care facility?

Have there been any problems between groups or between members of the nursing staff on each shift? If so, what are they?

What do you consider the major formal communication problem in your health care facility?

LEADERSHIP STYLES

A leadership style refers to the overall pattern of behavior a person uses in performing certain tasks. Styles of leadership vary, but each allows a person a choice in selecting the overall method in implementing the specific behaviors needed to accomplish a task. The selection of a leadership style determines the amount of control exercised as that style is enacted. For example, an authoritarian style of leadership is used when maximum control is the intent or goal of the person using that style. The opposite is true when the laissez-faire leadership style is operative, which infers the absence of control (or minimum control) by the person exercising it. Midway between these extremes is the democratic style of leadership, in which the degree of control varies and alternates between the style user and the members of the group.

In health care facilities, the amount of control and interaction used between a nursing team leader and the nursing team members are determined by the size, structure, and values of the health care facility [1]. If a large, complex health care facility values procedural efficiency over human needs, the most likely style of leadership to be used is an authoritarian style, because efficient task achievement supersedes input from the nursing staff or any interactions that may contribute to this goal. With this in mind, determining the effectiveness of the leadership styles used by other nurses within a health care facility is an important factor. Assessment questions to consider are:

What is the predominant leadership style used by your head nurse? By your supervisor? By
   your director of nursing service? Are the styles appropriate for the task, situation, or staff?
What is the nursing staff's response to the style used by your head nurse? By the supervisor?
   By the director of nursing service?
To what extent does control play a part in the leadership style used by your head nurse? By
   the supervisor? By the director of nursing service?
Is your head nurse flexible in the use of her style of leadership? In other words, does she
   adjust her style to meet the needs or tasks of the nursing staff? If not, what is the nursing
   staff's response?

SOURCES OF REWARD OR ACKNOWLEDGMENT

One of the methods a health care facility uses to attract and keep its nurses lies in its ability to reward. The ability to reward is a source of organizational power that is often used to spur increased job performance. Reward power is based upon the way the nursing staff perceive the health care facility's ability to reward them for their work. Within any setting, rewards assume a variety of substantive forms: pay increases, promotions, public commendations, more attractive work assignments, and bonuses. When reward power is used exclusively it does not produce a consistent increase in job satisfaction [2]. Nevertheless, the use of reward power is a persuasive factor in maintaining a stable work force and is equally persuasive when it is withheld, thus eliminating nursing staff no longer perceived as useful or desirable to the health care facility and its goals. Assessment questions to consider are:

What kinds of reward or acknowledgment are given by your health care facility?
Who gives rewards in your health care facility?
What kinds of behavior does your health care facility reward?
Are the rewards given uniformly or are certain people rewarded more than others?
What are the effects of being rewarded on the nursing staff?

What are the effects on the nursing staff when they are not rewarded or when rewards are less than expected? Are rewards expected periodically?

What is the effect on the nursing staff's quality of work when rewards are nonexistent or less than expected?

CATEGORIES OF ASSESSMENT IN INFORMAL ORGANIZATIONAL STRUCTURES

Informal organizational structures exist in every formal organization. They are structured according to the needs of its members and occur when people working within a formal organization do not feel their needs are being met by the existing structure. Informal groups emerge when existing organizational structures are unwilling or unable to give people more information about their work, increase their social contacts, and coordinate and collaborate with them in accomplishing a task [2]. These factors serve as the common bond that unifies informal groups in order to meet and satisfy common interests and needs.

Informal structures are loosely organized, their responsibilities less clear cut, and their goals less specific. Because informal structures result from a deficit within a formal organization, they generally represent a truer picture of the organization's actual working structure. Assessment questions to consider are:

Is there an informal structure or group in your health care facility?

Is the informal group small? Large?

What appear to be the common bonds and interests that unify this informal group?

What differences exist between the formal structure of your health care facility and its informal structure?

How does the informal structure of your health care facility function? Does it have any goals? Any responsibilities?

Which is the more accurate picture of your health care facility, its formal structure or its informal structure?

TYPES OF COMMUNICATION

Since personal relationships form the basis of informal organizations, social interaction with the participants provides a rich source of information about how these informal groups establish the link between achieving their need satisfaction and organizational goals. The method most often used is referred to as "the grapevine." Unhampered by the slow, often impersonal formal channels of communication, grapevines are active, influential, quick, personal, and flexible. They are also often inaccurate. Nevertheless, their usefulness should not be underestimated because they can be skillfully manipulated either to correct the shortcomings within an organization's formal structure or escalate inaccuracies and create or perpetuate dissatisfaction within the working environment. Because grapevines constitute informal channels of communication, it is important to observe and listen to others in a health care facility as they engage in this type of communication and appraise its impact among the nursing staff. Assessment questions to consider are:

"Who sits with whom at meals and coffee breaks, day after day? (Observe with whom people choose to sit at meetings and staff development programs.)

Which people carpool together, socialize together? (Listen for people who continually support or oppose one another on issues.)

Which subgroups interact with ease?
Which subgroups avoid one another?
Who always supports new ideas?
Who always criticizes new ideas?
Who neither supports new ideas nor offers constructive criticism?
Who speaks out in the various subgroups?
Who listens?" [4]
Is there a grapevine in your health care facility?
How accurate is it?
Who are the persons who seem to have all the "latest news"? Do they share their sources of
    information?
Who generally "hangs around" after important meetings?
Are you part of the grapevine? If so, how did you become involved?
Are there co-workers who are not a part of the grapevine and refuse to participate in it? If so,
    what are the reactions of the nursing staff to their stand?
How does the grapevine correct the shortcomings in your health care facility?
Does the existence of a grapevine in your health care facility escalate difficulties?

LEADERSHIP BEHAVIORS

Leadership behaviors are action-oriented. They are the day-to-day activities nurses use to
achieve health care goals. How nurses perceive and operationalize their job is unique and, to
a certain extent, defies categorization. Thus, while a nurse may have a preferred style of
leadership (e.g., authoritarian, democratic, laissez-faire) it is *how* that nurse activates specific
behaviors within that style that is important. To paraphrase a familiar saying, "It's not the
leadership style that counts as much in achieving a goal, it's what you *did* to get there that
does."

Nurses, however, cannot activate leadership behaviors effectively when they are not aware
of what they actually do in this regard or choose not to use what they do recognize in
achieving health care goals. The leadership behaviors of nurses are strengthened to the
extent that each nurse is consciously aware of and uses those specific behaviors that facilitate
goal achievement. In Part II of this book, Yura, Ozimek, and Walsh identified four major
process components of nursing leadership: deciding, relating, influencing, and facilitating.
They selected specific human actions (i.e., behaviors) that were descriptive of each process
component and classified them so nurses could be more effective using leadership behaviors in the achievement of health care goals.

Recognition of specific leadership behaviors takes place where they most often occur—
with the patient or client. They become viable behaviors when nurses share with each other
what behaviors were effective in the course of giving nursing care. As this supportive
exchange occurs, greater opportunity exists for a repository of behaviors to accumulate, and
subsequently enables each nurse to become a more effective practitioner. Assessment
questions to consider are:

What leadership behaviors do you use in your professional practice?
What leadership behaviors do your co-workers use in their professional practice?
Do you compliment your co-workers when you see them use leadership behaviors effec-
    tively?
When is the last time you were told that something you did was done well? When was the
    last time you gave recognition to a co-worker about her leadership behaviors?

Do you seek out a co-worker for specific assistance in a certain area of leadership behavior because you know that she is good in that area? In other words, do you seek out a co-worker because she has special ability in one of the four components of nursing leadership?

What leadership behaviors of yours do you consider to be particular strengths?

In what ways are you developing or adding to your present leadership behaviors?

SOURCES OF REWARD OR ACKNOWLEDGMENT

Being rewarded is a form of feedback that indicates a positive regard for one's efforts within a particular health care facility. Because informal groups emerge as a response to a formal organization's inability to provide adequate communication, how and by whom rewards are given assumes special importance. Rewards extended to and received within informal groups are subtle in form. The sources for these subtle rewards generally come from co-workers (although they can also come from those in positional authority). Such rewards are not monetary. Rewards such as saying thank you or going out to lunch for a special occasion bolster self-esteem, cement group cohesiveness, and sustain the intrinsic satisfaction persons receive from their job.

When monetary rewards are insufficient or nonexistent, then subtle forms of reward and acknowledgment from co-workers assume special importance. Each cannot be used alone, nor is each an indicator of success without the other. How a person is accepted by co-workers and how a person is included in group activities and is acknowledged by patients are some important sources of reward. Although many nurses are internally motivated and receive personal satisfaction from the tasks they accomplish well, personal satisfaction alone is not in and of itself an adequate source of compensation. Assessment questions to consider are:

What kinds of rewards or acknowledgment do members of the informal group give to each other?

How strong is the group's support system?

Is the informal group's support system effective and helpful to others?

What are the common forms of reward or acknowledgment given by your patients or clients? What effect does this have on you? Is this a primary source of gratification for you?

Are you accepted by your peer group and included in their activities?

SOURCES OF POWER

Each nurse has potential power; that is, the ability to influence and change the behavior of others to a specified end. Power is an intrapersonal energy resource that manifests itself through personal relationships. Because the need for social contact is a precipitating factor in the emergence of informal organizations, the inevitability of potential power energizing into an active part of human interactions assumes all the more importance in a working environment. Two sources of power that are particularly suited as interactional energizing agents within a health care facility are expert power and referent power [2].

In nursing, *expert power* is professional credibility. That credibility is based upon a nurse's ability to demonstrate valid knowledge and skill in implementing her nursing practice. If other members of the nursing staff perceive that their co-worker does indeed have valid knowledge, skill, and ability, they will acknowledge her as a competent practitioner whom they respect. In other words, she will have established herself as a professional nurse with expert power. The potential power within her now is activated within the health care facility and is acknowledged in interactions with others.

Referent power is a more subtle source of power. Its subtlety stems from a person's ability to attract others on the basis of personal qualities alone. Personal qualities may include good humor, thoughtfulness, integrity, and honesty. Whatever they may be, these are the qualities that persuade and influence other nurses. Nurses who have referent power are admired by their colleagues, and their personal qualities are not only valued but are a source of attraction and identification for other nurses.

Consciously affiliating or aligning oneself with a nurse who has either expert or referent power or both is useful. Before that usefulness can be tested, the existence of expert or referent power needs to be assessed by the nurse who wishes to acquire them. This comes about through active involvement in the day-to-day activities of the health care facility. As this is done, new knowledge can be acquired, more skills can be refined, and new, strong peer relationships can be developed. These are the power sources all nurses need to have. Assessment questions to consider are:

Who among your co-workers do you consider has expert power? What specifically leads you to that conclusion?
How do your co-workers respond to a co-worker who is acknowledged to have expert power? How do people in positional authority respond?
How did your co-worker achieve expert power? Have you asked?
Does your head nurse have expert power? Is she acknowledged as such by the nursing staff?
What are you doing to achieve expert power?
Do your co-workers seek you out for help with a particular skill or piece of knowledge?
Who among your co-workers do you feel has referent power? What specifically leads you to that conclusion?
In what ways do your co-workers relate to the person with referent power? Do they identify with her?
What kind of influence do you perceive this nurse has upon your co-workers?
Are those nurses you have identified as having both expert and referent power in fact one and the same person? Different persons? Are they part of the informal group or are they in positional authority?
Are you consciously associating with those co-workers who have expert and referent power? If so, what impact has this association had on your professional practice? If not, what prevents you from doing so?

REFERENCES

1. Bernhard, L. A., and Walsh, M. *Leadership: The Key to the Professionalization of Nursing.* New York: McGraw-Hill Book Company, 1981, pp. 47–49.
2. Deep, S. D. *Human Relations in Management.* Encino, Calif.: Glencoe Publishing Co., Inc., 1978, pp. 92–106, 72–74, 129–135.
3. Hardy, M. E., and Conway, M. E. *Role Theory: Perspectives for Health Professionals.* New York: Appleton-Century-Crofts, 1978, p. 76.
4. Schweiger, J. L. *The Nurse as Manager.* New York: John Wiley and Sons, 1980, p. 21.
5. Swansburg, R. C. *Management of Patient Care Services.* St. Louis: C. V. Mosby Co., 1976, p. 216.

BIBLIOGRAPHY

Claus, K. E., and Bailey, J. T. *Power and Influence in Health Care: A New Approach to Leadership*. St. Louis: C. V. Mosby Co., 1977.

Donnelly, G. F., Mengel, A., and Sutterley, D. C. *The Nursing System: Issues, Ethics and Politics*. New York: John Wiley and Sons, 1980.

Epstein, C. *The Nurse Leader: Philosophy and Practice*. Reston, Virginia: Reston Publishing Co., 1982.

Yura, H., Ozimek, D., and Walsh, M. *Nursing Leadership: Theory and Process* (2d ed.). New York: Appleton-Century-Crofts, 1981.

37 Organizational Process and Bureaucratic Structure

Ann Marriner

ORGANIZATION GROWS out of a need for cooperation. We shall consider both the process of organization and the structures involved.

ORGANIZATIONAL PROCESS

Organization is a process by which a manager develops order, promotes cooperation among workers, and fosters productivity. Activities analysis, decision analysis, and relations analysis are tools that can be used to determine what structure is needed. *Activities analysis* is the study of the work to be done and its order of priority, how it can be clustered, and the relationship of tasks to one another. *Decision analysis* is the investigation of the decisions to be made, where in the structure they should be made and by whom. *Relations analysis* looks at the contribution each person makes to the organization with special attention to whom he works with, to whom he reports, and who reports to him.

Organization is a logical process which involves defining the agency's mission or objectives; establishing policies and plans; clarifying the activities necessary to meet the objectives; organizing the activities for best utilization of available human and material resources; delegating to appropriate personnel the responsibility and authority necessary to do the activities; and grouping personnel vertically and horizontally through information systems and authority relationships.

ORGANIZATIONAL STRUCTURE

Although planning is the key to effective management, the organizational structure furnishes the formal framework in which the management process takes place. The organizational structure should provide an effective work system, a system of communications, identity to individuals and to the organization, and it should consequently foster job satisfaction. Agencies contain both informal and formal structures.

INFORMAL STRUCTURE

The informal organization comprises personal and social relationships which do not appear on the organization chart. This might include a group which usually goes to coffee together,

Reprinted with permission by *Supervisor Nurse: The Journal for Nursing Leadership and Management*, July 1977.

works together on a particular unit, or takes a class together. Informal organization is based on personal relationships rather than a respect for positional authority. It helps members meet personal objectives and provides social satisfaction. People who have little formal status may gain recognition through the informal structure. Rather than being commanded through organizational assignment, informal authority comes from the follower's natural respect for a colleague's knowledge and abilities.

Informal structure provides social control of behavior. The control can be either internal or external. If pressure is intended to make a member conform to group expectancies, it is internal. Kidding a member about her dirty shoelaces would be an example. An attempt to control the behavior of someone outside of the social group, such as the supervisor, is external control.

The informal structure has its own channels of communication, which may disseminate information more broadly and more rapidly than the formal communication system. Unfortunately, the "grapevine" may contain rumors which are not authenticated. The best way to correct an invalid rumor is for the supervisor to give accurate information. It is better not to state that she is correcting the rumor, for in doing so she may strengthen it; the facts she has given may be seen primarily as a subterfuge to refute the rumor.

The informal organizational structure is important to management. The supervisor should be aware of its existence, study its operating techniques, and use it to meet the agency's objectives. It will help her to avoid antagonism.

FORMAL ORGANIZATION

The formal organizational structure is defined by executive decision as a result of planning. It can be diagrammed to show the relationships among people and their positions. It describes positions, task responsibilities, and relationships. The two basic forms of formal organizational structure are the hierarchic or bureaucratic model and the adaptive or organic model.

BUREAUCRATIC STRUCTURE

A hierarchy or bureaucracy is an organizational design to facilitate large scale administration by coordinating the work of many personnel. It is associated with subdivision, specialization, technical qualifications, rules and standards, impersonality, and efficiency. In Figure 37-1, which illustrates a typical bureaucratic hierarchy, the supervisors are responsible to the director of nursing. She in turn must answer to the hospital administrator, who is accountable to the board of directors. The supervisor also has authority over those below and they are accountable to her.

DUAL MANAGEMENT

Dual management separates technical and administrative responsibilities. It has a hierarchy in which technical professionals make the technical decisions and control technical matters and another hierarchy in which supervisory management make the decisions about such issues as personnel and budget. This dual hierarchy gives equal status to managers and to technical professionals. It provides a set of titles and job descriptions for each hierarchy.

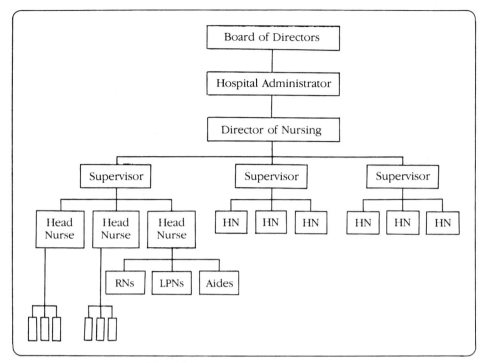

Figure 37-1. Bureaucratic hierarchy.

PRINCIPLES OF ORGANIZATION

Certain principles of organization help to maximize the efficiency of the bureaucratic structure.

LINES OF AUTHORITY

The organization should have clear lines of authority running from the highest executive to the employee who has the least responsibility and no authority over others. There should be unity of command. Each person should have only one boss. Each person should know to whom he reports and those responsible to him.

The authority and responsibility of every individual should be clearly defined in writing. This reduces role ambiguity as one knows what is expected of him and what his limitations are. This prevents gaps between responsibilities, avoids overlapping of authority, and helps to determine the proper point for decisions. Although many people do not feel it is necessary to have their responsibilities in writing, it can be revealing to have them write what they believe their functions to be and then note the duplicated efforts and the jurisdictional disputes. It is not uncommon, when someone leaves an agency, for no one to know exactly what the person did. Under such circumstances, it can be difficult to justify replacement and confusing to offer a meaningful orientation to the new person.

DEFINITION OF ROLES

A clear definition of roles is necessary for effective delegation but does not guarantee it. Role clarity allows the employee to know what is expected of him, to whom he reports, and to whom he goes for help. Role ambiguity leads to anxiety, frustration, dissatisfaction, negative attitudes, and decreased productivity. Although job descriptions increase productivity and satisfaction, they should not be so exact that innovation is discouraged.

DELEGATION

Supervisors should delegate responsibility to the lowest level within the organization where there is enough competence and information for effective performance and appropriate decision making. Ordinarily, increased delegation and general rather than close supervision increases effective performance, production, and employee satisfaction.

The employee should be given formal authority commensurate to the responsibility delegated. It is not uncommon for supervisors to delegate authority and then undermine it by making decisions that were supposedly delegated. For example, if the head nurse is responsible for the quality of care given on her ward, she should not have to accept a member to her team who has been hired without consulting her. In turn, the head nurse should not tell a patient that he can have a bath at a certain time without consulting the person assigned to give that bath. Preferably the nurse's aide and her patient will determine when various routines can be performed in accordance with the doctor's orders and the team leader's rationale.

The delegation of responsibility should be accompanied by accountability. Most effective control systems are probably those which provide feedback directly to the accountable person as this seems to increase motivation and provide direction. When this information is passed through a supervisor as performance evaluation rather than guidance, it tends to be nonfunctional and only infrequently contributes to improved performance. This delegation of functions with accompanying responsibility and accountability is particularly difficult for the supervisor because she remains responsible for the actions of her subordinates. She remains as responsible as her subordinates for their performance or the neglect of their duties. Consequently the span of control principle becomes important.

SPAN OF CONTROL

There is a limit to the amount of coordination that can be done by one person. It is dependent upon several factors. One can coordinate more similar than dissimilar positions. The more the positions are interdependent, the more coordination is involved. The span of control needs to decrease as the complexity of the subordinate's tasks increases. The stability of the agency should also be considered. If the agency has been functioning in a similar manner for a long time, the problems which arise have probably been solved before and coordination is less difficult than in a changing situation where many new problems arise. The span of control is not likely to be uniform throughout an organization. Top level managers of positions which are interdependent and dissimilar will likely have a smaller range of control than lower level supervisors who are coordinating people doing similar tasks in a confined area. The span of control should not be so wide that the supervisor does not have time to deal with human relations aspects such as giving workers individual attention, communicating information about the agency's policies, and listening to any suggestions, grievances, and problems. On the other hand, she needs a large enough span of control to keep busy, so that she won't interfere with delegated responsibilities just to have something to do.

Three types of divisions are commonly used to define span of control: (1) function or process, (2) product or service, and (3) region. Function is associated with specialization which may apply to individuals and to departments or divisions. For example, one nurse may pass medications and do treatments, another may just start IVs, or the nurse's aides may give the baths and change linens. There may be a surgical nursing division with departments for specific types of surgery. It is preferable that if a person is responsible for more than one type of responsibility that they be similar. Efficiency is maximized if a person predominantly does the tasks she can do best and for which her proficiency will consequently continue to increase, but she may become bored. It is not uncommon to find individuals within our organization who are assigned several unrelated tasks. Although that may work for some people in given situations, it is not considered good organization and their replacements are not as likely to be successful. It is more viable to hire personnel to fill the organizational structure than to change the structure to fit personnel.

Having individuals doing the same or similar tasks and divisions with specific functions can help expand the range of control. Similarly, having departments providing specific services, such as cardiac intensive care, or producing certain products can influence the structure. Organization by geographical location becomes increasingly viable when operations are scattered. Many agencies use a combination of these methods. For instance, a school of nursing may be organized according to campuses (regional divisions), according to undergraduate, graduate, and continuing education (product division), according to in-patient, out-patient, medical-surgical, maternal-child, or some other service division. The school may have individual faculty members assigned to teach according to specialization (functional division).

The organizational structure should be flexible to permit the necessary expansion and contraction in response to changing conditions without disrupting the basic design. It should also be kept as simple as possible, since additional levels of authority complicate communications and too many committees may impede progress.

DISADVANTAGES OF THE BUREAUCRATIC STRUCTURE

There are disadvantages to the bureaucratic model. It may be detrimental to healthy personality patterns by predisposing the authoritarian leadership style, increasing insistence on the right of authority and status, and fostering a pathological need for control. If the superior does not have the technical competence of her subordinates, she may feel insecure and fear her subordinates. Autocratic behavior may become a defense mechanism through the use of power and fear strategies over subservients and the enforcement of norms through arbitrary or rigid rules. The use of rewards and punishment to get desired behavior may alienate personnel. Self-serving behavior patterns may develop through competition for the advancement of individual interests. A certain aloofness can result from the specialization that leads to impersonality. Personnel also may develop a ritualistic attachment to routinization, become attached to subgoals, and show resistance to change.

BIBLIOGRAPHY

GENERAL

Albers, Henry H. *Principles of Management: A Modern Approach.* New York: John Wiley & Sons, Inc., 1974.

Haimann, Theo, and William G. Scott, *Management in the Modern Organization.* Boston: Houghton Mifflin Company, 1974.

Kast, Fremont E., and James E. Rosenzweig. *Organization and Management: A Systems Approach.* New York: McGraw-Hill Book Company, 1974.

Koontz, Harold, and Cyril O'Donnell. *Principles of Management: An Analysis of Managerial Functions.* New York: McGraw-Hill Book Company, 1972.

Krazmier, Leonard J. *Principles of Management: A Programmed-Instructional Approach.* New York: McGraw-Hill Book Company, 1974.

McFarland, Dalton. *Management Principles and Practices.* New York: Macmillan Publishing Co., Inc., 1974.

ORGANIZATIONAL PROCESS

Cohen, Michael D., James G. March, and Johan P. Olsen, "A Garbage Can Model of Organizational Choice," *Administrative Science Quarterly,* 17 (March 1972), 1-25.

Muther, Richard, and Ray J. DeMoor, "Planning an Organization Structure," *S.A.M. Advanced Management Journal,* 38 (January 1973), 28-33.

Tersine, Richard J., and Max B. Jones, "Models for Examining Organizations," *Journal of Systems Management,* 24 (September 1973), 32-37.

ORGANIZATIONAL STRUCTURE

Ansoff, H.I., and R.G. Brandenburg, "A Language for Organization Design: Part I and Part II," *Management Science,* 17 (August 1971), B705-B731.

Forrester, Jay W., "A New Corporate Design," *Industrial Management Review,* 7 (Fall 1965), 5-17.

Gerwin, Donald, and Wade Christoffel, "Organizational Structure and Technology: A Computer Model Approach," *Management Science,* 20 (August 1974), 1531-1541.

Jaques, Elliott, "Organizational Structure and Role Relationships," *Nursing Times,* 67 (February 4, 1971), 154-157.

Lawrence, Paul R., and Jay W. Lorsch, "Differentiation and Integration in Complex Organizations," *Administrative Science Quarterly,* 12 (June 1967), 1-47.

Schaefer, Marguerite, "How Should We Organize?" *Journal of Nursing Administration* (February 1976), 12-14.

Schollhammer, Hans, "Organization Structures of Multinational Corporations," *Academy of Management Journal,* 14 (September 1971), 345-365.

Shetty, Y.K., "Is There a Best Way to Organize a Business Enterprise?" *S.A.M. Advanced Management Journal,* 38 (April 1973), 47-52.

Smith, David, "Organizational Theory and the Hospital," *Journal of Nursing Administration,* 2 (May-June 1972), 19-24.

Stevens, Barbara J., "Nursing Management and the Sense of Structure," *Journal of Nursing Administration,* 4 (July-August 1974), 57-59.

INFORMAL ORGANIZATION

Graham, Gerald, "Interpersonal Attraction As A Basis of Informal Organization," *Academy of Management Journal,* 14 (December 1971), 483-495.

Odiorne, George S., "Put Cliques to Work for You," *Nation's Business*, 46 (August 1958), 50-53.

BUREAUCRATIC STRUCTURE

Anthanassiades, John C., "The Distortion of Upward Communication in Hierarchical Organizations," *Academy of Management Journal*, 16 (June 1973), 207-225.

Bennis, Warren, "The Coming Death of Bureaucracy," *Think* (November-December 1966), 30-35.

———, "Organizational Developments and the Fate of Bureaucracy," *Industrial Management*, 7 (Spring 1966), 41-55.

Brinkerhoff, Merlin B., "Hierarchical Status, Contingencies, and the Administrative Staff Conference," *Administrative Science Quarterly*, 17 (September 1972), 395-407.

Landsberger, Henry A. "The Horizontal Dimension in Bureaucracy," *Administrative Science Quarterly*, 6 (December 1961), 299-332.

Maniha, John K., "Universalism and Particularism in Bureaucratizing Organizations," *Administrative Science Quarterly*, 20 (June 1975), 177-190.

Read, William H., "The Decline of the Hierarchy in Industrial Organizations," *Business Horizons*, 8 (Fall 1965), 71-75.

DUAL MANAGEMENT

Evans, Peter B., "Multiple Hierarchies and Organizational Control," *Administrative Science Quarterly*, 20 (June 1975), 250-259.

Ritti, R. Richard, "Dual Management—Does It Work?" *Research Management*, 14 (November 1971), 19-26.

38 The Role of Power in the Nursing Profession

Dalton E. McFarland and Nola Shiflett

THE IDEA OF POWER

To many professionals, "power" is an undesirable word, connoting dominance and submission, control and acquiescence, or one person's will over another's. Lasswell even goes so far as to state that anyone interested in power is sick and that the interests of "political man" result from the displacement of private conflicts onto public issues [1]. To Zaleznik and Kets DeVries, however, leadership *is* the exercise of power, and it is dangerous and misleading to equate the need for power with illness [2]. Working from a psychoanalytical framework, they view power-oriented behavior in the context of total personality development and character structure, with power having both normal and pathological expressions. Like any human attribute, it can be benevolent or malicious, used or abused, inspiring or stifling.

For the purposes of this article, power is defined as the influence of a person or a group such that others obey or conform. Those toward whom power is directed either accept its use as legitimate and appropriate or reject it and accept the consequences. Acquiescence by members of an organization makes power a legitimate form of influence on their work behavior, and generally there is little or no question about acquiescence. However, an indifferent or rebellious person may fail to carry out the demands of a power figure and then must accept the consequences. Some people comply with lip service or sub rosa forms of resistance. Others express concerns or reservations about the power figure's actions, in which case the outcome is subject to negotiation, testing the balance of power. If a power-holder fails to gain acquiescence, his power base will be weakened or destroyed, so he is likely to invoke sanctions against the resisters.

Power as defined above is the strongest of several forms of influence, including authority, leadership, and control, which must be considered together in order to understand power fully. *Influence*, the broadest of these terms, can be regarded as an interpersonal relationship or a group effect that is not necessarily based on power or authority. It can derive from friendship, for example, or other psychosocial phenomena, as well as from power.

Authority is a type of power that resides in expertise or in delegation of responsibility within an organizational framework. In either case, current management theory treats authority as a form of power that subordinates make legitimate by their acceptance. Power and authority are thus closely coupled; together they make an organization coherent and move it toward its goals.

Control means that an organization's performance or its members' behavior is meeting standards that the leaders, administrators, or other power-holders have determined to be

Copyright © 1979 Nursing Resources, Inc. *Power in Nursing*, Volume 7, Number 2, 1979.

desirable. Control is thus one objective of power. Smith and Kaluzny, following Mechanic [3], treat power as synonymous with influence and control, based on a definition of power as "any force that results in behavior that would not have occurred if the force had not been present" [4].

Leadership is a broad form of influence that cuts across the others. Tracing the development of power, authority, and influence in the context of leadership, one readily notes that these terms are often used loosely and even interchangeably; universally accepted definitions of these terms are not yet possible. The writers of the articles in this book and in other sources adapt their definitions to their particular purposes. The definitions we present in this article provide a good frame of reference for understanding power in nursing, but there is ample opportunity for interested persons to dig more deeply into their complexities.

POWER AND PERSONALITY

Increasingly, power is analyzed in a psychological framework. Although there are other approaches to the study of power, we are just beginning to understand the role of personality in organizations. For example, acquiescence to or acceptance of power implies submissiveness, docility, or the desire to be dominated. Yet Zaleznik and Kets DeVries note countervailing forces in the organizational context; authority figures are temporary and must therefore meet at least the major commonly held goals, and there are many ways to live with authority and other forms of power [5]. Also, Follett's "law of the situation" determines, along with inner personality conflicts, the behavior of a given power-holder and of those who are subject to that power [6]. Follett advocates "power with" people in preference to "power over" people.

In another major psychological study, McClelland classifies power orientations into four stages according to the individual's ego development [7]. He also classifies power according to its source and its object. McClelland considers the four stages to be progressive along a scale of social and emotional development or maturation, although each stage may have its own pathological form. Within each stage he also describes ways in which females achieve a feeling of power in a different way from males. The stages are:

STAGE I: "IT" STRENGTHENS ME

Adults in this stage are infantile—still totally dependent on another as their source of strength. Their preferred status is to be a client or close associate of a powerful person. If pushed to a pathological extreme or deprived of the association, these persons develop hysterical symptoms and may no longer feel in control of themselves; they turn to a dependence on food, drugs, or religion.

STAGE II: I STRENGTHEN MYSELF

Persons at this stage feel powerful through control of their bodies or possessions. They may focus on body-building exercises or on acquiring material possessions. They may feel in control through understanding what makes people tick or how systems operate. The pathological response at this level is obsessive compulsiveness.

STAGE III: I HAVE IMPACT ON OTHERS

The person at this stage derives feelings of power through controlling others. This person is competitive and may try to outwit or outmaneuver others or give them things in order to control or dominate them. The pathology of this stage may lead to "smothering" love, crime, or personal violence.

STAGE IV: "IT" MOVES ME TO DO MY DUTY

Persons in this stage may subordinate their personal goals to a higher authority or make decisions based on the good of the organization. The pathology of this stage is labeled "messianism," meaning that the person can no longer distinguish between personal views and higher authority in the form of God, state, or organization.

We now encounter a dilemma. Zaleznik and Kets DeVries state that, "So long as interest in power can remain attached to universal ideals, the risks of abusing power diminish" [8]. But according to McClelland, power plays based on collective authority carry a far more dangerous potential than power plays based on individual authority [9]. While the pathology of Stage III may result in a few murders, the pathology of Stage IV may lead to holy wars.

TYPES OF POWER

Power derives from multiple sources that may operate simultaneously. Wieland and Ullrich describe five sources of power: legitimate, reward, coercive, expert, and referent [10]. *Legitimate power* is the authority vested in a role, position, or office that is accepted and recognized by the members of the organization; it can be called positional authority. *Reward power* is based on the power-holder's use of positive sanctions, which may be as simple as a compliment or as complex as monetary benefits. *Coercive power*, the opposite of reward power, involves negative sanctions, such as threats of harm, punishment, or withheld rewards; this is the most visible form of power. *Expert power* is founded on the power-holder's valid knowledge or information. *Referent power*, the most subtle form, is based on attractive personal characteristics that lead others to emulate or please the attracting person. All of these sources are available to the nurse administrator in the hospital. Planned use of these sources of power can be called a power strategy, which requires careful consideration of the probable consequences in the specific context.

Derivative forms of power can also be useful to the nursing administrator, such as *associative power*, which comes from close association with a powerful individual or group. Nurses, for example, acquire power from members of the medical staff, or from administrators with whom they work. Another derivative form is the power that the lower participants of a hierarchy may have over the higher members. For example, the nursing administrator may have power over the hospital administrator through 1) control of resources that the administrator is dependent upon; 2) control of others' access to the administrator; 3) control of techniques, procedures, or knowledge that are vital to the administrator; or 4) personality attributes such as charm, likeableness, or charisma that the administrator considers desirable in a subordinate. Note that this same type of power can be utilized by staff members in relation to the nursing administrator.

Derivative forms of power are less certain to attain results than other forms, and some derivative powers may not be considered legitimate. Wieland and Ullrich state that "lower participants may circumvent or manipulate the organizational hierarchy by using various forms of power that are not legitimate" [11]. Also, a derivative power may be legitimate in some circumstances but not in others.

We shall first analyze power in nursing at three interrelated levels: (1) the power of the individual nurse, (2) power within organizations, and (3) power of the professional in society. We shall then analyze the problem of integrating these levels of power.

POWER AND THE INDIVIDUAL NURSE

"Nurses are the least political of all the people in health care work." This statement by a nurse reveals the dichotomy between the ideals of service nurtured by professionalism on the one hand and the necessity of coping with bureaucracy on the other. The power game is a game of politics from the point of view of the individual in an organization. Yet little in a nurse's training today teaches the art of politics or strategies for using power. Her training focuses on clinical expertise and on competencies for patient care, overshadowing or ignoring the skills and insights needed for coping with life in an organization. This gap in training has been noted by Kramer, who attributes to "reality shock" the large numbers of nursing graduates who are leaving the profession. In nursing school they are taught humanism, individual thinking, and treatment of each patient as an individual, but they find the real world of nursing vastly different, even opposite, from what they were taught. As a result, nurses are shocked to find that they don't have any control or say in the organization. Their feelings of powerlessness are disturbing to them [12].

If Kramer is right in alleging that feelings of powerlessness are pervasive among nurses, it may be not only because their training is not sufficiently oriented to reality, but also because the profession has not sufficiently brought the strength of group power to bear on the use and distribution of individual power, which always occurs unevenly in organizations. Those who seek to acquire it differ in their success and in their perception of the sources on which they can draw. Power is also temporary and continually shifting, in accordance with changing pressures and tensions. There are no guarantees of permanent power, though it may last longer if it is earned or sanctioned as legitimate, leading to acquiescence by the less powerful.

Power relationships among individuals are often highly situational, that is, contingent on specific factors that may not be present elsewhere. A good illustration is a lower participant who has more effective power than someone with greater formal authority and status. In one such case, a nurse found herself helpless when an escort employee wheeled a patient to the laboratory and left him there for over an hour. The nurse, who could not get the patient treated or returned, expressed intense feelings of helplessness and frustration.

The power of the individual nurse is increasing; her health care role now incorporates greater recognition of her expert power. In many hospitals nurses have sought and acquired more responsibility and have transferred many routine or clerical duties to others. Moreover, greater autonomy and independence have followed from more appropriate training and from greater trust by administrators and patients. For example, in most coronary care units, specially trained nurses now have the authority to administer drugs and defibrillation on their own initiative, which has resulted in decreased mortality rates. Patients accept nurses as the source of primary care in ambulatory clinics, also, and there are expanded roles for nurses in anesthesia and in handling patients with chronic diseases [13].

In addition to expanding their use of expert power, nurses can increase their power in two ways: (1) by accepting it as a normal element of human interaction, and (2) by acquiring power from a broader range of sources. According to Martin and Sims, power tactics are important and, whether they are good or bad, are worth discussing in their own right. No one can entirely avoid using power tactics; the aim is to use them effectively. This requires practice, based on continuing observation and analysis of the interplay of forces in the organization. Martin and Sims assert that it is neither immoral or cynical to recognize the actual daily practices of power. They present eight possible tactics: (1) alliances, (2) maneuverability, (3) communication (control of information), (4) compromise, (5) negative timing (withholding action), (6) self-dramatization, (7) confidence (decisiveness), and (8) guarding against friendship or other commitments that might limit the acquisition or use of power [14].

These and other tactical maneuvers should be used with discretion, according to their appropriateness for the individual and for the context. Important as it is, power is a means and not an end in itself. Achieving power for its own sake, without regard for the organization, peers, or patients, is a hollow victory.

POWER AND SEX ROLES

One aspect of individual power is particularly relevant to nursing: the male-female dichotomy in relation to power. While the field of nursing is 90 percent female, administrators and physicians are predominantly male. History and mythology are replete with references to male suspicion of female powers, resulting in fear, distrust, and superstition about women as sorcerers, witches, or temptresses. One result of these historical traditions is a deep-seated male need to dominate.

The female administrator faces the problem of overcoming the views of male managers who limit the roles of women in the belief that they are inferior and therefore cannot be good managers. Male-female role stereotypes exacerbate the problem. At a seminar for male managers conducted by the National Association of Bank Women, the 21 participants were divided into two groups. One group was asked to list adjectives descriptive of a good manager, the other group listed adjectives describing the ideal woman. As shown in Figure 38-1, only three of the adjectives for the ideal woman were also mentioned in the list for a good manager: flexible, intelligent, and decisive. These results indicate why the typical male manager does not consider the "ideal woman" as a good bet for management [15].

The fact that so many nursing directors are women is significant for the nature and scope of their power. McClelland argues that power needs and expressions are different for females as compared to males [16]. This conclusion is based in part on certain female characteristics: lack of assertiveness, concern with interdependence of people rather than things, and more concern for complex circumstantial concepts. He also states that sexually determined expectations shape female behavior, especially in deriving satisfaction through giving. These sexual differences are illustrated by the woman in Stage I who lists men as her inspiration, has more precious possessions, lends more things, and has more frequent illness symptoms than the man. The Stage-II woman is more concerned than the man with loss of voluntary control and with freedom *for* rather than freedom *from*. She shows in every way possible that she is in charge, not in need of help of any kind, and free to control her own life. The Stage-III woman with a high desire for power is active and assertive like the man, but demonstrates more liking for new experiences (except regarding sexual matters, about which she is highly secretive) and less need for affiliation with groups. These women tend to be inward looking and to have a feeling of oneness with the world. The Stage-IV

The Ideal Woman	Good Manager
Attractive	Intelligent
Wealthy	Aggressive
Educated	Objective
Supportive	Decisive
Flexible	Reliable
Intelligent	Flexible
Mature	Motivated
Tolerant	Pressurized
Decisive	Sensitive
Open-minded	Responsible
Frugal	Trustworthy
Loving	Considerate
Gentle	Imaginative
Soft-spoken	Goal-oriented
Good conversationalist	

Figure 38-1. Comparison of descriptions of the ideal woman and the good manager. (Source: Daniel A. Polk, "Women in the Corporation," *National Association of Bank Women Journal* [September/October 1977], p. 20. Published by the National Association of Bank Women, Inc. Reprinted by permission.)

woman, like the man, joins organizations and tends to share her deeper feelings with mates and friends. These women are secure in their own identity and feel free to assume desired roles in family or business. McClelland concludes that "power motivation apparently helps women develop into higher stages of maturity, just as it hinders men" [17].

McClelland believes that sex role is a key variable in determining how the power drive is expressed, for men and women channel their drive for power in different directions. A wealth of psychological research indicates significant differences in ideas about male and female traits. Both sexes generally characterize males as strong, hard, heavy, and assertive, and females as small, weak, soft, and light. Women are regarded generally as having opposite characteristics from men, and descriptions of female traits tend to have a negative tone. Despite these differences in perception, however, McClelland acknowledges that women display special characteristics that make them valuable members of organizations. They pay attention to the details of what is going on around them and modify their behavior accordingly. They care more about personal relationships. Their motor skills are superior to those of men. They prefer situations in which interdependence is important [18]. Rather than attempting to emulate the tougher qualities of men, women power-seekers may do better to draw upon their own special strengths.

Martin observes that nurses are now involved in a major battle, the central issue of which is power. The struggle is unequal because of the sex-role stereotype that females are less competent than males; if women are considered naturally inferior to men, not even education can bring them onto an equal plane. Women's self-fulfillment is blocked by ascribing to them circumscribed, supportive, subservient, or other secondary roles. As a result, the expansion of nursing's functions in health care is blocked. Hence the power struggle, in which nursing may find support in the various women's rights movements [19].

Part of the problem in this struggle stems from women's lack of power in the bargaining process. Power is in itself a reward, but some degree of power must be attained if one is to bargain successfully for more. The woman who violates female role-performance expectations is penalized by peers, superiors, and even family members [20].

According to Donovan, "The organizational behavior resulting from the fusion of the individual and the organization will be altered substantially and for the good wherever there is growth and increased awareness of nurses as persons" [21]. The nurse's experience is bound to be enlarged by attention to personhood, involvement in political activity, and the women's liberation movement. Increased growth and self-awareness among nurses can greatly increase their power potential.

The influence of the feminist movement in nursing has been substantial. It is likely that this movement in support of nursing causes will strengthen the power base of the administrative nurse by forcing confrontations with male-dominated sectors of the hospital. Wilma Scott Heide gives evidence of this possibility in her introduction to Ashley's analysis of the feminist movement in nursing:

Many men in medicine, health care and hospital administration have kept nurses powerless and inhibited the growth of nursing as a caring profession.
The real power to change lies beyond nursing's historically tragic drama of dependence and the artifices of ladylike powerlessness.
Feminist nurses invite and welcome other health care practitioners to create the kind of world where the power of love exceeds the love of power. [22]

QUESTIONS OF ETHICS

Korda describes a "jungle" approach to the acquisition and use of power. He sees it as basically physical—a matter of domination and territorial control. It helps to be tall, to have some overwhelming physical feature, and to control a strategic space such as a corner office. In meetings, powerful people do not leave early, and they force rivals to sit on their left. A large office is more powerful than a small one, and the power figure places furniture between himself and visitors. Korda's book contains many aphorisms, pontifications, and bits of advice but provides few guidelines for answering the ethical questions that are implied. To him the desire for power is what keeps most people working [23]. The power tactics in Buskirk's manual are described simply and illustrated [24]. Both books make fascinating reading, but the reader should be cautious and avoid a mechanical approach to power.

Playing the power game raises the question of the ethics involved in various strategies and tactics. Each nurse must assess the extent to which her actions become undesirably manipulative or calculating and the extent to which others may be hurt. Power tactics are not inherently or necessarily unethical, but some may be in certain contexts.

The ethical implications of power tactics cannot be overemphasized. The use of any tactic has consequences that affect the game, as well as other people, their jobs and careers. People in organizations hold strong expectations about the uses of power and will use counterstrategies to limit another's power that exceeds or runs counter to their expectations; power that is primarily directed toward satisfying selfish interests is suspect. Many persons try hard to redistribute the available resources to their own advantage, and the powerful are not always above brutality toward others. Yet power also has its obligations. People expect power-holders to help them out, to use power wisely, with judgment and discretion, and in the interests of the organization. A person who flaunts or uses power for its own sake will inevitably run into countervailing forces, including painful stress.

POWER IN THE ORGANIZATIONAL CONTEXT

Most professionals, including nurses, nowadays work within organizations [25]. These organizations provide structured job opportunities, resources, planning, goals, and clientele, which are important elements in the nurse's power base. To acquire increased power and authority, therefore, nurses need a sophisticated experiential knowledge of organizational processes and the behavior of people within them.

Organizations find professionals notably harder to deal with than other types of workers because they band together through kindred interests, which gives them the power of alliances and coalitions. Furthermore, professionals value autonomy, independence, and peer evaluation more than organizational values such as loyalty, conformity, obedience, or subservience and therefore cannot be treated like other employees, for their work means more to them than the tenets of bureaucracy. The struggle between loyalty to the profession and loyalty to the organization presents a dilemma, which the nurse can meet by developing a careful sense of her priorities, according to the situation.

Both professional and organizational loyalties are necessary. But nurses should recognize that their individual power is enhanced if higher power figures in the institution delegate legitimate authority to them. Thus a basic route to increased individual power is through climbing the administrative hierarchy, earning power through effective task performance.

The first step in acquiring positional authority is to come to grips philosophically and emotionally with the necessity for high-quality nursing administration. Not every nurse desires administrative power, but those who do must accept a new way of life, particularly in the eventual decline of active clinical skills but also in new duties, which demand new skills. The administrative nurse must come to terms with her inner conflicts concerning personality, her professional ideals, and the needs of the hospital. But for those who are so disposed, the work can be enormously rewarding.

Accepting an administrative role that one dislikes weakens one's power, because the ingredients for leadership are missing. Awareness of the sources, uses, and abuses of power is vital to the astute nursing administrator, yet some are reluctant to participate in a game played by the rules of power. It is an asset to be able to play the game with skill, although it is helpful to wear the mantle of power lightly, to use it sparingly, and to remain cautious in demonstrating it. But those who do not have power or are unwilling to use it risk losing the confidence and respect of their subordinates. To shun power entirely is to be a weak and ineffective leader.

The nursing administrator's position and title confer on her a legitimate power that is generally recognized throughout the organization. There may be disagreement about the precise scope of her power, but it is usually adequate for solving problems within the nursing department. Beyond the department itself, her power is less, for a department is more homogeneous and coherent than the organization as a whole.

The nursing administrator also has substantial reward and coercive power, based on her formal rights to hire, evaluate, promote, or discharge individuals. These activities, of course, are not substitutes for skillful leadership and motivation. If the administrator bears in mind that this power is only part of her continuing relationship with those whom she supervises, there is less danger of relying excessively on one power source or of using power for its own sake.

EXPERT POWER

The nursing administrator gains expert power from two sources: professional knowledge and administrative skill. But this duality poses an inner conflict, for the two types of expertise are not always compatible. The nursing administrator faces erosion in her clinical nursing skills, although at the same time she gains in administrative skills. Lambertsen suggests a compromise: that the nursing administrator need not be an expert clinical nurse but rather should have "an ability to make or to interpret decisions about the nursing needs of individuals, families, or other social groups" [26]. But Erickson states, "If more than superficial knowledge of nursing care practice is essential to this centralized accountability for administration of the composite activities comprising the nursing department . . . then a nurse is needed as the top-level administrator of the department" [27].

Aydelotte also recognizes this conflict: "The director of nursing is in a unique place in the organizational structure of a hospital. She is not an executive in the full sense, nor is she solely a practicing professional. She provides professional expression for the particular group she represents by initiating and encouraging innovation in its practice, by conducting research. . . . Concomitantly she exercises influence in determining goals and policy, and in directing the movement of her professional group toward departmental and institutional goals" [28]. However, one of the authors of this article found in his research that the nursing administrator has difficulty in resolving the twin pressures of the two roles [29]. She idealizes the role for which she has the least time (nursing) and resents the role that makes urgent demands on her time and energy (administration).

One takes up a profession out of fascination for its potentials for fulfillment. The nursing administrator feels, not unrealistically, that her professional role must suffer because of the immediacy of administrative burdens. She feels she has been "diverted" into administration and tends to feel guilty about neglecting her profession, the erosion of clinical skills, and the loss of close patient contact. For some people, such as a hospital administrator, administration is the profession of first choice; in nursing, it is often the result of circumstances or opportunity. The nursing administrator continues to be filled with nostalgia for the work she has given up. Unless she can reach a compromise and resolve the dilemma within herself, others will detect her confusion, and her power will be reduced and leadership weakened.

REFERENT POWER

The nursing administrator may or may not be an attractive person with enough referent power to induce others to emulate her. If she develops hostile, defensive personality patterns, her referent power is diminished.

Ideally, the nurse with a high power motivation has matured to Stage IV of McClelland's model and has enough inner resources to feel secure in her own identity and to show concern for other individuals. She is able to sublimate her personal desires to the good of the institution and to make decisions based on rational evaluation of the total situation. Emotional maturity is thus a vital part of her power base.

ASSOCIATIVE POWER

The nursing administrator has access to associative power through her contacts with general administration and with the medical staff. Physicians are clearly the superordinate power source in the health care field. Lambertsen stresses the need for coordination: "It is vital . . .

that nursing care services be coordinated with medical care services and that the congruent roles of physicians and nurses be recognized" [30]. For this to occur, there must be frequent contact and communication between nursing and medicine at all levels, thus giving the director of nursing an opportunity to utilize her associative power.

The nurse administrator also has frequent contact with higher administration and, in fact, should be a vital part of the top administrative team. Schulz and Johnson suggest "a participative management scheme, which would also utilize such techniques as management by objectives. Moreover, we suggest that a management team concept would be appropriate for most hospitals. In this arrangement the nurse administrator would essentially function as a partner with the hospital administrator and physician members of the team" [31].

But however desirable, coordination, cooperation, and collaboration do not provide lasting solutions in power struggles. As professionals, the hospital administrator, the physician, and the nursing administrator have been trained to preserve their autonomy wherever possible and to give ground grudgingly when that autonomy is under fire. But harmony and conflict can coexist; indeed the hospital may be enriched by power relations that generate innovation, adaptiveness, and change through negotiated conflict.

LOWER-PARTICIPANT POWER

The astute nursing administrator will recognize but not fear the power of her subordinates. Nurses constitute the largest health care group, usually about 60 percent of the hospital personnel. As Bowman and Culpepper state, "Nursing's greatest resource is people. For too long nurses have underestimated the power they have in being the largest group of health professionals in the nation. If nurses as a group mobilized for patient advocacy, they could radically change the picture of health care delivery in the United States" [32].

The power of subordinates is collective, for in a one-to-one relationship the superior wins, though perhaps only in the short run. The nurse administrator must relate effectively to staff members individually and as a group since, "The power of a leader, and hence his effectiveness, is dependent upon the willingness of his subordinates to accept and support him" [33].

The nursing administrator can utilize subordinate power very effectively for the benefit of patients and her institution. Lambertsen states, "The potential and actual dimensions of the role of the nursing service administrator in achieving coordination of patient care are limitless. It is her key role and the reason for the existence of her position. Administrators of nursing services are a crucial group, for it is only through creative leadership at this level that the goals of nursing care for patients and families can be realized" [34].

DEPENDENCY AND THE NEGOTIATED ORDER

Dependency is a key aspect of power. In this context, nurses and other professionals are relatively dependent on hospitals and other organizations for clients, rewards, and opportunities to develop themselves, continue their careers, and minister to the sick. This is a constraint on the nurse's power. On the other hand, the organization is highly dependent upon its nursing staff and the individual nurse's capabilities, although if there is a large supply of nurses, the organization may regard any individual as dispensable. Nurses derive power from their expertise through the availability of alternative opportunities; they may leave one organization for another, return to nonadministrative duty, avoid organizational life by going into private practice, or even leave the profession.

Administrators often dislike the independence that professionals display, and many of them fear the power that groups can wield in the formal structure. Those who believe in an autocratic or even a benevolent management style find it difficult to accept group-participative structures, yet every administrator must work in and through groups as well as with individuals. Therefore nursing leaders and administrators, to be effective, must give special attention to forms of power that derive from group situations. Preferably leaders use this power responsibly and within appropriate boundaries and for the good of the organization rather than for personal prestige and status [35].

Within the organization, power shifts continually among individuals and among groups; it is distributed by negotiation. In addition to a personal role, the individual also has roles in both the group and the organization, so intergroup power is a key concept, because individual power derives largely from membership in a group. For most nurses, the staff of a department or floor unit in a hospital is the primary group, and the hospital as a whole represents a secondary attachment. Both alignments are important and are intertwined to some extent. The route to greater power for the individual nurse, therefore, is to develop strategies for participating in the power negotiations among different groups.

The three main groups involved in the hospital inter-group power system are the administration, the medical staff, and the nursing staff. An individual, such as a nursing administrator, may belong to more than one group at the same time. The three groups function with each other under a balance of power that represents a negotiated order. The general character of this order remains generally stable over time, although specific issues or events may cause temporary realignments [36]. Each of the three centers is itself a cluster of power centers that may or may not correspond to departments or other structural units. Here too, there is a generally stable pattern, but one that reflects realignments of the negotiated order over time.

To participate effectively in this negotiated order, nurses need group leaders who have enough personal and positional power to represent their constituencies. Balance of power among the groups is maintained only by continuous surveillance and by solving the problems of power distribution. If power is not evenly distributed among key groups, it can result in lower morale or the malfunctioning of the groups that are losing ground. The main determinants of intergroup power are: (1) whether a group (such as nursing) can successfully cope with and control uncertainty; (2) whether the group can provide substitutes for the activities and services of another group, and (3) whether the group is important as an integrative mechanism with other groups [37].

The ability to reduce uncertainty confers power on the group by creating dependencies. If future events are hard to predict, if tasks are relatively unstructured, and if information is uncertain, a group may gain power by developing coping activities that reduce uncertainty for other groups. In nursing, coping activities can be used to achieve an effect on power. Future conditions can be portrayed as uncertain; task performance can be made ambiguous, and normal flows of information can be disrupted or made uncertain. Such coping activities, however, can also provide a positive potential source of power for nursing because of the close working relationship between nursing and other departments of the hospital.

There is an inverse relationship between substitutability and power. That is, the more difficult it is to find substitutes for a group's services and resources, the greater that group's power is. In complex systems this power ensues from the effects that occur if services or expertise needed by other units or persons are withdrawn. Withdrawal of services may sometimes be effective as a threat rather than an actuality, but power wanes if the threatened action never occurs. Actual withdrawal is disruptive if there are no satisfactory substitutes for the services denied, causing the target group to try to avoid its occurrence. In nursing there is partial substitutability for the services of RNs to the extent that LPNs, nurses' aides, or candy stripers can fulfill some of their functions during periods of conflict. This substitutability, in addition to questions of professional ethics, makes withdrawal a relatively undesirable source of power and therefore one that must be used only as a last resort.

A group's integrative importance depends on the extent to which its resources or activities are connected to the resources or activities of other groups and the impact on the organization's performance if the group were eliminated or performed poorly. From this perspective, nursing has a high degree of integrative impact, which strengthens its power.

The negotiated order resulting from the interaction of groups may be produced through tacit or explicit agreements covering exchanges or interactions to take place over time. Another way is by structuring the group so as to include the dissenting or disruptive persons from other groups, which permits surveillance of their opposition and provides an opportunity to indoctrinate them and persuade them to go along with the power center. This strategy, called co-optation, risks giving the opposition opportunities for counterefforts conducted from the inside. Thus incorporating dissenting forces has a price, since those forces must see some advantages in their inclusion.

A third way to negotiate intergroup power relationships is through the political strategy of a coalition, that is, two or more groups joining forces to achieve mutually desired goals. An organization almost always requires a dominant coalition to provide direction, control, conflict resolution, and common goals. In a hospital, for example, administrators, medical staff, and nursing may form a coalition to dominate the rest of the organization, or any two groups may attempt to dominate the third. However, coalitions tend to break down as the interests and strategies of the member groups change.

Power within the organization should ultimately be viewed as an influence process that is shaped by the context of the organization, its formal and informal group structure, and the power of individual members. These components are in a state of dynamic equilibrium, with interdependent elements; changes in one sector can be expected to produce changes in one or more of the other sectors.

The power of the individual nurse and of the nursing staff is therefore closely related to the nature and goals of the organization. In this connection, King notes that no other group of health professionals provides services in such a wide variety of organizations—schools; industries; official and voluntary agencies; hospitals of various size, purpose, and ownership; nursing homes; extended care facilities; model cities programs; neigborhood health clinics; and crisis, drug, and alcohol centers [38].

This range of organizational settings poses two problems for nursing in relation to power. The first is that, for nursing generally, power is highly diffused among sub-groups which may disagree with one another over key issues that affect them differently. The second is that individual nurses and nursing administrators must be alert to great differences in the contexts within which power is sought and applied.

The nurse's multiple spheres of influence can provide opportunities for increased power, but they can also lead to diminished power unless the nurse overcomes the problems of communication and physical separation that otherwise may prevail.

Nursing's organizational power base develops from each individual's investment in the goals of the organization, and the structure of the organization reflects and facilitates this power base, with power taking the form of control over outcomes in which all members of a coalition have an investment [39]. Therefore the decisions of a group or its leader tend to be consistent with its base of power [40].

As health care organizations lose more and more of their autonomy to external groups such as government agencies, review boards, planning councils, and the like, the sources of internal power may become eroded. The organization becomes relatively powerless within its own domain and in attempts to change the domain. The power of nursing in the organization is therefore in danger of declining in strength, so nurses should examine the power relationships that prevail for professionals in society as a whole [41, 42].

POWER, SOCIETY, AND NURSING

Nursing relates to other groups in society through its status as an emerging professional occupation and through interaction with other parts of the health care system. Professional attributes influence nursing's role in health care, but these attributes in turn are conditioned by the values and beliefs pervasive in society.

Nursing works within an implied social charter that gives the profession visibility, legitimacy, and power. At the same time, society constrains and regulates nursing through laws, customs, and expectations to assure responsible performance of the profession's work. Peer review and control of educational requirements and of admission to practice are devices used jointly by government units and the profession to provide a regulated field of endeavor serving important social or human needs.

Society not only makes demands, it also provides resources for meeting them; the public interest is protected by government agencies at the federal, state, and local levels. The decision-making mechanisms are inordinately complex and growing more complicated almost daily.

Nursing is not fully established as a profession in the narrowest sociological definition of the term, which holds that there should be specialized knowledge, formal training, an organized association, ethical codes, and autonomy. For nursing, the missing ingredient is autonomy [43], defined as the right of self-determination and governance without outside control. Individual practitioners are self-regulating and have control over their work functions. However, sociologists recognize that many occupations, including nursing, are emerging as professions, and these are technically considered "qualifying associations." Jones and Jones believe that nursing is in a strong position to consolidate its strengths and achieve ultimate autonomy [44].

Individual autonomy is promoted by the collective autonomy inherent in the concept of a profession [45]. Christman argues that nursing staffs should have parity with the medical and administrative staffs, thus freeing nurses from hierarchical controls, requirements for permissions and consultations, and excessive supervision [46]. He argues also that nurses should have direct relationships to and responsibilities for their patients. Nevertheless, complete autonomy would require greater independence from physicians and thus may not be attainable; Christman's concept appears difficult to put into operation [47].

The debate over autonomy is somewhat academic in that it represents an ideal, and it is only one of many criteria defining an occupation as a profession. Other criteria should be recognized, such as skilled training, service orientation, and the like. The focus of any field, including nursing, is the attitudes of its practitioners. Nursing's status as an emergent profession is to be found in the attitudes, philosophies, beliefs, and behavior of its members.

In practice, nursing has a degree of autonomy and independence, coupled with social and ethical guidelines for achieving society's ends. According to Freidson, the leaders of an occupation persuade the establishment that its members possess a technical competence so important to the public and so special that no other occupation with the same domain but with lesser competence or integrity should be legitimized [48]. This is how the "license and mandate" of the profession are obtained.

A profession unites its members by maintaining a communications system, by providing a focus for identifying with each other and with the group, and by providing services, such as educational opportunities, publications, job placement, and so on. An organized profession also has maintenance and self-protective functions, such as legislative lobbying and working through political and social channels to acquire and maintain benefits for its members. It regulates admission through an examining board.

Although the existence of a health care crisis can be argued, there is little doubt that accelerating medical technologies and service demands are creating pressure on various parts of the system. As cohesive, identifiable groups within the health care system work for the interests they deem important, their activities, beliefs, values, and philosophies will often be in conflict with those of other groups. Hence power is important in enabling the nursing profession to relate to the other groups. In the years ahead the profession will be immersed in struggles with the other power centers to protect and enhance its power in society as well as in the system, whose parts will continually be reshaped to meet society's changing and developing needs [49]. As a well-organized profession, nursing can serve both society and its members well, provided that it exercises legitimate power with appropriate ethics and competent practices.

Neither the existing power centers nor the decision mechanisms are set for all time. Although it is difficult to predict future power shifts, one can understand their nature by examining the history of the past few decades. According to Ginzberg, three innovations have led to important power shifts in the health care system: the improved education and training of increasingly more specialized physicians, the improved capabilities of hospitals to provide effective therapy, and the growth of new financial systems through insurance and governmental programs. This transformation of modern medicine has brought changes in the relative power of interest groups. Early power centers, such as the American Medical Association, philanthropic groups, and state and local governments, have suffered a relative loss of power, while the power of nursing, biomedical research, the educational establishment, the federal government, labor unions, and commercial and nonprofit insurance channels has increased [50].

From a societal point of view, this loosely structured, diverse power system with its multiple points of decision making poses difficult problems of control and of responsiveness to consumer needs. Nursing along with other health care groups is likely to be involved in conflicts with consumers, other providers, and government bodies. There are also conflicts within the health care system in the changing roles of nurses versus those of physicians, nursing paraprofessionals, and administrators.

Using conflict and change constructively entails paying attention to the way the power game is played. In such struggles, the outcomes are most likely to depend on control of resources, such as people, money, knowledge, facilities, technology, and so on; a large factor will be the flow and allocation of dollars.

INTEGRATION OF POWER CONCEPTS

We have examined power relationships in nursing at three levels: the individual, the organization, and society, categories that reflect the usual research design. But for a fuller understanding of power we need an integrative model that relates the findings from the three levels of analysis. Kemelgor has developed a linkage model for power showing the key interdependencies [51]. This model, shown in Figure 38-2, suggests areas of research that could result in important payoffs for nursing administration. He concludes that interdisciplinary research is required to trace sequences and cause-and-effect relationships and to take account of human variability inherent in the power process.

All this suggests that power is a fruitful area of research for nursing administrators, one that can yield practical benefits as nurses become more aware of their potential for a constructive role in the power systems in which they work.

Figure 38-3 shows the interrelatedness of social, group, and personal systems, in all of which power is a main element. These systems are dynamic, meaning that a change in one is very likely to generate changes in the others. There is a divisive tension in organizations, in part resulting from the conflicting interests of individuals and groups and from competitive struggles among them. To offset these tensions and hold the organization together, certain members, usually administrators, are charged with responsibility for coordination and control. Those who have power may thus be either the cause of divisiveness or the corrective agents. Stability results when power is wisely directed toward organizational purpose and when the power strategies are balanced so that the dominant coalitions or power centers are aware of their limitations. Thus power is both the social glue that holds the organization together and the source of its dynamism, which can lead to conflict, divisiveness, and change [52].

The emergent role of nurses in health care organizations is one of coordination and integration. Staff and head nurses, for example, coordinate through feedback—that is, through communication leading to adaptation in contingencies, as contrasted with coordination through rigid scheduling, specialization and other forms of standardization [53]. Coordination by feedback is provided mainly through the nurse's professional status, with a considerable amount of discretion. Also, the professional nurse's crucial position in the network of communication and coordination increases her opportunity and capacity to absorb uncertainty. This in turn yields power through the effects of decentralization of authority on the influence structure of the organization [54].

Arndt and Huckabay believe that nursing administration should have an integrative role in the total system [55]. Their systems concept of integration holds that administrators must see any one change as the first of a series of changes within the system or even of change of the whole system. Administrators should know that symptoms are rarely problems and that the effectiveness of the system cannot be measured according to one criterion, ignoring others.

If the political aspects of an organization are cohesive, well understood, and well managed, they can provide an integrating force. Rather than believing that politics is "dirty," we consider it a force for good in the health care system, because the task of ordering means to ends can help the administrator and other power figures act more humanely. To recognize political processes is to recognize the systems nature of an organization. To deny the existence of a health care system, as some researchers do, is to deny that it is, in part, a political entity [56].

Coalitions provide balance of power and thus a degree of integration. Balance reflects agreement, if only temporary, over the legitimate distribution of power among constituent groups, and authenticates the coalition's norms and role prescriptions. An unbalanced relationship is unstable, for it encourages members of an organization to use power in such a way that they reduce their cost of meeting the demands of other power centers. Power networks in a coalition are generally complex, with many variations in the interaction

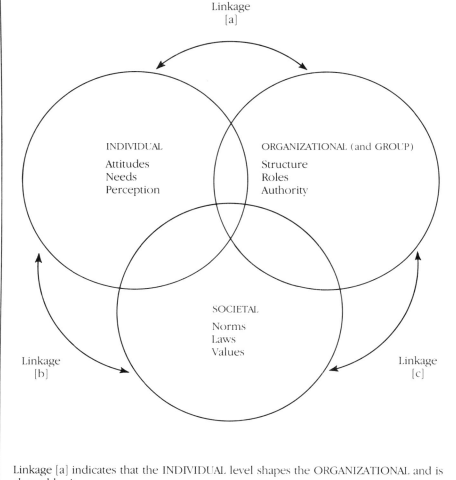

Linkage
[a]

INDIVIDUAL

Attitudes
Needs
Perception

ORGANIZATIONAL (and GROUP)

Structure
Roles
Authority

SOCIETAL

Norms
Laws
Values

Linkage
[b]

Linkage
[c]

Linkage [a] indicates that the INDIVIDUAL level shapes the ORGANIZATIONAL and is shaped by it.

Linkage [b] indicates that the ORGANIZATIONAL level shapes the SOCIETAL and is shaped by it.

Linkage [c] indicates that the SOCIETAL level shapes the INDIVIDUAL and is shaped by it.

Figure 38-2. The inherent linkages between the various levels in the power process. (Source: Bruce H. Kemelgor, "Power and the Power Process: Linkage Concepts," *Academy of Management Review* 1 [October 1976], p. 144. Used by permission.)

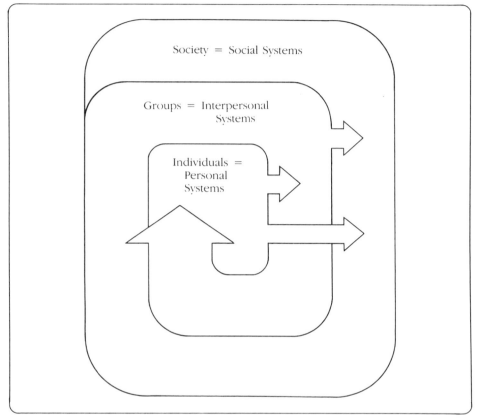

Figure 38-3. Dynamic interaction systems. (Source: Imogene King, *Toward a Theory of Nursing.* New York: John Wiley & Sons, 1971.)

patterns, the relative status, and degree of dependency of its members, and in the use of rewards to influence the distribution of power with respect to these elements [57]. Nursing leaders should be aware of the ebb and flow of coalitions and of alignments of the weak and the strong. In coalitions involving physicians or administrators, nursing leadership can be a force for maintaning an effective balance.

CONCLUSION

In a complex organization, *power, authority,* and *control* have great impact on nurses' careers and on the performance of nursing functions. Therefore the nurse leader needs to think carefully about such questions as: What is the nature of power in this institution? How is power organized, used, and distributed here? How can I gain sufficient power, control, and authority to do my job? How do I use power and authority? Within a large system, nurse leaders are involved in various kinds of power strategies, so they must be attentive to such phenomena as coalitions, caucuses, power shifts, cliques, and an array of power games. A nurse administrator must seek ways to gain, retain, and even trade off power in order to be an effective member of the organization [58].

These questions are especially important if the nurse is to be an agent of change for the better. As Alexander has succinctly stated:

The power structure is an important part of our culture that affects significantly the number and range of alternatives that are available to individuals in an organization. There are no easy or even reasonably successful ways to effect a broadening of alternatives available to those in positions of no power. If nurses or other groups have no power within the organizational structure to effect necessary change, they have the alternative of working with external forces to effect these changes. The rational nurse-leaders who are agents of change should recognize its limits and should seek to understand the way those who control the situation organize it to their thinking. [59]

While power is by no means the sole motivation in the nursing profession, it is a fact of life which influences the ability of the profession to develop, grow, maintain itself, and achieve its primary missions in patient care.

REFERENCES

1. Lasswell, H. *Psychopathology and Politics.* New York: Viking Press, 1960, p. 104.
2. Zaleznik, A., and Kets DeVries, M. F. *Power and the Corporate Mind.* Boston: Houghton Mifflin, 1975, p. 8.
3. Mechanic, D. Sources of power of lower participants. *Administrative Science Quarterly*, 7:351, 1962.
4. Smith, D. B., and Kaluzny, A. D. *The White Labyrinth.* Berkeley: McCutcheon, 1975, p. 182.
5. Zaleznik, A., and Kets DeVries, M. F. 1975, pp. 71–72.
6. Metcalf, H. C., and Urwick, L. *Dynamic Administration: The Collected Papers of Mary Parker Follett.* New York: Harper & Row, 1940, chap. 4.
7. McClelland, D. C. *Power: The Inner Experience.* New York: Irvington, 1975, chap. 2.
8. Zaleznik, A., and Kets DeVries, M. F. 1975, p. 3.
9. McClelland, D. C. 1975, p. 21.
10. Wieland, G. F., and Ullrich, R. A. *Organizations: Behavior, Design, and Change.* Homewood, Ill.: Richard D. Irwin, 1976, p. 248.
11. Wieland, G. F., and Ullrich, R. A. 1976, pp. 251–252.
12. Kramer, M. *Reality Shock: Why Nurses Leave Nursing.* St. Louis: C. V. Mosby, 1975.
13. Rushmer, R. F. *Humanizing Health Care: Alternative Futures for Medicine.* Cambridge, Mass.: M.I.T. Press, 1975, pp. 99–102.
14. Martin, N. H., and Sims, J. H. Thinking ahead: power tactics. *Harvard Business Review*, 34:25–29, 1956.
15. Polk, D. A. Women in the corporation: one man's view. *National Association of Bank Women Journal*, 53:20, 1977.
16. McClelland, D. C. 1975, p. 75.
17. McClelland, D. C. 1975, p. 95.
18. McClelland, D. C. 1975, pp. 81–90.

19. Martin, L. L. View from the Firing Line: Family Nurse Practitioner in California. In Bullough, B. (Ed.), *The Law and the Expanding Nursing Role*. New York: Appleton-Century-Crofts, 1975, pp. 95–117.
20. Epstein, C. F. Ambiguity as Social Control: Consequence for the Integration of Women in Professional Elites. In Stewart, P. L., and Cantor, M. G., *Varieties of Work Experience: The Social Control of Occupational Groups and Roles*. New York: John Wiley & Sons, 1974, pp. 26–38.
21. Donovan, H. M. *Nursing Service Administration: Managing the Enterprise*. St. Louis: C. V. Mosby, 1975, p. 118.
22. Heide, W. S., introduction to Ashley, J., *Hospitals, Paternalism, and the Role of the Nurse*. New York: Teachers College Press, 1976, pp. v–viii.
23. Korda, M. *Power: How to Get It, How to Use It*. New York: Random House, 1975.
24. Buskirk, R. A. *Handbook of Managerial Tactics*. Boston: Cahners Books, 1976.
25. Hughes, E. C. *Men and Their Work*. New York: Free Press, 1958, p. 133.
26. Lambertsen, E. C. A greater voice for nursing service administrators. *Hospitals*, 46(7):101–108, 1972.
27. Erickson, E. H. Are nurses needed for administration or management in hospitals? *J. Nurs. Admin*. 4(3):20–21, 1974.
28. Aydelotte, M. D. Administration and directors of nursing. *Hospitals*, 48(23):61–63, 1974.
29. McFarland, D. E. *Managerial Innovation and Change in the Metropolitan Hospital*. New York: Praeger, 1979.
30. Lambertsen, E. C. 1972, p. 104.
31. Schulz, R., and Johnson, A. C. *Management of Hospitals*. New York: McGraw-Hill, 1976, p. 105.
32. Bowman, R. A., and Culpepper, R. C. Power: Rx for change. *Am. J. Nurs*. 74(6):1056, 1974.
33. Divincenti, M. *Administering Nursing Service*. Boston: Little, Brown, 1972, p. 48.
34. Lambertsen, E. C. 1972, p. 108.
35. Alexander, E. L. *Nursing Administration in the Hospital Health Care System*. St. Louis: C. V. Mosby, 1972, p. 205.
36. Strauss, A. et al. The Hospital and Its Negotiated Order. In Freidson, E. (Ed.), *The Hospital in Modern Society*. New York: Free Press, 1963, pp. 147–169.
37. Ivancevich, J. S., Szilagyi, A. D., and Wallace, M. J., Jr. *Organizational Behavior and Performance*. Santa Monica, Cal.: Goodyear, 1977, pp. 249–251.
38. King, I. M. The Health Care System: Nursing Intervention Subsystem. In Werley, H. H. et al. (Eds.), *Health Research: The Systems Approach*. New York: Springer, 1976, pp. 51–60.
39. Emerson, R. M. Power-dependence relations. *American Sociological Review*, 27:31–41, 1962.
40. Crandall, N. F. Power, Influence, and Organizational Decisions. In *Proceedings of the 8th Annual Meeting Southeast Division*. American Institute for Decision Sciences, 1978, pp. 71–73.
41. Pugh, D. S. et al. The context of organization structure. *Administrative Science Quarterly*, 14:91–114, 1969.
42. Jacobs, D. Dependency and vulnerability: an exchange approach to the control of organizations. *Administrative Science Quarterly*, 19:45–59, 1974.
43. Maas, M. L. Nurse Autonomy and Accountability in Organized Nursing Services. In Stone, S. et al. (Eds.), *Management for Nurses: A Multidisciplinary Approach*. St. Louis: C. V. Mosby, 1976, pp. 45–46.
44. Jones, R. K. and Jones, P. A. *Sociology in Medicine*. New York: John Wiley & Sons, 1975, p. 159.
45. Maas, M. L. 1976, pp. 35–36.

46. Christman, L. The autonomous nursing staff in the hospital. *Nurs. Admin. Quart.* 1:37–44, 1976.
47. Freidson, E. *Profession of Medicine: A Study in the Sociology of Applied Knowledge.* New York: Dodd, Mead, 1970, pp. 63–66.
48. Freidson, E. The Impurity of Professional Authority. In Becker, H. et al. (Eds.), *Institutions and the Person.* Chicago: Aldine, 1968, p. 32.
49. Ginzberg, E. Health Services, Power Centers, and Decision-Making Mechanisms. In Knowles, J. H. (Ed.), *Doing Better and Feeling Worse: Health in the United States.* New York: W. W. Norton, 1977, p. 203.
50. Ginzberg, E. 1977, pp. 203–205.
51. Kemelgor, B. H. Power and the power process: linkage concepts. *Academy of Management Review,* 1:143–149, 1976.
52. Smith, D. B., and Kaluzny, A. D. 1975, pp. 180–183.
53. March, J. G., and Simon, H. A. *Organizations.* New York: John Wiley & Sons, 1958, pp. 160–161.
54. Heydebrand, W. V. *Hospital Bureaucracy: A Cooperative Study of Organizations.* New York: Dunellen, 1973, pp. 210–211.
55. Arndt, C., and Huckabay, L. M. D. *Nursing Administration: Theory for Practice with a Systems Approach.* St. Louis: C. V. Mosby, 1975, p. 277.
56. Donovan, H. M. 1975, pp. 44–45.
57. Emerson, R. M. 1962, pp. 40–41.
58. Leininger, M. The leadership crisis in nursing; a critical problem and challenge. *J. Nurs. Admin.* VIII:32, 1974.
59. Alexander, E. L. 1972, p. 162.

39 Exercising Leadership Behaviors in a Bureaucratic Structure

Geoffry McEnany

INTRODUCTION

I see myself as an explorer moving through a series of journeys that will provide me with new insights about myself as a professional nurse. This chapter tells about an exploration I undertook into a bureaucratic structure as a senior nursing student at the University of San Francisco School of Nursing.

At the University of San Francisco's School of Nursing, all senior nursing students are required to be enrolled in a fourteen-week course in nursing leadership with corresponding theoretical and clinical components designed to assist students in developing knowledge and skill in the use of leadership behavior. Students are encouraged to develop independence and latitude in its development. One of the focal points of this course was to understand how the bureaucratic health care delivery system functions and how that functioning affects the well-being of patients and clients. Access to such a system affords nursing students a variety of channels through which they may develop their leadership abilities.

The basis for my clinical "exploration" is the use of two theoretical frameworks; the Yura, Ozimek, and Walsh framework for nursing leadership, and Orem's self-care model, adapted by Underwood, for use in the care of psychiatric clients.

THE TERRITORY

The "Tenderloin" is a rundown section of San Francisco bordered by the financial and business districts of the city. It is a community both bizarre and contradictory, home for many of the city's indigent peoples—refugees, poor families, destitute elderly, the homeless "street people," and, at the same time, home for thousands of transient, affluent tourists who temporarily reside in its many "chain" hotels. The seemingly transient atmosphere of the Tenderloin is deceptive; one can easily be fooled by the endless array of bars, peep shows, adult book stores, and massage parlors. As a newcomer to the Tenderloin, I had to allow myself to look beyond the derelicts that line the streets and the "bag ladies" who finger the contents of refuse containers with the discriminating eye of an expert shopper. Survival is the name of the game and fear is the universal feeling in this environment that is both life-sustaining and life-threatening. Hardship, isolation, aloneness, and, most of all, debilitating loneliness make the Tenderloin an encapsulated hell for many of its residents. This is where I would spend fourteen weeks and where—good or bad—I would learn about nursing leadership.

THE BUREAUCRATIC MAZE

The Tenderloin teems with resident hotels, bars, and flop houses. A circuit of social supports such as meal programs for the poor, senior citizen centers, and a variety of health care delivery agencies located in the area attempt, sometimes against overwhelming odds, to meet the physical and mental health needs of its residents. My clinical experience began in one of these agencies, a city-funded outpatient mental health center for the elderly.

The mental health center was housed in a small building wedged between the auspicious and imposing San Francisco Mint and an inauspicious and unimposing San Francisco fire station. On a mild day, the sidewalks of this short street are lined with defenseless, helpless men in varying degrees of intoxication to whom the street offers a few moments of uninterrupted oblivion.

At first glance, the clinic appeared ordinary; clients waited to be seen in a small, innocuous waiting room just inside the front door. A series of offices lined the long corridor leading to the rear of the clinic. Downstairs, more windowless offices completed what must have seemed like a maze in a rabbit warren.

How do I begin to make sense out of the physical and mental maze that I see and feel? This feeling began in a meeting with the director of the agency. I was handed several organizational charts, all of which seemed complex and unintelligible. But as the director droned on I began to see that *he* understood them—*he* saw the relationship between one line and another—*he* understood their function. I was overwhelmed by the realization that there was validity to my feeling that I was "low man on the totem pole." This is where I felt I would always be if I did not make a concerted effort to "know my local maze."

I wondered with great concern how I would ever be able to exhibit leadership behaviors when everyone in the clinic seemed more of a leader than I. Scanning the organizational charts, I saw where nursing had been placed; in a minuscule box in the lower right hand corner of one of the charts. So much for professional status. There was only one staff nurse, and he was ultimately accountable to eight people in management positions. All but one of the eight positions were filled by professional, non-nursing personnel. "Welcome to the land of bureaucracy," I thought to myself.

Following my meeting with the director, I met the staff of the mental health center. Employees of the center consisted predominantly of social workers, paraprofessionals, and psychiatrists. The sole staff nurse explained the functions of the clinic, its role in the community, and the clinical duties of the staff. The roles of the various staff members appeared to overlap considerably. For example, the staff nurses' functions were similar to social workers and paraprofessional mental health workers. Nevertheless, all nonadministrative personnel worked to help elderly psychiatric clients maintain their ability to live as independently as possible in the community. Home visits to clients were routinely done by staff members in an effort to assess clients' psychosocial status, provide supportive therapy or crisis intervention, and collect data on an ongoing basis to maintain updated plans of treatment. When the needs of a client exceeded the resources of the mental health center, the staff would frequently make referrals to other community agencies to ensure that the social and medical needs of the clients were met.

Clients seemed well cared for, in the traditional sense of caring. From what I observed, the agency's staff were doing their jobs insofar as the caretakers were rendering services *for* the client. However, I noticed a moderate degree of passivity on the part of clients as they were processed through a very complex system. The caretakers were doing *all* of the work while clients relinquished their responsibility for their care to others; those who are being helped were being rendered helpless by the helpers!

The initial concerns I had regarding my role and objectives for nursing leadership began to dissolve as my assessment progressed. Nursing, in my estimation, did not offer anything unique to the system of care delivery in the clinic except for medication administration; the void in the delivery of care was disturbing. Clients' charts were medically oriented, and nursing care plans were nonexistent. Client "treatment plans" were created by physicians and were used by all caretakers. The specialized services that nurses *could* offer were being disregarded; nurses functioned as just another cog in the bureaucratic machinery, offering a homogenized version of care that mirrored the work of other non-nursing professionals in the clinic. How could a professional nurse survive this bureaucratic maze? Already I felt overwhelmed and stifled.

Further examination of the system was essential. I proceeded to learn more about the work in which nurses were involved with clients, as well as the role of the nurse in interagency collaboration, because it would lend a balanced perspective of the overall functioning of the nurse within the agency. For the next three weeks, I accompanied the clinic nurse on home visits, to interagency meetings, and spent a substantial amount of time observing the agency and the people it served.

Upon completion of my assessment, I identified three needs for the clinic nursing personnel and their clients:

1. Nursing services needed to be clearly differentiated from other disciplines within the clinic.
2. A philosophical or theoretical framework to guide nursing care delivery needed to be established which emphasized self-care, not the perpetuation of chronicity in psychiatric clients within the community.
3. A method was needed to ensure the consistency of care delivered to clients by nurses.

Thinking I had a solid idea of some of the needs of the clients and staff, I began to formulate a plan that I hoped would yield a change in the system. As I began the change process, I realized how David must have felt as he faced the giant.

GETTING IT ALL TOGETHER

I decided that the framework for nursing care delivery which suited my outlined needs for the agency and its clients was the "self-care model," adapted by Underwood from Orem's universal theory on self-care. Underwood's adaptation essentially contours the category of the Orem model to the needs of institutionalized psychiatric clients. Underwood's adaptation did not include psychiatric clients within the community. I felt that this would be a golden opportunity to see if this model could be used effectively outside an institutional setting. The self-care categories are:

1. Demand for air, food, fluid
2. Elimination
3. Body temperature and personal hygiene
4. Rest and activity
5. Solitude and social interaction [1]

Frequently, psychiatric clients experiencing internal disorganization lose some or all of the abilities to discern their basic needs in the five areas outlined in Underwood's model. In such instances, the role of the nurse is to assist the client in regaining his self-care abilities.

This type of nursing intervention minimizes the clients' dependence on health care support systems while maximizing their potential for maintaining independent living.

The central focus of nursing using the self-care model is teaching. Implementing the self-care model involves accurate assessment of the clients' deficits in self-care activities, mutual goal setting between client and nurse, planning methods for how the goals will be met, and evaluating the clients' ability to follow through with actions necessary to meet the self-care goals. As the client becomes more independent in his abilities to care for himself, "hands on" nursing intervention is withdrawn; the nurse supports the client's ability to care for himself and offers appropriate feedback as he does so.

Positive reinforcement and support are essential if self-care is to be successful. Using the self-care approach, I was essentially asking clients to relinquish their dependence on caretakers. In all likelihood, this approach would be met with resistance from clients. Substituting meaningful reinforcements as a client moves toward independence in self-care would become my primary role.

The list of needs I had formulated from my assessment of the agency and clients made me feel that I had made it to first base in my clinical experience. I was *sure* that they would give me an opportunity to exhibit nursing leadership behavior. Within the Yura, Ozimek, and Walsh framework of nursing leadership, I felt that I had thoroughly completed the requirements of the *deciding* component of leadership, that is, I felt I had a sound basis for making judgments and that basis rested on my knowledge and skills. I was now ready to embark upon the work of the *relating* component, a leadership component based on establishing productive relationships [2].

The director of the clinic, my preceptor, and I met to discuss the possibility of using Underwood's self-care framework in delivering nursing care. During our meeting, I presented the administrator and the nurse with copies of data-base assessment tools, samples of care plans and medication teaching plans developed by Underwood for implementing self-care nursing. I explained the function of the tools and discussed my belief that using the self-care model could vastly improve nursing care. The director listened and my preceptor supported my plan with nods and affirmative statements. When I had completed my presentation, the clinic director continued to pensively examine the written information I had provided on self-care. After a moment's pause, he told me that my plan would be "taken under consideration."

A week later, the director asked to meet with me again; I sat in the office feeling like I was waiting for a judge to deliver a verdict. After what felt like a moment of agonizing silence, the director told me that I could implement the self-care model with clients in my care *only*, providing "it did not interfere with the present functioning of the clinic system." He asked that at the end of my fourteen-week experience the model be reassessed for future use with agency clients. In the meantime, however, I was given the opportunity to present the self-care model to the agency staff during a team conference. Possibly because of the large number of professional, non-nursing personnel present, the degree of interest was varied. The group cautiously supported the idea of change, much to the distress of the clinic director. I was not surprised that many staff members did not overtly support my plan, in light of the director's resistance to change.

During several confidential conversations with my preceptor, prior to the team conference, I was warned of a malignant conditon among clinic caretakers coined as "professional suffocation." What this amounts to is, "Do not make waves if you want to survive in the system." Introducing change is considered unleashing a tidal wave at the clinic, especially since it involves pointing out inadequacies in the present mode of operations at the agency.

In turn, this may be perceived as threatening by the administrator, who has the power to make life difficult while on the job for those who rock the boat. The second lesson in bureaucracy became evident: small changes in the system can be considered major victories.

During my weekly home visits with clients, I began to introduce the concept of self-care by discussing methods of how they could begin to take more responsibility for themselves in their daily living. I developed nursing care plans in accordance with the self-care model and the data I gathered from my visits. These plans would serve as the basis for "nurse-client contracts," which I hoped would make clients more accountable for their own care.

Having completed all of the preparatory work in making "all systems go," I felt that I was now ready to put my plan into action. The task ahead was to use the leadership component of influencing, which, according to Yura, Ozimek, and Walsh, involved my knowledge, skill, and ability to establish relationships in working to achieve the nursing care I had planned [3].

FROM PLANS TO ACTION

For the next ten weeks, I provided feedback to various members of the agency staff about the progress of my clients and my efforts in using the self-care model. Very few members of the staff inquired about the effectiveness of self-care nursing. Discussion with some staff members gave me insight into their silence, which confirmed my suspicions: the director had reservations about making major changes in the role of nurses in the clinic. By virtue of my presence, I symbolized a conflict in the system, and staff were very careful in offering support of my work, for fear of being perceived by the director as siding with my cause. Realizing how this dynamic could affect the chances of nursing personnel's use of the self-care model after I completed the lab, I seized every opportunity available to reinforce my beliefs about the model. My preceptor became a very important person as I asked him to convey verbal progress reports about my use of self-care nursing during his weekly meetings with the director. Because I did not have access to weekly conferences with the director of the clinic, I saw this utilizaton of my preceptor as the best method of influencing the administration.

During this period, I found that a positive attitude, coupled with humor, was an indispensable tool in effecting change and humanizing a rigid system delightfully.

I found several approaches that were helpful in assisting my clients to assume more responsibility in self-care. Informal "contracts," written and signed by the client and nurse, proved beneficial to the client. The "contracts" served as reminders to clients to follow through with self-care in the absence of the nurse. For example, "Mrs. B.," a depressed client, had deficits in self-care in the category of Personal Hygiene, but was not fully aware of her need for improvement in this area. She and I negotiated a contract that spelled out what she needed to do every day to take care of hygiene needs. Sometimes the contract took the form of a daily checklist that we had mutually developed. During subsequent home visits, the checklist was reviewed and modified according to Mrs. B.'s ability to follow through with meeting the tasks independently. For clients with more severe limitations, a checklist proved futile. In those instances, a referral for a homemaker or home health aide who could visit daily to physically or verbally assist the client was more appropriate.

Using the *influencing* component of nursing leadership, self-care was accomplished in a variety of ways. When needs were identified by the client or myself, and mutual goals were established, I encouraged my clients to assume more responsibility in problem solving. For example, "J.W.," an eighty-one-year-old socially isolated woman, needed to improve her self-care in the area of solitude/social interaction. With J.W., I assisted her in seeking out resources in the community and had her make the contacts with the community resources independently. I found that using self-care techniques helped to reinforce the client's belief that he is *functional* and *effective* in his abilities. Nurses are often *too* ready to do something *for* the client that he can do for himself.

THE RESULTS

During my final week at the mental health center, I met with the agency director as planned to discuss the results of using the self-care model and its possible use by agency nursing personnel. I sat in the office alone and was acutely aware of the absence of supporting staff members. I realized that the meeting would yield a decision about implementing the self-care model; this was my opportunity to facilitate utilization of the framework by nursing personnel in the agency. I felt like an attorney about to present a case.

The advantages of self-care nursing, its acceptance by my clients, and examples of clients' behavioral changes as a result of the use of self-care principles were discussed at length. I distributed samples of actual nursing care plans, the data base, medication teaching forms, and related self-care literature to the director, who carefully examined the material and asked questions about my impressions of how the model worked with the agency's client population, i.e., what were the advantages, disadvantages, and problems encountered in using the self-care framework. I had the feeling that I was being placated and that the director's questions were an attempt to feign interest. I was certain that a decision had already been made concerning the future use of the self-care model in the agency, and if my perceptions were accurate, the outcome would be negative.

The final judgment rested on the director of the clinic; other input from nursing personnel was not considered at this point because "the choice rested in the hands of the administration." Once again, I waited with anticipation for the decision. After several minutes of verbal accolades about the model and its success in improving care, the director declined its use as a permanent feature in the mode of operation at the clinic. I was politely told that the self-care framework would involve major transitions in the functional role of the clinic nurse as outlined by his/her job description. In addition, care plans would have to substitute for the current treatment plans, ". . . and what would doctors think of the nurses' formulating plans for clients' care?" I diplomatically defended what I had done for fourteen weeks, stating that nurses knew nursing, and that psychiatrists and social workers were best prepared for the work of their own disciplines; to assume otherwise would be ridiculous. The director sat behind the large desk in the office, in silence, faintly smiling, yet not offering any futher discussion about the topic at hand. Another lesson about bureaucracies emerges: Never assume that a bureaucratic system will readily accept change.

Looking back at those fourteen weeks, I came to the conclusion that I did not give adequate time to the leadership component of *deciding*; I needed to give the clinic staff more time to observe, analyze, and plan for the use of what the agency director called "a radical change of approach to the role of nursing in the clinic." In fourteen weeks, I was trying to undo and reconstruct many years of practice, security, and tradition. Given the vested interests accumulated by each staff member and the threat that changes of this kind would impose, success was impossible in the time that I had. As a result, my attempt to facilitate change, as outlined in the Yura, Ozimek, and Walsh framework of nursing leadership, was unsuccessful [4]. If I had it to do over again, I would have incorporated change theory more actively in my plans. In addition, I would have taken more time to keep the clinic staff more informed and involved in the progress of individual clients and their self-care. Perhaps by doing this, more ongoing feedback would have been available to the director. In retrospect, this may have been a factor contributing to the negative response toward implementing self-care nursing in the clinic.

Despite my disappointment about the agency's decision, I felt good about the fact that my clients had begun to learn alternative behaviors to counteract the effects of chronicity. The elderly people with whom I worked gained substantial satisfaction from realizing that they *could* control their lives more independently. As their nurse, I realized that I had met my own objectives, and it was a great feeling to be able to withdraw my "hands on" care of clients, appreciating that they could accomplish many of the tasks of living without assistance. Clients' responses to the self-care approach were generally favorable. Depressed or socially isolated people especially seemed to appreciate what the model offered to them. As one old woman told me at the end of the fourteen-week experience, "I feel as though I can do things that I haven't done in a long time. . . . I guess that I just needed to show myself that I'm not just an old, useless lady."

Conversely, some clients had shown less overt success with self-care nursing. One instance particularly stands out in my mind. "G.E.," a seventy-two-year-old schizophrenic man, lived with his forty-year-old mentally retarded son in a single room in the Tenderloin and was my most challenging client. Despite using medications to control his psychosis and delusions, he was convinced that he would never return to normal life. He had not left his room in six months when I met him and was extremely rigid in his methods of coping. Several weeks were consumed in developing a fragile trust with this man, and attempts to assist him in improving his self-care were most unsuccessful. His chronically disorganized behavior was not to be changed by a mere fourteen-week trial of self-care nursing. His son, however, whom I looked upon as half of an inseparable dyad, was interested in proving how well he could care for himself. Weekly he would tell me how many times he had bathed, washed his clothes, and taken rides on the cable cars. The son's attempt to interest his father in similar activities usually precipitated an argument between the pair.

The dynamics of the clients I worked with were fascinating, and I believe that my attempts at promoting self-care in the Tenderloin were not in vain.

IN RETROSPECT

My journey through a bureaucratic structure has concluded. My exploration of its structure and my role in it helped me find what I was looking for in the Tenderloin; this experience in nursing leadership was nothing less than rich. There is no product I can show you—nothing visible or concrete to demonstrate. What this journey gave me was an opportunity to explore a process. It was through that process that I learned about a phenomenally powerful system. I allowed myself to experience the sense of powerlessness that so many of the "underdogs" in the network so frequently feel. At the same time, I chose to confront "the system" with all its attendant power in what I believe was a very important cause: the client, without whom the bureaucratic system would be rendered impotent. In that respect, advocacy assumed greater meaning. It meant that I needed to be an advocate not only for my clients but for my profession as well.

Self-assurance, determination, assertiveness, and perseverance are no longer words that simply decorate the nursing literature I read. They have meaning for me as I have pursued a goal in this journey through a bureaucratic structure. I was not totally successful in implementing self-care nursing in the Tenderloin. Yet, I was successful in learning what it meant in terms of my professional and personal growth. I have become more aware of my strengths and my imperfections. They are the keys to leadership because they allow me to become more in touch with my internal sources of power. When this occurs, I can externalize my strength and put it to work where it counts the most—with my clients.

REFERENCES

1. Underwood, P. "Facilitating Self-Care." In Patricia Pothier (ed.). *Psychiatric Nursing.* Boston: Little, Brown and Company, 1980, pp. 117–118.
2. Yura, H., Ozimek, D., and Walsh, M. *Nursing Leadership—Theory and Process* (2nd ed.). New York: Appleton-Century-Crofts, 1981, p. 103.
3. Ibid., p. 104.
4. Ibid., p. 105.

SUGGESTED READINGS

Anna, D., Christensen, D., Hohon, S., Ord, L., and Wells, S. "Implementing Orem's Conceptual Framework." *Journal of Nursing Administration,* November 1978, pp. 8–11.
Fenner, K. "Developing a Conceptual Framework." *Nursing Outlook,* February 1979, pp. 122–126.
Hunn, S. "Self Care Medication Teaching Plan" (pamphlet). San Francisco: Langley Porter Institute, 1979.
Joseph, L. S. "Self-Care and the Nursing Process." *Nursing Clinics of North America,* Vol. 15, No. 1, 131–142, March 1980.
Mullin, V. "Implementing the Self-Care Concept in the Acute Care Setting." *Nursing Clinics of North America,* Vol. 15, No. 1, 177–190, March 1980.
Orem, D. *Nursing—Concepts of Practice.* New York: McGraw-Hill, 1971.
Smith, M. C. "Proposed Metaparadigm for Nursing Research and Theory Development." *Image,* Vol. 11, No. 3, 75–79, October 1979.

Questions to Part IV

1. How would you improve formal communication within your health care facility?
2. Identify one problem you would like to see corrected in your health care facility. How would you initiate this correction through formal channels? Through informal channels?
3. What kind of a health care facility do you prefer working in? Give specific reasons.
4. In retrospect, after assessing your health care facility, which aspect should have been assessed more closely?

Index

Index